# THE
# Athlete's Guide
# to Diabetes

## Sheri R. Colberg, PhD

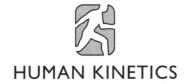

HUMAN KINETICS

**Library of Congress Cataloging-in-Publication Data**

Names: Colberg, Sheri, 1963- author.
Title: The athlete's guide to diabetes / Sheri R. Colberg, PhD.
Other titles: Diabetic athlete's handbook.
Description: Champaign, IL : Human Kinetics, 2020. | Revision of: Diabetic athlete's handbook. | Includes bibliographical references and index. | Identifiers: LCCN 2018039302 (print) | LCCN 2018040032 (ebook) | ISBN 9781492588733 (epub) | ISBN 9781492588726 (PDF) | ISBN 9781492572848 (print)
Subjects: LCSH: Diabetic athletes—Handbooks, manuals, etc. | Diabetes—Exercise therapy—Handbooks, manuals, etc.
Classification: LCC RC660 (ebook) | LCC RC660 .C4747 2020 (print) | DDC 616.4/62062—dc23
LC record available at https://lccn.loc.gov/2018039302

ISBN: 978-1-4925-7284-8 (print)

This publication is written and published to provide accurate and authoritative information relevant to the subject matter presented. It is published and sold with the understanding that the author and publisher are not engaged in rendering legal, medical, or other professional services by reason of their authorship or publication of this work. If medical or other expert assistance is required, the services of a competent professional person should be sought.

This book is a revised edition of *Diabetic Athlete's Handbook*, published in 2009 by Human Kinetics.

The web addresses cited in this text were current as of September 2018, unless otherwise noted.

Senior Acquisitions Editor: Michelle Maloney
Managing Editor: Julie Marx Goodreau
Indexer: Alisha Jeddeloh
Permissions Manager: Martha Gullo
Graphic Designer: Julie Denzer
Cover Designer: Keri Evans
Cover Design Associate: Susan Rothermel Allen
Photographs (cover): Christian Petersen/Getty Images (football); Bryn Lennon/Getty Images (cycling); Hannah Peters/Getty Images (skiing); Doug Benc/Getty Images (golf)
Athletes on the Cover: Patrick Peterson (football), Mandy Marquardt (cycling), Kris Freeman (skiing), Michelle McGann (golf)
Photographs (interior): © Human Kinetics, unless otherwise noted
Photo Asset Manager: Laura Fitch
Photo Production Manager: Jason Allen
Senior Art Manager: Kelly Hendren
Illustrations: © Human Kinetics, unless otherwise noted
Production: Westchester Publishing Services
Printer: McNaughton & Gunn

Human Kinetics books are available at special discounts for bulk purchase. Special editions or book excerpts can also be created to specification. For details, contact the Special Sales Manager at Human Kinetics.

Printed in the United States of America

10  9  8  7  6  5  4  3  2  1

The paper in this book is certified under a sustainable forestry program.

**Human Kinetics**
P.O. Box 5076
Champaign, IL 61825-5076
Website: www.HumanKinetics.com

In the United States, email info@hkusa.com or call 800-747-4457.
In Canada, email info@hkcanada.com.
In the United Kingdom/Europe, email hk@hkeurope.com.

For information about Human Kinetics' coverage in other areas of the world, please visit our website: **www.HumanKinetics.com**

E7437

For my loving husband, Ray Ochs, and my three amazing sons—may you all stay healthy, happy, and active.

# Contents

# Part II   Guidelines for Specific Activities   185

# ——— Foreword ———

**M**ake no mistake about it: diabetes is a complex, chronic disease that is more complicated than most. Exercise and sport involve complicated physiological processes and doing them with a disease like diabetes makes them that much more challenging to manage. This reality should not stop you from exercising, getting fit, or competing at whatever level you choose. In fact, as Dr. Sheri Colberg has written, diabetes should be your reason to exercise. The tremendous array of health and mental benefits that exercise and fitness bestow on you usually outweighs the risks, but you need to tackle the challenges with an understanding of what is going on in your body.

Like any athlete, the athlete with diabetes deserves to be surrounded by a group of experts and resources that can help you achieve your goal—to optimize health and performance and to compete at your desired level. With a firm foundation and a solid support team, you will be well on your way to successful completion of your goals. Over the last 2 decades, awareness of the needs of athletes with diabetes has grown considerably, as has the number of people with diabetes who are demonstrating tremendous toughness and perseverance in tackling their incredible metabolic and management challenges. Multiple resources exist now to assist you in achieving your goals. Some resources have come and gone over time, but the book you are now reading has become a consistent force for education and diabetes management. Now, with her third edition of this guide, Dr. Colberg has made many outstanding and timely updates that make this resource another absolute necessity for both physically active individuals and athletes with diabetes.

The entire guide has been heavily revised and significantly updated with particular attention to very pertinent and timely subjects such as fat adaptation and fuel use, novel technologies, nutrition, and sports medicine topics for the young and aging athlete with diabetes. And, once again, Dr. Colberg successfully taps into one of the greatest resources out there: the wisdom and experience of athletes and exercisers with diabetes from around the world. Hundreds of real-life examples provide the reader with ample opportunity to explore the stories of a remarkable array of athletes with diabetes around the globe. Again, the sheer number of you who are out there giving it your all every day is one of the most astounding and inspiring aspects of this book.

You can do whatever you want to do in the face of diabetes, provided that your efforts do not put your health at risk. You can achieve whatever it is that you set your sights on: from greater long-term health through fitness to competing in the Olympics, and everything in between. Ultimately, integrating diabetes and exercise is all about self-management. It mandates continual learning and empowerment to free you from reliance on an already overtaxed system of health care delivery. Excellent resources exist to empower you, including this outstanding update of *Diabetic*

*Athlete's Handbook*. Enjoy reading and rereading it and learning from one another. And keep displaying the tremendous perseverance and toughness that make you and your efforts extraordinary.

Matthew Corcoran, MD
Founder & President, Diabetes Training Camp Foundation

# —— Preface ——

Diabetes treatment has gone through dramatic changes in the past few decades. At present, corresponding with the third iteration of this book, being an athlete with diabetes has become even more mainstream. But you can never learn enough about managing diabetes with exercise, and gaining expertise in new sports and activities through the experiences of others with diabetes is invaluable. One of the primary purposes of this book is to enable anyone with diabetes of any type to feel empowered enough to be active without having to be fearful of losing control of diabetes management.

I received a diagnosis of diabetes myself at the age of 4 in 1968, back in what I call the dark ages of diabetes. I went through childhood, adolescence, and early adulthood without benefit of a blood glucose meter. I have participated in a variety of sports and physical activities over the years, many without ever knowing what my actual blood glucose level was. The list of sports is long, and it includes swimming, running, racquetball, soccer, tennis, weight training, gymnastics, volleyball, cycling, aerobics, dancing, stair climbing, hiking and backpacking, canoeing, football and equipment managing, snowshoeing, cross-country and downhill skiing, horseback riding, sailing, snorkeling, and skydiving! I did most of these sports while feeling less than my physical best: without a meter or the ability to adjust my insulin doses to compensate, my blood glucose was usually either too high or too low.

While I was growing up, doing any kind of exercise made me feel better overall and more in control of my diabetes, even though at the time I did not have enough knowledge about the physiology behind my condition to understand why. I began exercising regularly on my own and through team sports as a preteen, and I have continued being active on an almost daily basis throughout my adulthood. It was not until I obtained a blood glucose meter that I realized how much better I could feel during exercise with my blood glucose in a more normal range. But even with a meter, managing my diabetes during activities has been a trial-and-error learning process.

When I got my first meter, few guidelines or books were available to offer any guidance. I eventually learned how to manage my blood glucose for my usual activities, but every time I tried a new or unusual activity, it was like I had to start all over again. When back in 1990 I first attended a meeting of the International Diabetic Athletes Association (IDAA, which became the Diabetes Exercise & Sports Association, or DESA, and later part of InsulinDependence before that organization went under), I met many other active people with diabetes. It struck me then that I could use the experiences of others to help shorten my own trial-and-error process.

From this point, I eventually got the idea and motivation for the book *The Diabetic Athlete*, published in 2001, which included many real-life examples from IDAA members (obtained via a postal questionnaire). For the 2009 version of that book, reborn as the *Diabetic Athlete's Handbook*, I posted my diabetic athlete questionnaire on my website, and I received replies from active people with diabetes from around the world. For this latest edition—*The Athlete's Guide to Diabetes*—I used the power of social media to again get athletes from everywhere around the world to share their exercise expertise via an online survey.

The current edition includes 15 athlete profiles in total, which highlight the accomplishments and training regimens of a variety of athletes with type 1 diabetes. The number of included activities has expanded to 165, including sports and activities such as curling, pickleball, sprint cycling, cricket, powerboat racing, and even race car driving. It also addresses the latest trends and advancements in management regimens, including low-carbohydrate eating for athletes, the latest insulins and diabetes medications, continuous glucose monitoring (CGM) systems, and closed-loop insulin delivery systems. This book is a compilation of updated experiences to help you manage your blood glucose better while playing sports, exercising for fitness, or just being more active in general.

Part I of this book covers the basics about exercise, physical activity, and fitness. Knowledge is power when it comes to managing diabetes. I have researched this topic for years—all through my childhood, and while earning a doctoral degree in exercise physiology from the University of California at Berkeley, and ever since. Although you do not need a PhD to understand how your body adapts to exercise, you do need to understand the basics to make safe changes in your diet and medication, and this book will teach you those.

Part II of this book is more experiential in nature and can help you reduce the trial-and-error needed for participation in almost every conceivable sport or physical activity. It is arranged into five chapters by type of activity. Each chapter gives general recommendations for diet and medication changes for each sport or activity, along with real-life examples from athletes with diabetes who participate in them. No one-size-fits-all solution applies to blood glucose management during exercise because everyone is unique. But these chapters provide you with many examples that can give you a place to start when figuring out what works best for you personally.

I believe that combining this basic information (the *why* of exercise) and experiential information (the *how* of exercise) can help everyone better understand how to maintain normal blood glucose levels during (and after) any physical endeavor. Whether you are interested in just recreating or want to be a serious competitive athlete, it is time to get out there and go for it!

# ── Acknowledgments ──

I would like to thank all the people who helped me update this book yet again so that I can continue to make a difference in the lives of active people with diabetes. This list includes the wonderful members of my extended professional and social diabetes family (you know who you are) who are full of information themselves. I am especially grateful to the nearly 300 athletes with diabetes who completed my online survey and answered my follow-up questions because without their input, I would not have had many real-life and sport-specific examples to share. For any of you whose examples I could not fit into the book, I apologize and again thank you for taking the time to share all that you do. Finally, I would like to acknowledge all the hard-working people at Human Kinetics, including Michelle Maloney, Julie Marx Goodreau, Sue Outlaw, Martha Gullo, Jenny Lokshin, and countless others who work behind the scenes.

# I

# The Athlete's Toolbox

# 1

# Training Basics for Fitness and Sports

If you are already an avid exerciser, you are undoubtedly aware of the benefits of exercise for your physical and mental health and diabetes management. If you are just starting to get more active, you have a lot of positive changes to look forward to. Exercise can help you build muscle and lose body fat, suppress your appetite, eat more without gaining fat weight, enhance your mood, reduce stress and anxiety levels, increase your energy level, boost your immune system, keep your joints and muscles more flexible, and improve the quality of your life. For many with diabetes, being physically active has made all the difference between managing diabetes or letting diabetes control them.

## DIABETES: THE BASICS

With diabetes, your body lacks the capacity to adequately regulate your blood sugar—otherwise known as *blood glucose*, the primary sugar circulating in your blood. Normally, after you eat a meal the food gets digested and broken down into easily absorbed molecules such as glucose. Glucose is a simple sugar that comes mostly from carbohydrate in your diet, and it is critical to have enough glucose, because your brain and nervous system use it as their primary fuel. When your blood glucose level drops below 65 milligrams per deciliter (mg/dL)—or 3.6 millimoles (mmol/L), if you live outside the United States—you experience *hypoglycemia*, or low blood glucose ("a low"). You are likely already familiar with the effect that hypoglycemia has on your ability to think straight and react normally: if you ever found yourself saying, "I know what $2+2$ equals, but I just can't think of it," you were probably low.

In a healthy individual without diabetes, the normal fasting range for glucose is now 80 to 99 mg/dL (4.4 to 5.5 mmol/L); when the blood glucose level starts to rise, an organ in the abdomen called the *pancreas* senses the increase and releases the hormone *insulin* to help lower the level. Insulin works by binding to receptors on cells in muscle and fat tissues, the primary places where glucose can be stored. If you have diabetes, either your pancreas has reduced capacity to release insulin (causing a relative or absolute insulin deficiency) or your insulin does not work well to remove the excess glucose from your blood (insulin resistance, which occurs mostly in muscle). In either case—or when both are the case—your blood glucose rises too high after you have eaten, or when you get stressed out, or when you are ill, or at other times. Your liver is the organ responsible for making sure that you have enough glucose in your blood.

> *Your liver can become insulin resistant, leading it to release too much glucose, especially overnight when you go a long time without eating.*

Although you may find it easier to function with your blood glucose a little too high compared with too low, you should take any precautions you can to avoid the long-term health problems that can result from elevated blood glucose over time. Among the possibilities are heart disease, premature death, nerve damage, amputations, joint problems, vision loss, kidney failure, birth defects in your offspring (if you are a female), and more. Keeping your blood glucose as close to normal as possible is the best way to prevent many, if not all, of these potential health issues. That is where regular exercise, a healthful diet, effective use of medications, and a blood glucose meter or other glucose monitoring device come in handy.

## DOES THE TYPE OF DIABETES YOU HAVE MATTER?

Over the years diabetes has been classified in various ways, including by age of onset (juvenile onset versus adult onset), insulin requirements (insulin-dependent or non-insulin-dependent), and by roman or arabic numerals. The last major revision of the classifications occurred in 1997 when the American Diabetes Association (ADA) recommended calling the two main types "type 1" and "type 2" diabetes to minimize the confusion caused by labeling an adult with a "juvenile" disease.

The debate over the best way to classify diabetes into types has yet to end. The ADA still recognizes diabetes as "a group of metabolic diseases characterized by hyperglycemia resulting from defects in insulin secretion, insulin action, or both," and they also state that chronic elevations in blood glucose can cause health issues that are seen in all types. The recent controversy is more focused on how many types actually exist; some groups recommend five diabetes categories, and others as many as 11. The argument is that having extra classifications may lead to more personalized and effective treatments in the future based on whether autoimmunity, insulin deficiency, insulin resistance, or a combination of these are contributing causes.

At present, we still only have two main diabetes types, but whether you use insulin has a bigger impact on your response to exercise than the type of diabetes you have. Exercise can throw a curveball when it comes to blood glucose management. The risks and precautions can vary somewhat, so understanding the differences among types is important before we get into the nitty-gritty of exercise and the specific recommendations for managing blood glucose with regimen changes.

## Type 1: Always Insulin Requiring

Type 1 diabetes is the less common form, comprising only about 5 to 10 percent of all cases. This type usually has an autoimmune basis: the immune system has gone awry, destroying most or all of the insulin-making capacity of the pancreatic beta cells. When you have type 1 diabetes, you must take insulin to survive. The typical symptoms of type 1 include the "polys" (polyuria, polydipsia, and polyphagia, otherwise known as excessive urination, thirst, and hunger), unexplained weight loss, and unusual fatigue. All these symptoms are related to having an elevated blood glucose level caused by a lack of insulin in the body.

The teenage years are when type 1 diabetes is most commonly diagnosed, which is why it used to be called *juvenile diabetes*. However, most people living with this type in the long term are over the age of 18. In fact, more than half of all new cases of type 1 diabetes are now being diagnosed in adults of all ages. In adults, the onset of symptoms is generally much slower than it is in young people; as a result, it may be managed for a while without outside insulin if the body is still making at least some of its own. Being misdiagnosed at first with type 2 diabetes is common, and you may initially respond well to oral diabetes medications, which can further confuse the diagnosis. (But you are not likely to be as insulin resistant as someone who has type 2 diabetes usually is.)

You can request antibody tests be performed to help make the diagnosis of type 1 diabetes. This could be helpful because early treatment with insulin helps preserve your remaining pancreatic beta cells for a little longer. However, some people who appear to have type 1 diabetes do not have any evidence of autoimmunity, one of the reasons additional categories have been proposed. At some point, if your blood glucose continues to rise over time, even when you are exercising like a fiend, it is time to consider injected or pumped insulin as your friend, not your foe.

*Requiring daily insulin makes exercising trickier because both insulin and physical activity can independently (but additively) lower blood glucose. You may need to alter your insulin and carbohydrate or other food intake for exercise to avoid lows (or highs).*

## Type 2: Insulin Resistant With an Overworked Pancreas

Although many consider it a more easily managed condition, type 2 diabetes should not be taken lightly. It often goes undiagnosed for 5 or more years, so when you are diagnosed with it you may already have some diabetes-related health problems. Generally, its onset is caused by a combination of insulin resistance and loss of insulin production over time, which leaves your pancreatic beta cells unable to keep up with insulin demands. So long as your pancreas can still make enough insulin to overcome your resistance to it, you will not develop type 2 diabetes.

*It is possible to have enough insulin resistance to have prediabetes, which is when your blood glucose levels are above normal but not high enough to reach a diabetes diagnosis.*

Many people who have type 2 diabetes end up eventually needing supplemental insulin to lower their blood glucose, although a variety of new medications may be equally effective in managing it. In women, a related type called *gestational diabetes* is commonly diagnosed during the last trimester of pregnancy; although it usually stops after giving birth, it greatly increases a woman's risk for developing type 2 diabetes later in life. Thus, insulin may also be necessary during pregnancy to manage blood glucose levels to prevent complications for both the mother and child.

We can think of insulin resistance as being analogous to a lock and key, where the cell's insulin receptor is the lock and insulin is the key. If the key fits into the lock and opens it, glucose can enter the cell (insulin sensitive). On the other hand, if the key does not fit the lock or goes in but fails to turn, the glucose stays in the bloodstream (insulin resistant). You want your insulin to work as efficiently as possible to get glucose into the cells—so that you need less insulin to get the job done.

The good news is that becoming more physically active makes your insulin work better. This explains why exercise and dietary changes early on are often effective in managing type 2 diabetes and, in many cases, reversing prediabetes. Insulin resistance often develops in people with type 1 diabetes as well, but it can usually be improved by similar lifestyle changes that subsequently lower insulin needs, such as being more active, choosing foods more carefully, losing weight, and managing stress.

# GETTING PHYSICALLY FIT IS THE BEST THING YOU CAN DO

Physical fitness has undeniable health benefits for everyone. If you exercise regularly, you will have lower risk for many health problems including heart disease, obesity, hypertension, type 2 diabetes, certain cancers, and other metabolic disorders. The usual health benefits of exercise apply to everyone and probably even more so when you have diabetes. Enhanced insulin action makes all types of diabetes easier to manage. The improvements that you can experience in your levels of cholesterol (more of the good type and less of the bad) and blood fats (triglycerides) can greatly lower your heart disease risk, which is already higher if you have diabetes. Regular exercise can lower systemic inflammation, reduce blood platelet stickiness, lessen the chances that blood clots will form, and lower your risk for heart attack or stroke. If nothing else, being active will help improve your ability to cope with stress and enhance your outlook on life and diabetes.

Much of what you may attribute to getting older—such as muscle atrophy or loss of flexibility in joints—really results from being inactive. Elevations in blood glucose can cause premature aging, accelerate heart disease, and lead to other illnesses. Regular exercise can keep you looking and feeling younger for longer and even greatly lower your risk of getting any diabetes-related complications. While enjoying your favorite physical activities, you can help maintain your long-term health—and that's a win–win situation!

*Exercise regularly to slow down aging, manage your blood glucose, reduce your risk of long-term complications, and feel stronger and better overall.*

# WHAT DOES IT MINIMALLY TAKE TO GET FIT?

How much and which types of exercise do you need to do to become fit? According to the latest guidelines (shown in table 1.1), all healthy adults ages 18 to 65 years (including most with diabetes) should engage in moderate intensity aerobic physical activity (e.g., brisk walking or bicycling on level terrain) for 30 to 60 minutes a day on 5 days each week (for a total of at least 150 to 300 minutes weekly), or vigorous intensity aerobic activity like running or uphill bicycling for 20 to 60 minutes a day on 3 days each week (for a total of at least 75 to 150 minutes weekly), or a combination of moderate and vigorous intensity exercise to reach the recommended volume. In addition, all adults will benefit from performing activities that maintain or increase muscular strength and endurance at least 2 days each week but preferably 3 days, along with regular flexibility training. You should do these planned activities in addition to your activities of daily living such as standing, casual walking, grocery shopping, or taking out the trash.

There are also recommendations for adults over 65 or anyone between 50 and 64 years old with chronic conditions or physical functional limitations (such as arthritis) that affect their ability to move or their physical fitness. Older adults should meet or exceed 30 minutes of moderate physical activity on most days of the week, but more humble goals may be necessary if you have arthritic joints or any other physical limitation. Just maintaining functionality is an important benefit

### Table 1.1 Weekly Recommended Physical Activity for Adults

| Healthy adults ages 18 to 65 |
| --- |
| • Do moderate aerobic training 30 to 60 minutes a day, 5 days a week (at least 150 to 300 minutes weekly), or vigorous aerobic training 20 to 60 minutes a day, 3 days a week (at least 75 to 150 minutes weekly), or a combination of both intensities to reach the recommended volume of exercise.<br>• Do 8 to 10 strength-training exercises, 8 to 12 repetitions of each exercise, at least 2 nonconsecutive days per week but preferably 3 days.<br>• For joint range of motion, include flexibility exercises for each major muscle group (a total of 60 seconds per exercise) on 2 or more days per week. |
| **Adults over age 65 (or 50 to 64 with chronic health conditions)** |
| • Aim to meet the recommended volume of aerobic training for all adults.<br>• Do 8 to 10 strength-training exercises, 10 to 15 repetitions of each exercise, 2 or 3 times per week.<br>• Perform flexibility training at least 2 or 3 days per week.<br>• To lower your risk of falling, practice balance or neuromotor exercises at least 2 or 3 days per week.<br>• Have a physical activity plan that allows you to be as active as possible, given your physical limitations. |

of activity for older people, and maintaining some level of fitness makes it easier to do everyday activities such as gardening, walking, or cleaning the house. For older people or those with limitations, strength training is especially important to prevent loss of muscle mass and bone strength, and working on flexibility will additionally help prevent limitations. Finally, anyone over the age of 40 needs to work on maintaining balance and staying on their feet, but balance and neuromotor training are particularly important for anyone with a higher risk of falling for any reason.

*In addition to exercising regularly, try to reduce how much time you are sedentary. Intersperse frequent, short bouts of standing and physical activity to break up your sedentary time and rev up your metabolism.*

# COMPONENTS OF AN EXERCISE TRAINING PROGRAM

Whether you are already a regular exerciser or just a beginner, several basic guidelines apply to improving your fitness level and managing your blood glucose. Keep in mind that fitness can be defined many ways. Your overall health and stamina benefit from aerobic or cardiorespiratory fitness—what we think of as conditioning resulting from prolonged aerobic activities such as brisk walking, jogging, cycling, swimming, rowing, and aerobic dance. Another form of fitness is muscular—related to both muscular strength and muscular endurance. Particularly if you are just getting started, your health care team or fitness professional can help you develop an exercise prescription with careful consideration of your diabetes management, complications, cardiovascular disease risk, personal fitness and health goals, and exercise preferences.

*An exercise program includes your exercise type (mode), how hard you work out (intensity), how long you are active (duration), how often you exercise (frequency), your total exercise amount (volume), and how quickly you advance (progression).*

## Mode: Picking Aerobic and Resistance Activities

If your main goal is to increase your maximal oxygen consumption ($\dot{V}O_2max$), cardiorespiratory fitness, or endurance capacity, your training should be *aerobic* in nature: involving the large-muscle groups performing rhythmic, prolonged activities such as walking, running, swimming, cycling, rowing, or cross-country skiing. Resistance training is not a usual means to increase $\dot{V}O_2max$, fitness, or endurance, but it is effective for increasing muscular strength and muscular endurance and preventing the loss of muscle mass with aging and inactivity. Such training can be done in a variety of ways, including using resistance training machines, free weights (barbells and dumbbells), resistance bands, and body weight as resistance. Any gains in your muscle mass from doing any type of training can increase your daily caloric needs and improve your insulin sensitivity. To reach optimal cardiorespiratory fitness, your exercise program must include an aerobic component, but to preserve your muscle mass and strength you should incorporate regular resistance training as well.

Another way to become more fit is simply to do a variety of activities, an approach known as cross-training. For example, you could run or cycle for 30 minutes and do some resistance training on Monday, Wednesday, and Friday; swim moderately for 45 minutes on Tuesday; and take a dance class on Saturday. Cross-training is really the key to avoiding overuse injuries, keeping your exercise fresh and fun, and achieving maximal overall fitness. When it comes to managing your blood glucose, this approach is also effective because each activity recruits different muscles altogether or the same ones in varying patterns, which results in wider use and enhanced fitness of your whole body. The only downside is that because you do each activity less frequently when you vary them, you will

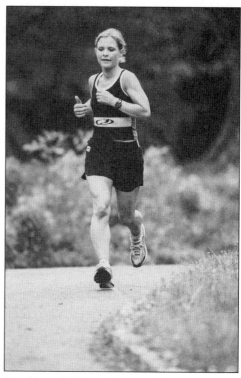

Aerobic activities such as running increase your endurance capacity and cardiorespiratory fitness.

likely not experience a training effect as pronounced as you can get by focusing on a single activity. One of the latest fads, CrossFit (which is definitely not for everyone), is an extreme example of a cross-training approach: the workouts incorporate elements from high-intensity interval training, Olympic weightlifting, plyometrics, powerlifting, gymnastics, kettlebell sports, calisthenics, strength athletics, and other exercises, varying by the day.

> *Most competitive and Olympic-level athletes vary either their activities or the intensity at which they do them on different days of the week, both for fitness and injury prevention.*

## Intensity: How Hard You Work Out

How hard you work out should reflect your training goals, such as whether you want to maximize your endurance performance or just expend some calories. But for improvements in cardiorespiratory fitness, you will need to do either moderate or vigorous intensity training. Vigorous activities will challenge you, resulting in rapid breathing and a greatly elevated heart rate. Some examples are race walking, jogging or running, bicycling uphill, gardening with a shovel, or playing competitive sports such as soccer or lacrosse. Moderate-intensity activities still make you feel as though you are exerting yourself, but your breathing will be less labored and your pace slower. Such activities include brisk walking, swimming at a moderate pace, or bicycling on level terrain.

## Intensity and Interval Training

Intensity and duration of exercise are interrelated. Usually you cannot keep higher-intensity exercise going as long as you can lower-intensity activities—but the greater the overload that the harder exercise provides, the greater the performance gains. If your goal is weight loss, doing an activity at a lower intensity for a longer duration may work better for you. In either case, consider your initial fitness level and exercise goals, your risk for joint or heart problems, any diabetes-related complications, and your personal preferences. If your workouts are too hard, you may stop doing them because of injuries (more on potential injuries and prevention in chapter 7) or loss of motivation.

If you cannot maintain a higher intensity to start, you can increase your fitness by doing intervals. During any activity, simply increase the intensity of your exercise for short periods (interval training) to gain more from it. For example, if you are out walking, speed up slightly for a short distance (such as between two light poles or mailboxes) before slowing back down to your original pace. During your workouts, continue to include these short, faster intervals occasionally and lengthen the intervals when you can. Performing intervals will not only improve your fitness and use up extra calories but also make you feel more fatigued at the end of each workout. Over the course of several weeks, you will be able to move faster and sustain a quicker pace for longer due to the extra conditioning from your interspersed faster or harder activity. The same principle applies to almost every kind of exercise that you do, from walking to cycling to gardening. In fact, even competitive athletes generally reach a plateau at a certain level unless they do some type of more intense interval training from time to time.

## Monitoring Exercise Intensity

You can monitor your exercise intensity in various ways. Heart rate (HR) is a measure of intensity because it is linearly related to how much oxygen your body is using, although your $\dot{V}O_2$max declines as you age. To be the most effective for cardiorespiratory fitness gains, your exercise should maintain your heart rate in a target training range. The recommended range is 40 to 89 percent of $\dot{V}O_2$ reserve or heart rate reserve (HRR), although when you are just starting out you may need to go as low as 30 percent.

Because it is hard to measure your oxygen use but easy to take your pulse, use the HRR method to determine a target heart rate that is more accurate and individualized. The American College of Sports Medicine (ACSM) recommends aerobic training intensity ranges using HRR as follows:

Easy = 30% to 39% HRR

Moderate = 40% to 59% HRR

Vigorous = 60% to 89% HRR

HRR equals your maximal heart rate minus your resting heart rate, so to figure out your own HRR-based target, you need to know both rates. Directly measuring your maximal heart rate is the most accurate, but you can also estimate it using either of the following formulas (valid only for adults). Generally, the first works well on people aged 20 to 40, and the second one is better for master athletes over 40 years of age:

$$\text{Maximal HR} = 220 - \text{Age}$$

$$\text{Maximal HR} = 208 - 70\% \text{ of Age}$$

For instance, using either formula to estimate maximal HR, a 40-year-old athlete would have a maximal heart rate of 180 beats per minute (220 – 40, or 208 – 28), although the two would differ slightly at other ages. For yourself, measure your resting heart rate upon waking before you get out of bed, then estimate your maximal heart rate using the first formula if you are 20 to 40 years old. Use the second formula if you are over 40. Multiply your estimated reserve first by 40 percent (the low end of the moderate range) and then by 89 percent (the high end of the vigorous range) before adding each back to your resting heart rate to determine your lower and upper limits (a moderate-to-vigorous intensity range of 40 to 89 percent of HRR).

$$\text{Lower range of HR } (40\%) = 0.40 \, (\text{Maximal HR} - \text{Resting HR}) + \text{Resting HR}$$

$$\text{Upper range of HR } (89\%) = 0.89 \, (\text{Maximal HR} - \text{Resting HR}) + \text{Resting HR}$$

If a 40-year-old athlete has a resting heart rate of 70, her HRR is 110 beats per minute (180 – 70). Her range is 40 to 89 percent of HRR added to her resting value, or 114 to 168 beats per minute. See table 1.2 for these calculations. As noted, a very deconditioned person can choose to start exercising at a lower range of HRR (30 to 39 percent, or an easy activity) to establish a baseline level of fitness before working out more intensely.

Another method to monitor intensity is the rating of perceived exertion (RPE) scale, a subjective measure of how hard you feel like you are working overall—including total body sensations like heart and breathing rates, sweating, and muscle fatigue. The rating should reflect how strenuous the exercise feels to you, encompassing your overall physical stress, effort, and fatigue rather than a single factor like leg pain or shortness of breath. The recommended range of RPE for optimal fitness gains is "somewhat hard" to "hard" (12 to 16 on the Borg category scale that ranges from 6 to 20). Working out below the range of 12 to 16 may not overload your cardiovascular system enough, and working above that range may limit how long you can keep going working aerobically.

An even simpler method to ensure that your exercise intensity is in the appropriate range is to use the talk test. If you are breathing too hard to carry on a conversation with an exercise partner, then your intensity is higher than necessary or recommended. And if you can not only talk but also sing a few phrases without breathing hard, you are exercising at an intensity that is too low for most fitness gains.

**Table 1.2  Sample Calculation of Target Heart Rate (HR) Training Ranges**

**Individual:** 40-year-old athlete
**Resting HR (RHR):** 70 beats per minute (bpm)
**Maximal HR (MHR):** 180 bpm (estimated using 220 – Age or 208 – 70% of Age)

Target **HR** = [(MHR – RHR) × Desired intensity)] + RHR

| | |
|---|---|
| **Low end of moderate HR range (40%)** | = [(180 – 70) × 0.40]<br>= [110 × 0.40] + 70<br>= 44 + 70<br>= 114 bpm |
| **Low end of vigorous HR range (60%)** | = [(180 – 70) × 0.60] + 70<br>= [110 × 0.60] + 70<br>= 66 + 70<br>= 136 bpm |
| **High end of vigorous HR range (89%)** | = [(180 – 70) × 0.89] + 70<br>= [110 × 0.89] + 70<br>= 98 + 70<br>= 168 bpm |
| **Target HR range (40%–89% HRR)** | = 114 to 168 bpm |

*Talk test:*

*Light (or easy): Can talk, sing, or whistle while doing the activity*

*Moderate: Can talk but not sing during activity*

*Vigorous: Short of breath or winded and unable to talk easily or sing*

## Hard and Easy Days

You may benefit from purposefully varying your exercise intensity from day to day, such as by doing hard and easy days of training. By alternating workout intensities (light, moderate, and vigorous), your body will gain both the enhanced fitness and strength benefits of hard workouts and the healing effects of greater recuperative time between intense workouts. Varying intensity in this manner also helps prevent overuse syndrome, which results from overstressing your body with repeated harder workouts and manifests itself as frequent colds, chronic tiredness, and joint and muscle injuries. A day of rest at least once a week is vitally important, even if on that day you simply do a different or low-intensity activity. But do not allow more than 2 days to elapse between workouts if you want to maintain your heightened insulin action, as we will discuss in more detail in the next chapter.

## Precompetition Tapers

As you near an athletic competition or an event such as a road race (even if you are doing it recreationally), consider how to cut back on your training to optimize how well you do and how good you feel when the big day arrives. How hard you work out is probably the most important factor in improving performance and maintaining your fitness level even when you cut your frequency or duration of exercise. Pre-event tapers (decreasing your training volume) can last from 1 day up to 1 week or more, and they are most effective if you maintain the intensity of your workouts while cutting their duration. With diabetes, although you may effectively maintain your fitness levels during pre-event tapering, be prepared to increase your insulin doses or reduce your food intake during a taper because you will be expending fewer calories and using less muscle glycogen and blood glucose. If you decrease your exercise intensity as well, you may need even greater regimen changes to keep your blood glucose from rising.

## Duration: Length of Your Workouts

The length of your workout usually depends on its intensity. The harder you work, the less time you must be active to gain the same benefits. You can get by doing about half the duration (75 minutes a week instead of 150) if you raise your intensity from moderate to vigorous. Although some improvements in endurance have been shown with extremely intense exercise (more than 90 percent of $\dot{V}O_2$max) lasting only 5 to 10 minutes, this type of exercise adds significantly to the risk for injuries and cardiovascular events, so it is less often recommended for most people. If you have diabetes, exercise that intense may also cause your blood glucose to rise.

You will generally expend more calories by exercising over a longer duration at a lower, more sustainable intensity. Although relatively modest amounts of physical activity will improve health, for weight loss and greater health benefits you may have to do more than the minimum of 30 minutes of moderate activity most days of the week. Your risk of getting an athletic injury increases, however, when your intensity and duration of exercise go up. The risk of injury among joggers has been found to be as high as 55 percent. Although more is often better, too much may result in injury, so respect your personal limits.

You can also break up your aerobic activity into smaller bouts during the day and achieve almost the same fitness gains. If you cannot currently work out for 20 to 30 minutes at a time without stopping, start with shorter bouts and work up to doing longer ones. If you are training for a prolonged event like a marathon, you undoubtedly will need to do some longer workouts, although not necessarily marathon-length ones. Similarly, an athlete training to participate in a 5K run (3.1 miles) may not benefit from workouts longer than an hour.

*Increasing your workout duration beyond 60 minutes does not increase your fitness gains enough to offset your greater risk of developing overuse or other orthopedic injuries resulting from longer-distance training.*

## Frequency: How Often You Exercise

Frequency is related to both intensity and duration of exercise. So mix it up— for example, you can meet the recommended guidelines by walking briskly for

30 minutes twice during the week and then jogging for 20 minutes on two other days. Athletes who train for a specific event or sport, however, may work out more often to get ready for an event even if their workouts are high intensity. The point of maximum benefit for most health benefits has not been established, but it likely varies with genetics, age, sex, health status, body composition, and other factors. Doing more than the minimum recommended (in frequency, intensity, and duration) further reduces your risk of developing inactivity-related chronic diseases like obesity and insulin resistance.

Generally, when you have diabetes your blood glucose will benefit from nearly daily and more consistent exercise. But with blood glucose monitoring and other methods of glycemic management available nowadays, you can still manage it even if you choose not to exercise every day. Besides, taking at least 1 day a week to rest (or at least to do easier activities) allows your body time to recuperate and may prevent overuse injuries such as tendinitis and stress fractures (see chapter 7). In any case, you can maintain your current fitness level with a minimum of 2 days per week of appropriately intense activity of adequate duration.

ACSM also recommends engaging in resistance training, along with flexibility training, a minimum of 2 to 3 days per week. You can gain or maintain strength by doing anywhere from 3 to 15 repetitions per set on each resistance exercise and 1 to 3 sets with at least 2 minutes of rest between multiple sets. Generally, doing 8 to 12 repetitions and 2 to 3 sets is recommended. Resistance training is essential to prevent loss of muscle tissue over time. Having more muscle will increase your metabolism and daily calorie use and can prevent fat weight gain while improving your insulin sensitivity. Proper training techniques for resistance work are discussed later in this chapter. Flexibility training is also essential in maintaining joint mobility and preventing injuries. If you are over 40 years old, include balance exercises most days of the week as well to lower your risk of falling.

## Volume: How Much Exercise You Get Overall

Your exercise volume is basically a reflection of how many calories you are expending— a function of the frequency, intensity, and duration of your workouts. In some cases, an equivalent exercise volume (such as exercising for 30 minutes every day or for 60 minutes every other day) appears to have a similar benefit to your blood glucose management. This is good news when you do not have the time or desire to be active every day but can make the time to do twice as much every other day. The same energy expenditure can alternately be reached by pumping up the intensity of whatever you are doing to expend the calories in less time. In some cases, adding in high-intensity intervals not only uses more carbohydrates but also increases your fitness faster and gives you options when it comes to choosing how to work out to meet your fitness and blood glucose management goals. The recommendation is to expend around 500 to 1,000 calories per week (with 1,000 being the equivalent of 150 minutes of moderate activity for most people, or a lesser duration of vigorous activity).

# Progression: How to Move Forward With Your Training

How fast you progress should be an individual choice. If you are just starting an exercise program, you will benefit from doing an initial conditioning phase lasting 4 to 6 weeks before moving on to an improvement phase lasting 4 to 5 months and then to a maintenance phase from 6 months onward. If you already have a higher level of fitness, you may shorten or skip the initial stage altogether. Keep in mind that you will make fitness gains more rapidly if you work out at the higher end of your intensity range (closer to 89 percent of HRR than to 40), but starting out at the lower end of the range is more prudent to avoid losing interest in working out or getting injured. It never hurts to err on the side of caution when ramping up your workouts and your total exercise volume.

> *Start out slowly and progress slowly, particularly if you are just beginning to get more active, are overweight or obese, or are dealing with any health complications that you might possibly aggravate with activity (such as arthritic knees).*

After you reach the maintenance stage, your progress will slow unless you continue to overload yourself by increasing your exercise intensity, duration, frequency, or a combination of these. According to the overload principle of training, you must continue to challenge your muscles and cardiovascular system to have further fitness improvements. Try not to increase your total exercise volume more than about 10 to 20 percent per week to avoid injuries.

## Resources for Active People With Diabetes

## Diabetes Motion

The mission of Diabetes Motion is to provide practical guidance about blood glucose management to anyone with diabetes, regardless of the type, who wants to be physically active. Whether you are new to exercise or a sports enthusiast, diabetes can get in the way of being active. This website provides free information that you can use to guide you on what to do, how to do it, and, most importantly, how to manage your diabetes safely and effectively for exercise. It also has links to exercise blogs on timely topics like CrossFit training, the effects of statins on exercise, and much more.

Founded by Dr. Sheri Colberg in 2014, a recreational athlete with over 50 years of practical experience with type 1 diabetes and decades of professional experience with diabetes and exercise, Diabetes Motion gives practical advice that is hard to come by elsewhere. In general, people who require insulin have to be more vigilant about managing their food intake and insulin doses along with exercising so they can avoid ending up with blood glucose levels that are too low (hypoglycemia) or too high (hyperglycemia). This means using a blood glucose monitor or continuous glucose monitor to keep on top of blood glucose changes. For more information, visit www.diabetesmotion.com.

# COMPONENTS OF AN AEROBIC WORKOUT

Having reviewed what components you need to consider in your exercise program, consider what to include in each workout. An aerobic workout consists of a warm-up, the main exercise, and then a cool-down (see figure 1.1). The warm-up and cool-down periods should consist of an easier activity that works the muscles and joints you will be using during the primary workout, such as a slow jog before and after a faster run. A good warm-up includes at least 5 minutes of an activity before the intensity is increased. An appropriate cool-down is 3 to 5 minutes of an easier activity after the harder one. Include some stretching before, during, or after each workout.

> *Take the time to warm up for at least 5 minutes before your aerobic exercise session, cool down for another 3 to 5 minutes, and stretch the major muscle groups involved in your activity either statically or dynamically to stay flexible and injury free.*

People with diabetes are at higher risk for heart disease and silent heart attacks, and proper warm-ups and cool-downs can also help prevent cardiac arrhythmias (abnormal heartbeats) or sudden cardiac events during and after exercise. A proper cool-down prevents blood from pooling in the extremities—one reason why you may feel dizzy or faint if you stop exercising suddenly. Also, you are more prone to dehydration when your blood glucose is above normal, especially while exercising in the heat. A combination of excess sweating and dehydration may cause

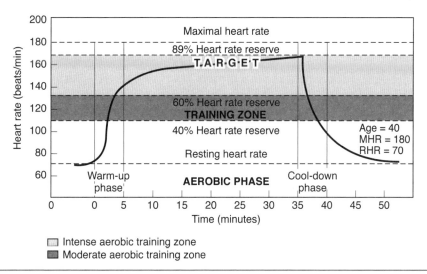

**Figure 1.1** Example of a vigorous aerobic workout for a 40-year-old person with a resting heart rate of 70 beats per minute.

fainting if you stop exercising abruptly without cooling down and allowing your body to redirect the blood flow away from your muscles and back to your central circulation.

# GETTING THE MOST OUT OF RESISTANCE TRAINING

Muscle-strengthening activities include a progressive weight-training program, weight-bearing calisthenics, or similar resistance exercises that use the major muscle groups. Ideally, you should do 8 to 10 exercises using your major muscle groups (in the upper body, thighs, and torso) on 2, but preferably 3, nonconsecutive days a week. Resistance training can be done many ways, including using resistance training machines, free weights, resistance bands, body weight as resistance, and more. Some examples of traditional strength-training exercises are overhead press, bench press, biceps and triceps curls, leg presses, leg extensions and curls, calf raises, and abdominal crunches. Core-strengthening and body-weight-as-resistance exercises include movements like planks, side planks, medicine ball twists, core ball transfers, bridging, lunges, wall sits, and burpees.

> *You will benefit from working on maintaining or increasing your muscular strength and endurance at least 2 nonconsecutive days each week, but preferably 3 days.*

Your strength gains will be maximized by doing 8 to 12 repetitions of each exercise to fatigue. If you are a novice at resistance work, you can start out with lighter weights or more flexible resistance bands that enable you to complete 1 or 2 sets of 12 to 15 repetitions on each exercise, but you should use enough weight or resistance to feel fatigued by the end of the last set. Although doing more reps using lower weights increases muscular endurance more effectively, lifting a greater resistance for fewer reps generally produces more of an overload on the muscle fibers and greater gains in muscular strength because all your muscle fibers will be engaged and will increase in size faster, and you will add more muscle mass. Larger muscles use more calories even at rest, improving your resting metabolism and insulin sensitivity.

The current guidelines do not provide a recommendation for a given number of sets of repetitions on each exercise. You can gain strength by doing only one set, but you will likely gain more strength by performing 2 or 3 sets of each. Alternatively, when doing more than one set per exercise, you can increase the weight or resistance on each successive set, slightly decreasing the number of reps each time the load increases (for example, from 15 reps on the first set to 10 on the second, harder set). If you have time for only one set, make it an intense, nearly maximal set that fully fatigues your muscles by the time you reach the last repetition in your desired range.

You may want to switch between easy resistance training days, when you do more reps with lighter weights, and hard days, when you lift heavier weights fewer times, depending on how motivated you feel on a given day and how much time you have. The only resistance-training principles that you absolutely need

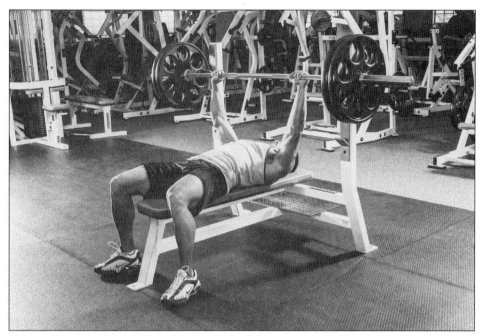

Include at least 8 to 10 resistance exercises using your major muscle groups on 2 or more nonconsecutive days a week.

to follow are (1) to work a particular area of your body (i.e., upper body) no more frequently than every other day, and (2) to train muscles with opposite actions on a joint equally, such as the biceps and triceps muscles of your upper arms or the quadriceps and hamstring muscles of your thighs. If you stop overloading your muscles, your strength gains will reach a plateau or start to reverse (atrophy). After you can do more than the number of reps that you are aiming for (i.e., if you can do 13 or more reps on your hardest set when your goal is 8 to 12), then you can increase the weight or resistance. If you do resistance training correctly your workout will never feel any easier, but you will know that you are getting stronger because you can lift more weight or handle a greater resistance.

## MAKING SURE YOU INCLUDE FLEXIBILITY TRAINING

Your workouts should also include a period of 5 to 10 minutes of static or dynamic stretching of the major muscle groups at least 2 or 3 days per week. This facilitates movement throughout the full range of motion of each of your joints, which can be limited by age-related changes in joints and worsened by elevations in blood glucose over time. The key to static stretching is to stretch to the point of discomfort, back off just a little bit, and then hold the stretch for 10 to 30 seconds. Avoid bouncing, which elicits the muscles' stretch reflexes, or you may end up contracting the muscles you are trying to relax.

*Stretch before, during, or after exercise at least 2 or 3 days per week or at any time your muscles feel tight. Warming up your muscles first works best before you do static stretches or do dynamic stretching that includes gentle movement.*

Stretching is usually easier after you have warmed up the muscles and joints and have increased blood flow to those areas, which is more the idea behind dynamic stretching. This type of stretching includes active movements like lunges, knee bends, and arm circles that work the full range of motion around your joints actively. Some studies have shown dynamic stretching to be more effective at preventing injuries than the more traditional static type, but the overall gains in motion around your joints are greater from doing static stretching.

People with diabetes form more *glycated end products* than normal. What happens is that "sticky" glucose molecules adhere to various structures in the body, including cartilage and collagen in joints, causing them to stiffen and lose their usual range of motion. Although everyone loses joint and muscular mobility with age, diabetes accelerates the usual loss of flexibility, especially when blood glucose levels remain higher and greater glycation of bodily structures occurs. The result is that people with diabetes are usually more prone to overuse injuries such as tendinitis (inflammation of the tendons connecting muscle to bone) and diabetic frozen shoulder, a condition characterized by limited and painful movement of the shoulder (see chapter 7). Your joint injuries may also take longer to heal properly.

# STAYING ON YOUR FEET WITH BALANCE AND AGILITY EXERCISES

In the past decade, a lot of research has been done on the importance of balance training, which can also include neuromotor exercises and agility training. It is important to stay flexible and do exercises that improve balance with aging. Having a strong core is important, but the best way to prevent falling (and possible injuries from falls) is to include some of this training as you age. When you have diabetes, your risk of falling is even greater, especially if you develop nerve damage in your feet. Both strength and balance training lower the risk.

When you think about it, staying balanced is an essential part of almost any physical training that you do. Unfortunately, the ability to balance yourself also diminishes with advancing age, and most people fall after losing their balance while standing or walking. The head, trunk, and arms constitute two-thirds of the body's weight, but with every step that weight is carried and supported mainly by the hip muscles of the stationary leg. If these muscles get weak, you may tilt to the side, and if you slip while you are already leaning, you are more likely to fall.

To avoid falls, work on strengthening the most important muscles for good balance at least 2 to 3 days per week, including exercises for the muscles that lift your legs to the side, lift your toes, and keep you moving forward—basically, work on your hip, knee, and ankle strength. The primary muscle that lifts the legs to the side is a gluteal (buttocks) muscle, the gluteus medius; the main toe lifter is the tibialis anterior, on the front of the shins. Your gastrocnemius muscle on the back of each calf keeps you moving forward. Minimally, include side leg raises, toe raises, and calf (or heel) raises to strengthen these muscles. Luckily, most resistance training and core bodyweight exercises double as balance training as well.

Balance practice can be as simple as practicing standing on one leg at a time. Hold onto or brace yourself against a table, chair, wall, or other sturdy object to start, but later on practice this using only one finger or no support at all. Once you get good at this exercise (on alternating legs), try it with your eyes closed to regain some humility. Other balance training can be done using balance equipment, agility exercises, Wii Fit balance exercises, exercises like the toe towel grab, cushion stand, sit-to-stand, heel-to-toe walking, and backward walking, or even tai chi, qigong, and yoga.

As you can see from this first chapter, you can undeniably benefit by getting and staying as fit as you possibly can, regardless of your current training state. The health rewards of your regular workouts will far outweigh any potential problems of having to consider exercise as an added (and often unpredictable) variable in managing your blood glucose levels.

## Athlete Profile: **Al Lewis, PhD**

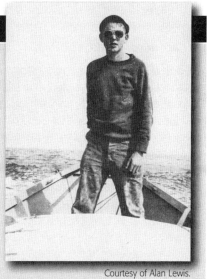

Courtesy of Alan Lewis.

**Hometown:** Victoria, British Columbia, Canada

**Diabetes history:** Type 1 diabetes diagnosed in 1938 (at age 4)

**Sport or activity:** During my preteen and teenage years, I did commercial fishing. In college (3 years at the University of Idaho, 2 years at the University of Miami), I was a competitive swimmer. I did master's swimming (Delta Retreads in Vancouver) until 2009 (at age 75), when I had an accident that forced me to have the lumbar region of my back fused. Since then, my activities have been gym based, biking, and hiking. Due to the back fusion, hiking poles are now standard equipment for my walking. This leads to intriguing comments from others like "Are you looking for snow?" or "Where are your snowshoes?" Needless to say, one develops pleasant but unique answers to these questions!

**Greatest athletic achievement:** The use of a "competitive approach" to diabetes (see more about Lewis' views on this topic in chapter 6).

**Current insulin and medication regimen:** Insulin pump (Humalog or NovoRapid) and frequent blood glucose checks.

continued ➡

*Al Lewis continued*

*Training tips:* Accumulate enough knowledge (not just information!) about your diabetes profile to understand and predict the changes in blood glucose that are likely to occur, first during workouts and second during competition. This needs to include the effect of the time of day.

*Typical daily and weekly training and diabetes regimen:*

▶ *Monday:* I wake up before 5:00 a.m., check my blood glucose, and eat a breakfast of yogurt, fruit, and milk. After taking a bus to the University of British Columbia (UCB), I do a gym workout on campus, including the stationary bike (10 minutes), then a Roman chair (hyperextension) series, followed by mat use for a cat–cow extension series, flat–arch exercise (1+ minute series), and stress and stretching exercises to address neck muscle strength and a shoulder cuff problem (caused by butterfly swimming damage years ago!).

▶ *Tuesday:* Day at the office working (my work is a continuing microscope study of copepod crustaceans as a semiretired oceanography professor).

▶ *Wednesday:* Repeat of Monday workout and schedule.

▶ *Thursday:* Day at the office working.

▶ *Friday:* Repeat of Monday and Wednesday workout and schedule.

▶ *Saturday:* Shopping.

▶ *Sunday:* Bike trip (with Carolyn, my wife)–weather permitting–to one of several locations. I am now using an electric assist bike, a result of the change in my mobility occurring after the back fusion.

*Other hobbies and interests:* Fly-fishing and wine making (primarily from red grapes).

*Good diabetes and exercise story:* The story is a dedication to two people. One (my mom) said that she would not allow diabetes to detrimentally affect what I wanted to do with my life; the other (a former U.S. navy officer) stated that if I was going to have my own vessel and work in the marine field I must take and pass the piloting course given by the U.S. Power Squadron. The March 9, 1949, letter from the commander of the Balboa branch of the U.S. Power Squadron commented that although I had passed the piloting examination I could not become a member until I was 16 (I was 15 at the time). However, that was enough to satisfy my father's seamanship requirements and for me to become a commercial fisherman. My boating picture was taken in 1950 on a 1-day fishing trip with a neighbor. The vessel was an 18-foot dory that I, along with one other at all times, fished between Newport Beach and Catalina Island. Since that time, I have had the pleasure–as well as the tribulations–of working on ocean-related projects of both an academic and a national/international nature. Yes, the negative role of diabetes has appeared at very rare times but has not had a detrimental impact on what is important to me. Mom would be pleased!

# 2

# Balancing Exercise Blood Glucose

**A**s everyone with diabetes knows, keeping your blood glucose in the normal or near normal range is a constant balancing act, especially if you use insulin. Adding exercise to the mix means one more variable to figure out, which can make the process feel overwhelming at times. However, the more you understand about what makes your blood glucose go down or up during exercise, the easier your levels become to manage, and the more confident you will feel about exercising when you have diabetes. Also, the special concerns—including pregnancy—that can complicate increased activity levels for women with diabetes are discussed at the end of this chapter.

## FACTORS IMPACTING YOUR EXERCISE RESPONSES

Whenever you contract your muscles, you increase your blood glucose use. This means you can develop hypoglycemia more readily during or after exercise. Your blood glucose response largely depends on how much insulin is in your bloodstream. If your insulin levels are high during an activity, your muscles will take up more blood glucose, and you will be more likely to experience a low. You might even experience later-onset hypoglycemia, which can occur up to 48 hours after exercise (more on this topic later in this chapter).

Conversely, doing any exercise when your blood glucose is too high and your insulin is low—especially when you have ketones, which are produced when your body tries to use fat as an alternative fuel—can cause your glucose level to rise even higher. Exercising under these conditions can bring on diabetic ketoacidosis (DKA), a condition that results from the combination of elevated blood glucose and insulin deficiency. Although ketones by themselves are not necessarily harmful (they also can result from fasting or a low-carbohydrate or low-calorie diet), DKA caused by insulin deficiency can make your blood very acidic and land you in the hospital. Certain types of exercise such as intense resistance workouts can raise your blood glucose levels as well, but you can learn how to effectively manage and prevent such elevations.

Many variables can potentially affect your blood glucose response to exercise, especially if you use insulin or certain other diabetes medications that cause insulin

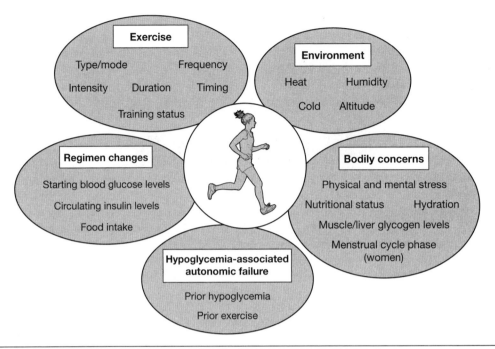

**Figure 2.1** A variety of factors have the potential to impact your blood glucose responses to exercise, especially if you use insulin.

release. Figure 2.1 shows some of the more important factors that could impact your blood glucose with activity. After you learn to manage these factors, or at least anticipate their effects, a somewhat predictable pattern will emerge, which can help you better anticipate your responses.

*Understand, predict, and manage the factors that can impact your response to exercise by checking your blood glucose before, (sometimes) during, and after workouts.*

You can manage some of these factors more easily than others, and this awareness can help you make more informed decisions about how to alter your diabetes regimen. Part II of the book provides more specifics about the potential effects of the environment, including the effect of individual sports and activities such as endurance sports (chapter 9), outdoor endurance–power sports (chapter 10), other types of outdoor power sports (chapter 11), and all outdoor recreation and sports (chapter 12).

# HORMONAL RESPONSES TO EXERCISE

The human body only has insulin to lower blood glucose but has five hormones that raise it (with some overlap). This hormone redundancy tells you that, at least from a survival standpoint, your body is desperate to make sure you do not run out of blood glucose; it is not as concerned about you having too much. Insulin is an important hormone for regulating your body's storage of fuels (carbohydrate, fat, and protein) after you eat. It tells your insulin-sensitive cells (mainly your muscle and fat cells but also your liver) to take up glucose and fat to store them for later as muscle and liver *glycogen* (the storage form of glucose) as well as stored fat. During exercise, any insulin in your bloodstream can make your muscles take up extra blood glucose. In people who have a pancreas that functions normally, insulin levels typically decrease during exercise, and levels of a hormone called *glucagon* (released from the alpha cells of the pancreas) rise to stimulate glucose release.

Your blood glucose levels are managed by your liver, which would normally respond to the relative amounts of insulin and glucagon (table 2.1). Insulin and glucagon released from the pancreas go directly to the liver via the portal circulation. After a meal, high insulin and glucose levels tell the liver to store glucose for later use; fasting overnight or doing extended exercise leads to glucagon signaling the liver to release glucose. How people with type 1 diabetes respond hormonally to exercise is a major issue: the insulin and glucagon at the level of the liver are seldom perfectly normal because their insulin is injected or pumped under the skin rather than released directly from the pancreas.

*People with type 1 diabetes have an altered hormonal response to exercise when their peripheral insulin is relatively high; lowering the circulating level of insulin helps normalize their hormone response.*

All exercise causes the release of hormones that increase the production of glucose by your liver and lower your muscular use, based on how long and hard you exercise. Easy and moderate activities only release a small amount of glucose-raising hormones (unless you do them for a very long duration), but intense exercise such as heavy resistance training, sprinting, or high-intensity intervals causes an immediate rise in your blood glucose and leads to an exaggerated release of hormones. These hormones include adrenaline (formally known as *epinephrine*) and *norepinephrine*, which are released by the *sympathetic nervous system* (allowing your body to respond to physical or mental stressors with an increased heart rate), as well as glucagon, *growth hormone*, and *cortisol* (see table 2.1). The effects of these glucose-raising hormones can easily exceed your body's immediate need for glucose, especially because high-intensity exercise may not last long. As a result, your blood glucose often rises during and after short bouts of intense activity.

*Intense exercise can cause a large increase in blood glucose because of your body's exaggerated release of glucose-raising hormones such as adrenaline and glucagon.*

You may be more insulin resistant immediately after intense exercise and for a few hours due to these hormones. In one study, after near-maximal cycling to exhaustion, one group of people with type 1 diabetes on insulin pumps experienced elevated blood glucose levels for nearly 2 hours. Similarly, in exercisers with type 2 diabetes, blood glucose also rose for 1 hour in response to maximal cycling, as did their insulin levels (because their bodies still produced their own insulin). You may

**Table 2.1   Hormones That Affect Blood Glucose**

| Hormone | Source | Main Actions |
|---|---|---|
| Insulin | Pancreas (beta cells) | Promotes blood glucose uptake into muscle cells and adipose (fat) cells (the latter mainly during rest); stimulates liver uptake and storage of glucose; inhibits fat release from adipose |
| Amylin | Pancreas (beta cells) | Supplements action of insulin by slowing digestion and absorption of glucose from food; blocks glucagon release; promotes early satiety (fullness after eating); cosecreted with insulin from functional beta cells but absent in type 1 diabetes and in individuals with type 2 who produce a little of their own insulin |
| Glucagon | Pancreas (alpha cells) | Stimulates liver glycogen breakdown and new glucose production from precursors to increase blood glucose; is affected by changes in the insulin-to-glucagon ratio at the liver |
| Epinephrine (Adrenaline) | Adrenal medulla | Stimulates muscle and, to a lesser extent, liver glycogen breakdown, and mobilizes free fatty acids from adipose cells |
| Norepinephrine | Adrenal medulla, sympathetic nerve endings | Stimulates liver to produce new glucose from available precursors; acts as "feed-forward" control of glucose during intense exercise along with epinephrine |
| Growth hormone | Anterior pituitary | Directly stimulates fat metabolism (release of free fatty acids from adipose) and indirectly suppresses glucose use; stimulates amino acid storage |
| Cortisol | Adrenal cortex | Mobilizes amino acids and glycerol as precursors for glucose production by the liver and releases free fatty acids for muscle use in the place of glucose (during fasting, starvation, and long-duration exercise) |

need some supplemental insulin to bring your blood glucose back down (albeit less than normal), or it may drop slowly over time on its own. After these hormones wane, your blood glucose may easily drop later when your body is working hard to restore the muscle glycogen you used during the activity. Be on the lookout for later-onset lows in these cases.

# ENERGY SYSTEMS AND ATP PRODUCTION

Your body has three distinct energy systems to supply your muscles with ATP (*adenosine triphosphate*), a high-energy compound found in all cells that directly fuels muscle contractions and movement. The three systems can best be considered a continuum: first one, then the next, and finally the third being revved up to produce ATP as you keep exercising. If you exercise for even 1 minute, you will end up using

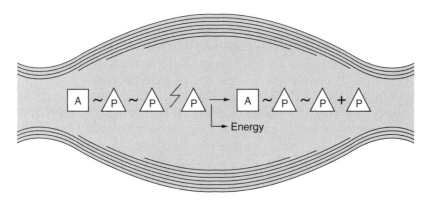

**Figure 2.2**   ATP directly provides all energy for muscular contractions by removing its last high-energy phosphate group.

all three to some extent. Depending on which energy system(s) you use, you may experience varying blood glucose responses during activities.

All three energy systems work by increasing the production of ATP, the only direct source of energy that your muscles can use. The breakdown of ATP directly fuels all contractions, as shown in figure 2.2. When a nerve impulse initiates a muscle contraction, calcium is released within your active muscle fibers, ATP energizes them, and they go into action. Without ATP, your muscles could not contract, and you would not be able to exercise—let alone move.

Muscle cells contain only small quantities of ATP ready for use—only enough to fuel an activity for about 1 second. To keep going longer, your muscles need ATP from another source right away. Although all energy systems can supply this, the rate at which they can do so varies. The fuels converted into ATP and the amount of time needed to produce it also differ by system. Because of these differences, your choice of exercise can affect your blood glucose responses. Learning more about the fuels that each of these systems uses can help you better understand why this happens and what to expect.

## ATP–CP System: Very Short Lived

For short and powerful activities, one energy system primarily provides all the requisite energy: the *ATP–CP system*. Also known as the *phosphagen system*, it consists of ATP that is already stored in muscle and *creatine phosphate* (CP), which rapidly replenishes ATP. This system does not use any oxygen for energy production, making it *anaerobic* (no oxygen required) in nature, as shown in figure 2.3. CP cannot fuel an activity directly, but the energy released from its rapid breakdown is used to resynthesize ATP for an additional 5 to 9 seconds after depletion of your muscles' initial 1-second supply of ATP.

In total, all your phosphagen stores (ATP and CP) can fuel an all-out effort for only about 10 seconds before being depleted. Any activity lasting less than 10 seconds is fueled mainly by phosphagens, including a power lift, 40-meter sprint, pole vault,

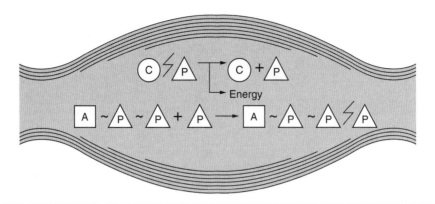

**Figure 2.3** Creatine phosphate (CP) provides energy to replenish ATP rapidly during 6 to 10 seconds of all-out effort.

long jump, baseball pitch or swing, or basketball dunk. Generally, these types of activities do not lower your blood glucose because glucose is not used to produce the energy. In fact, they can raise your glucose levels because they can cause an exaggerated release of glucose-raising hormones. You will not find yourself breathing harder during the first 10 seconds of exercise as this system does not need oxygen to operate. If you breathe harder after a short sprint ends, it is only because your body is using another energy system (the aerobic one) to recover.

## Lactic Acid System: Muscle Glycogen Use Only (and the Burn)

The second energy system, the *lactic acid system* (or *anaerobic glycolysis*) supplies the additional energy for activities that last longer than 10 seconds and up to about 2 minutes. Like your first energy system, the lactic acid system produces energy anaerobically (without using oxygen) through the breakdown of muscle *glycogen* (a storage form of glucose in the muscle), a process called *glycogenolysis*. After it has been released from storage, glycogen produces energy through the metabolic pathway of *glycolysis*, which forms lactic acid as a byproduct (as shown in figure 2.4). When you are resting, your muscle cells do some glycolysis, but because you are not using up much ATP, carbohydrates are processed aerobically (using oxygen) and not much lactic acid builds up.

Lactic acid (or *lactate*) gets a bad rap because you know when you are using this system—you start out planning to exercise for 30 minutes then feel like you cannot make it past the first 2! What is happening is that your muscles need a way to get more ATP after the first 10 seconds, and glycolysis proceeds rapidly to provide more, but not without the pain that makes you want to stop. This system soon becomes limited by the accumulation of lactic and other acids, which drop the pH of muscle and blood and cause the "burn" you associate with it. If you want to keep exercising, just hang on—the next energy system (aerobic) is gearing up to take over if you can just make it past the 2-minute mark.

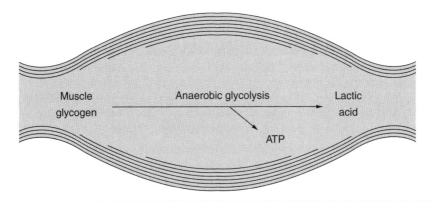

**Figure 2.4**   The breakdown of muscle glycogen results in ATP and lactic acid production and provides most of the energy for activities lasting 20 seconds to 2 minutes.

The lactic acid system derives only three ATP from each glucose molecule coming from muscle glycogen stores, which is a relatively small amount compared with the 37 to 39 ATP that may be made aerobically (via the third system) from each glucose molecule. Consequently, this system cannot supply the energy for prolonged exercise. Activities that primarily depend on this energy system include 800-meter runs, 200-meter swimming events, and stop-and-start activities such as basketball, lacrosse, field hockey, and ice hockey.

Many athletes also include some type of interval training in their weekly routines, which generally involves a metabolic adaptation derived from *lactate stacking*. When you do an intense interval lasting from 20 to 60 seconds, followed by an easier interval (or a rest), then another harder interval (and so on), each intense interval is focusing on using the lactic acid system and producing more acid, which starts to build up in your muscles and blood. You can push hard enough during repeated intervals that you build up more lactate than you can normally stand having in your muscles (due to the burn). Your body adapts to this type of training by becoming better at metabolizing it quickly in between the intense intervals. Your *lactate threshold* is the point at which lactate starts to accumulate in your blood during high-intensity work, which often corresponds with a big increase in your breathing (or feeling somewhat breathless). During intense intervals, lactate is being made without oxygen, but your body uses oxygen to process most of it during the easier work intervals. Some athletes aim for lactate levels of around 4 mmol/L when trying to work at their lactate threshold and 8 mmol/L or above when lactate stacking. Being more efficient at metabolizing lactate is always a good thing for your performance.

You also slip back into supplementing extra ATP using the lactic acid system, albeit temporarily, during longer activities whenever you pick up the pace or intensity (such as going uphill), at least until your aerobic system kicks itself up a notch to provide the extra ATP you need. The lactic acid system can even provide energy for your final kick to cross the finish line, assuming you have any muscle glycogen left at that point.

# Aerobic System:
# Using Any and All Fuels With Oxygen

Any activity you do lasting longer than 2 minutes continuously relies on the *aerobic energy system*, which can create ATP from an almost unlimited supply of carbohydrate, fat, and protein. These longer activities depend on aerobic production of energy using oxygen (see figure 2.5). Your muscles require a steady supply of ATP during sustained activities like walking, running, swimming, cycling, rowing, and cross-country skiing, which you usually do for longer than 2 minutes. Running a marathon or ultramarathon, doing an Ironman triathlon, or participating in successive full days of long-distance cycling or backpacking are extreme examples of prolonged aerobic activities.

The fuels you use during these extended activities are mainly a mix of carbohydrate and fat, with more fat being used during rest and a greater relative reliance on carbohydrate during exercise. Protein can help fuel activities, but it usually contributes less than 5 percent of the energy. The body does not store protein as it does carbohydrate and fat, so anytime you use protein as a fuel during exercise, you are breaking down a protein-based structure (like muscle) for energy or using amino acids coming from digested foods that have been converted into glucose. Your body may use slightly more protein (up to 15 percent) during extremely prolonged activities such as running a marathon or doing a triathlon or other ultraendurance event when your body is running low on carbohydrate stores.

Your body will rapidly begin to use more carbohydrate as soon as you start to exercise, and its contribution rises further with each tick upward in your exercise intensity. High-intensity or near-maximal activities use close to 100 percent carbohydrate. Muscle glycogen provides more of this carbohydrate (usually close to 80 percent) than blood glucose, unless you are already glycogen depleted from long-duration exercise or from being on a low-carbohydrate diet. The actual mix

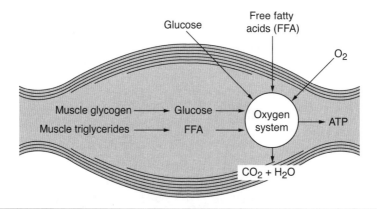

**Figure 2.5**   The aerobic system supplies ATP for longer-duration activities from carbohydrate and fat sources found in muscle or blood, plus a minimal amount of protein.

*At rest, your diet and your last bout of exercise affect the mix of fuels that your body uses, but it is typically about 60 percent fat and 40 percent carbohydrate. Your resting fat use can go higher if you eat few carbohydrates, are fasting, or have low muscle and liver glycogen stores.*

of aerobic fuels that your body uses during the activity depends on your training status, your diet before and during the activity, the intensity and duration of the activity, and your circulating level of insulin.

Hormones like adrenaline mobilize fats from fat cells (*adipocytes*), and those fats then circulate in your blood as *free fatty acids* that active muscles can take up and use during less intense activities. Your body will be able to use fats more during easy and moderate activities, along with some carbohydrates. Keep in mind that when your insulin levels are higher, your release of stored fat from adipose tissues can be impaired. The fats stored in the muscles themselves (*intramuscular triglycerides*) become more important in fueling your recovery from exercise or during prolonged exercise sessions (greater than 2 to 3 hours in length).

Remember that reaching the aerobic system requires that you first must use the other two systems. Both of your anaerobic energy systems (the ATP–CP and lactic acid systems) are important at the beginning of any longer-duration exercise before your aerobic metabolism gears up to supply enough ATP (as shown in figure 2.6). As mentioned, these first two systems are also important whenever you pick up the pace or work harder, such as when you begin to run uphill or sprint to the finish line of a race.

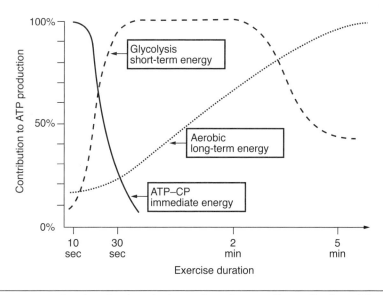

**Figure 2.6**   Your exercise duration largely determines the overall contribution of the three energy systems during an activity.

# USUAL BLOOD GLUCOSE RESPONSES TO ACTIVITIES

The way that your muscles make and use energy during physical activities, including how fast you move, how much force your muscles produce, and how long the activity lasts, can also affect your blood glucose responses. Other factors impact how your blood glucose ultimately responds to each unique exercise condition (refer to figure 2.1), but it is possible to make an educated guess about what to expect based on the release of glucose-raising hormones in response to differing types, intensities, and durations of activity.

Activities and sports that only use the first energy system (ATP–CP) are much more likely to raise blood glucose because they require a lot of power, especially when the duration is limited. If you primarily rely on the third system (aerobic), you will likely experience a decline in your blood glucose over time, depending on the time of day and your levels of circulating insulin (among other things). If you do activities that are a blend of intense (anaerobic) bouts and aerobic movement, such as playing soccer, basketball, or tennis, or undertaking high-intensity interval training or a CrossFit workout, your blood glucose is likely to stay more stable or even rise, depending on its intensity and the length of time of your workout (as shown in figure 2.7).

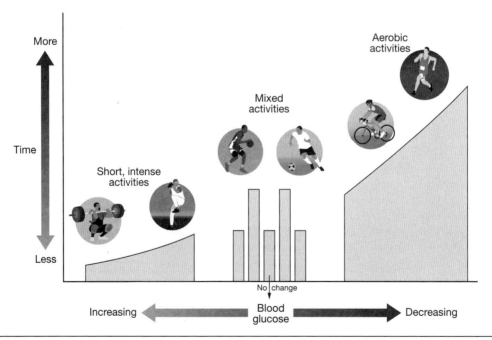

**Figure 2.7**   The type of exercise you do—and how long and hard you do it—often predicts the direction of your blood glucose responses.

# WHY YOU RELY ON CARBOHYDRATE DURING HARDER EXERCISE

At rest, you are already using about 40 percent carbohydrate to fuel your body's energy needs normally (or somewhat less if you are on a low-carbohydrate regimen), but as soon as you start to do any exercise, your carbohydrate use ramps up. How much its use goes up depends on your intensity: harder workouts will always require greater use of blood glucose and glycogen than easier ones, but even the easiest workouts use some carbohydrate. Muscle contractions stimulate the breakdown of glycogen in your muscles, along with glucose uptake from your bloodstream.

Why can't you just use fat as your only fuel if you are fat adapted from training on a low-carbohydrate diet? Because carbohydrate is more fuel efficient, meaning that your body gets more ATP out of it for a given quantity of oxygen breathed in. For that reason alone, carbohydrate is your body's number one choice of fuels when energy must be produced rapidly and aerobically (using oxygen) for longer than 2 minutes. Think of carbohydrate as being like a high-octane fuel, one that gets you more miles to the gallon. It takes less oxygen to get energy out of carbohydrate than from fat (or protein). When your body needs more ATP at a faster rate even while you are in an aerobic training range, you will use carbohydrate preferentially. If it is not available in sufficient amounts, you can use more fat, but ATP is produced more slowly from fat, and your pace will likely suffer somewhat.

Carbohydrate is critical for preventing exercise *fatigue*, which is simply defined as the inability to continue exercising at the same intensity. If you have to slow down at all, even if you can still keep going, you have by definition experienced this. Fatigue is often caused by depletion of glycogen stores in the muscles that you are using, resulting in "hitting the wall" or "bonking" that is common in longer-distance events. Reaching that point while doing a moderate exercise pace usually takes longer than 90 minutes, but it can happen sooner during vigorous or near-maximal activities because they are more dependent on carbohydrate as a fuel. Your muscles use some blood glucose along with glycogen, sometimes more glucose than usual depending on your insulin levels (more on this topic in chapter 3). But you will also start using blood glucose at a faster rate when your glycogen stores start to get low, and that is when you really have to watch out for lows. If you deplete your muscle and liver glycogen, especially if you have not eaten much for a while, you will likely have to stop or slow down what you are doing.

> *If you exercise long enough, your body will use up most or all of your stored carbohydrate. Starting with adequate muscle glycogen stores helps prevent both early fatigue and hypoglycemia, as does supplementing with some carbohydrate during exercise.*

By taking in some carbohydrate during exercise, you can keep your blood glucose stable for longer and prevent fatigue. Carbohydrate is digested and absorbed more quickly than either protein or fat; it usually starts to hit your bloodstream within 5 minutes. The amount you need depends on how long and hard you are exercising,

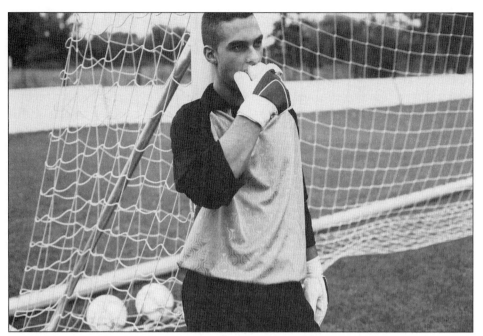

Taking in carbohydrate or other food during exercise may enhance performance in some events and keep your blood glucose from dropping excessively, especially when your insulin is higher.

what time of day it is, and how much insulin is in your system. You will need to monitor your blood glucose to figure out the appropriate amount (if any) for each different activity that you do, especially if you are exercising when your insulin levels are too high.

Even athletes without diabetes have been shown to improve their performance by ingesting carbohydrates during long events, and their bodies can use up to about 80 grams per hour while doing moderately intense activities like cycling and running. Some have suggested that with diabetes you may need to take in up to 60 grams of carbohydrates per hour if you have not adjusted your insulin doses down, but the actual amount will be affected by the intensity and duration of your activity as well as your starting blood glucose level. For most activities, 20 to 30 grams of carbohydrates is more than enough to prevent hypoglycemia, particularly if your insulin levels are relatively low during the activity (such as when you have only basal insulin in your body).

Refer to table 2.2 for some general suggestions for increasing your carbohydrate intake (with no insulin decrease) during aerobic exercise of different intensities and durations. For activities lasting more than 1 hour, continue to supplement with 30 to 60 grams of carbohydrate per hour to prevent hypoglycemia and enhance performance. Up to 75 grams per hour may be necessary to prevent lows when your insulin levels and intensity are higher. On the other hand, intense (near-maximal), short-duration exercise may cause your blood glucose to increase and will not require you to supplement with anything (you may need to take some insulin instead).

**Table 2.2    Carbohydrate Increases for Aerobic Activities in Grams**

| Duration (min) | Intensity[a] | Pre-Exercise Blood Glucose in mg/dL (mmol/L) | | | |
|---|---|---|---|---|---|
| | | <100 (5.6) | 100–150 (5.6–8.3) | 150–200 (8.3–11.1) | >200 (11.1)[b] |
| 30 | Easy | 5–10 g[c] | 0–10 g | 0–5 g | None |
| | Moderate | 10–20 g | 10–20 g | 5–15 g | 0–10 g |
| | Vigorous | 15–30 g | 15–30 g | 10–25 g | 5–20 g |
| 60 | Easy | 10–25 g | 10–20 g | 5–15 g | 0–10 g |
| | Moderate | 20–50 g | 20–40 g | 10–30 g | 5–20 g |
| | Vigorous | 30–75 g | 30–60 g | 15–45 g | 10–30 g |
| >60 | Easy | 10 to 20 g of carbohydrate per additional hour | | | |
| | Moderate | 20 to 40 g of carbohydrate per additional hour | | | |
| | Vigorous | 30 to 60 g of carbohydrate per additional hour[d] | | | |

[a]Easy activities are defined as less than 40%, moderate 40% to 59%, and vigorous 60% to 89% of heart rate reserve (refer to chapter 1 for guidance on how to calculate your exercise intensity).
[b]For a starting blood glucose above 250 mg/dL with moderate or high ketones, you may need a dose of rapid-acting insulin to lower glucose during an activity, not any extra carbohydrate.
[c]You should consume rapidly absorbed carbohydrates except possibly after the first hour when a mixture of carbohydrate sources or other foods may be helpful.
[d]You may need up to 75 grams per hour to prevent lows when you have higher insulin levels.

# HOW MUCH INSULIN YOU HAVE ON BOARD MATTERS—A LOT

As mentioned, in people without diabetes and in most people who have type 2 diabetes, insulin levels in the blood fall during exercise and glucagon (released from the alpha cells of the pancreas) stimulates your liver to produce more glucose. If you have to inject or pump insulin, however, your body cannot easily lower your circulating levels when you start to exercise. Having too much insulin on board can be bad news: it stimulates your muscles to take up more glucose from your bloodstream and inhibits your fat tissues from releasing their stored fat for use as an alternate fuel. You will hear a lot more about how athletes try to manage their insulin levels in the examples of specific sports and activities found in part II of this book.

Muscle contractions also stimulate blood glucose use, and the effect is additive, meaning that higher insulin levels can double the glucose-lowering effect and rapidly cause you to get low during exercise. Excess insulin keeps your fat cells from releasing free fatty acids, making less fat available as an alternative fuel for muscles. Note that if you exercise with higher blood glucose levels, you may use slightly more glucose and less glycogen as fuel.

> *The amount of insulin you have on board (in your bloodstream) during exercise is critical in determining how well you perform and whether your blood glucose stays stable.*

But you need to have some insulin in your body during exercise. If you have too little, your body will be missing the normal counterbalance to the rise in your glucose-raising hormones, and you could end up with blood glucose elevations (*hyperglycemia*) instead. A fine balance is required because if your insulin levels are too high, they can severely inhibit the release of these hormones and you can end up low. Adrenaline mobilizes stored fat and causes muscle glycogen breakdown, and glucagon increases glucose production by your liver. Without these (and especially with too much insulin on board), your muscles can take up more glucose than your liver produces, as shown in figure 2.8. In one study, intense cycling done with extremely low circulating insulin led to hyperglycemia and exaggerated *lipolysis* (mobilization of fat), whereas the same exercise repeated with too much insulin on board resulted in hypoglycemia and reduced fat release. To perform optimally, you need some insulin in your body to counterbalance the release of glucose-raising hormones, but not so much insulin that your blood glucose drops excessively.

## Timing of Exercise and Insulin Levels

The timing of exercise may also play a big role in your body's responses. For instance, you are much less likely to experience low blood glucose if you exercise before breakfast, especially before taking any mealtime insulin. At that time of day, you have only your *basal* insulin (the insulin that covers your body's need for insulin at rest, separate from food intake) on board, so your circulating levels will generally be low, but you usually have higher levels of cortisol, a hormone that increases your insulin resistance, to compensate. If you exercise right before other meals during the day, your insulin levels will also be lower at those times (but often higher than first thing in the morning, prebreakfast).

Aaron Kowalski, a runner from Somerville, New Jersey, agrees: "You can't get low without insulin in your system, meaning hypos can be avoided by being vigilant with insulin on board. Insulin on board is king!" Similarly, Lauren Bongiorno from

| Plasma insulin level during exercise | Liver glucose production | Muscle glucose uptake | Blood glucose |
|---|---|---|---|
| Normal exercise level | ⇧ | ⇧ | → |
| Markedly decreased | ⇧ | ↑ | ↑ |
| Above normal | ↑ | ⇧ | ↓ |

**Figure 2.8** Your blood glucose response to exercise is greatly affected by circulating insulin levels, which can alter how much your liver releases and how much your muscles use.

New York City does not like to run with any active insulin on board. If she needs even a slight correction before running, she will cut it back 50 percent, knowing that her blood glucose will drop. Kelly Butler from Menifee, California, also knows this phenomenon well. She usually only exercises in the mornings to avoid dropping and finds she only gets a low if she had to take more insulin overnight in response to a high; the higher insulin remaining in her system causes her blood glucose to plummet at a time of day when it normally does not.

Personally, I find it annoying that my blood glucose usually rises if I do any type of exercise first thing in the morning, and it feels like a crapshoot to try to guess how much insulin I might have to dose with before working out fasted if I want to prevent a rise. It really depends on how insulin resistant I am on any given morning and how I choose to work out. So my preference is to exercise later in the day before meals or at least 2 hours after my last dose of *bolus* insulin (taken for meals or correction). It is a personal choice really, but it is good to know what you can usually expect your blood glucose to do.

If you choose to exercise after breakfast and taking rapid-acting bolus insulin, your dose may affect whether you get low. In one study, exercisers with type 1 diabetes did 60 minutes of moderate cycling starting 90 minutes after taking their regular dose and eating breakfast. To prevent lows, they reduced their prebreakfast insulin by 50 percent and took no basal. How much they had to reduce their morning insulin bolus was far less than they needed in the afternoon for a similar workout. Long story, short: if you often develop lows during exercise, you might be better off exercising before taking any insulin to cover breakfast or starting activities longer after eating.

Anyone with type 2 diabetes who still makes insulin is also more likely to have glucose levels drop if exercising after breakfast or another meal (as opposed to before) because of the insulin released in response to eating; although if you make your own insulin you usually will not get hypoglycemic during exercise done at any time of day. Keep in mind that if you exercise long enough without eating, whether you have diabetes or not, you can develop hypoglycemia because you will be running low on liver glycogen after fasting overnight. So, for example, running a marathon in the morning without eating anything will not help you finish it well. Even athletes without diabetes can develop lows under those conditions.

> *You are less likely to develop hypoglycemia when exercising moderately in the morning before breakfast or whenever your insulin levels are lower (such as before other meals when you have not had any bolus insulin for a few hours).*

## Regulating Your Insulin Levels During Exercise

Physical activity is one of the main causes of hypoglycemia in people with insulin-treated diabetes. Exercising with low levels of insulin is indeed a much more normal physiological response. To lower your insulin on board during exercise, you may need to reduce your premeal insulin boluses taken within 1 to 2 hours of when

**Table 2.3  General Bolus Insulin Reductions Before Aerobic Activities Based on Duration and Intensity**

| Duration (min) | Intensity (%) | | |
|---|---|---|---|
| | Easy | Moderate | Vigorous |
| 30 | 0–25 | 25–50 | 50–75* |
| 60 | 25–50 | 50–75 | 50–100 |
| 120 | 25–75 | 50–100 | 75–100 |

*Note:* These premeal insulin changes assume that you are not eating extra food to compensate and that exercise starts within 1 to 2 hours after the bolus. You may need less or no insulin reduction if starting after that. For insulin pump users, basal rate reductions during an activity may be greater or lesser than these, whether done alone or with reduced boluses. You may also need insulin reductions (bolus and basal) after activities to prevent later-onset lows.

*For intense, near-maximal exercise, you may need an increase in rapid-acting insulin (rather than a decrease) to counter the effects of glucose-raising hormones.

you start an activity. Table 2.3 gives some general recommendations for rapid- or short-acting insulin boluses given for meals and corrections, not basal ones. (Basal insulins can also be reduced, but for guidelines on doing so, refer to the recommendations for individual sports in part II.)

How much insulin you have in your system between your exercise sessions can also affect how well you do during your next workout. You may end up restoring less muscle glycogen after exercise (or at any time) if you do not have enough insulin or your insulin action is diminished. Although your muscles can take up glucose and restore glycogen without much insulin for the first hour after an intense or long bout of exercise, after that you need to have enough insulin to facilitate adequate glucose uptake and glycogen storage. If you end up not storing as much glycogen, the next time you exercise your body may get fatigued much more quickly, especially if having low glycogen levels causes you to take up more blood glucose. Keeping your blood glucose closer to normal after exercise helps you restore glycogen more effectively than if your glucose runs high during that time. So you will likely need some insulin after exercise for any carbohydrate that you eat, albeit a reduced dose.

# HOW TRAINING AFFECTS THE FUELS THAT YOUR BODY USES

Aerobic training improves the capacity of your body to metabolize both carbohydrate and fat, which generally results in greater use of fat, slower depletion of muscle glycogen, and reduced reliance on blood glucose after your muscles have adapted. The training effect on fuel utilization is evident when you have diabetes: you will find that you either need less carbohydrate for the same activity (done at a similar pace or the same absolute intensity) after several weeks of training or not need to lower your insulin as much.

Some of these training adaptations occur because of a lesser release of your glucose-raising hormones during easy or moderate exercise. People without diabetes have the same training effect, but it is harder to see because their blood glucose levels hardly fluctuate. Insulin release usually goes down during exercise (if you make some or all of your own), but training actually causes it to decrease less. As a result, after training your body uses less glucose and muscle glycogen and more fat when you do the same intensity of exercise—all of which results in more stable blood glucose levels and less chance of getting low.

This change in fuel use (more fat and less carbohydrate) explains why you may need more carbohydrate to maintain your blood glucose when you first start doing an activity but less after training doing an activity for several weeks. But if you work out harder to reach the same relative intensity (e.g., running faster after training compared to your initial training pace), your carbohydrate use during the activity can be nearly as high as before even though you will be able to use slightly more fat than before training during that faster pace. This training effect is sport specific, which means that if you have been running but then decide to try a new activity like swimming, your blood glucose will probably drop more during swimming until you are trained in that sport as well.

*After training for several weeks, your blood glucose should drop less during that activity compared with when you first started doing it.*

# HOW EXERCISE AFFECTS INSULIN ACTION

When you are physically trained, you will likely have heightened sensitivity to insulin, which allows your muscles to take up glucose more easily at rest with lower levels of insulin. This effect is especially evident in people with type 2 diabetes or anyone else who is more resistant to insulin (such as those with type 1 who have "double diabetes," or symptoms of both types).

*Regular physical activity improves blood glucose levels by increasing your insulin action right afterward, for up to a day or two, and overall.*

Right after a workout, your insulin action is higher while you are taking up glucose to restore muscle (and liver) glycogen. You may need to reduce your basal levels of insulin and doses for meals to compensate to avoid getting low later on. Because you check your blood glucose, you are more aware of changes in your insulin action than anyone without diabetes. You will need less insulin during and after exercise, particularly during the window of opportunity for maximal rates of glycogen repletion that occur during the first half hour and up to 2 hours after exercise (and potentially for up to 48 to 72 hours afterward).

Over the long haul, training improves your insulin action by increasing your muscle mass—in effect, giving you a larger "glucose tank" in which to put excess glucose after meals. Trained athletes generally have low levels of circulating insulin,

## Resources for Active People With Diabetes

# Connected in Motion

Connected in Motion fosters a community of people living with type 1 diabetes so that they may inspire one another to live without limits. It creates a culture of support and engagement through peer-based, experiential diabetes education, sport, and adventure (including slipstreams and outdoor adventure events). By motivating individuals to take charge of their health today, it strives to improve the quality of life for people with diabetes now and tomorrow.

Founded in 2008 as a space for adults with type 1 diabetes to connect in an environment that feels different from a traditional support group, this organization currently operates programs throughout North America, bringing people with diabetes of all ages together to create a thriving community. Find out more about their programs and events on their website at www .connectedinmotion.ca.

---

despite being extremely insulin sensitive. However, insulin action begins to decline without exercise in as little as 1 to 2 days, even if you are usually active. Many athletes report that their total insulin requirements increase after 2 to 3 days without their regular exercise (such as when they are too busy to exercise, injured, or ill). Their normal daily insulin doses are set for regular activity, so it is only on days when they are not as active that they need to adjust their insulin.

Although insulin action can stay higher for 2 to 72 hours after an activity, one study of runners with type 1 diabetes found no change in insulin sensitivity after a marathon. In spite of 50 percent glycogen depletion, they were no more insulin, sensitive on the day after the marathon than on a resting day before it, and they were using more fat. These findings are similar to those in all marathoners and likely are the result of the excessive muscle damage caused by long-distance events, which keeps you from restoring glycogen until your muscles are fully repaired.

As you can see, many factors affect your ability to manage blood glucose during and after a workout. Keep in mind that you will tend to lower your blood glucose more when participating in new or unusual activities, but the intensity and duration of your exercise will also affect your glucose use. Intense activities may temporarily raise your levels but can cause them to fall later when your muscle glycogen is being restored, so be vigilant then to prevent lows. The reward of exercise training, though, is that you will lower your overall insulin needs with regular workouts of any type. Taking less insulin means less likelihood of an error on the side of causing hypoglycemia.

## DEALING WITH HYPOGLYCEMIA AND EXERCISE

Experiencing bad low blood glucose reactions lowers the quality of life of people with diabetes. Even the fear of such lows is enough to increase your anxiety levels.

However, you can do several things to lower your risk, including becoming more aware of the possible symptoms of hypoglycemia.

## Recognizing the Symptoms of Hypoglycemia

You need to know all the possible symptoms of lows, both at rest and during exercise, to detect and treat them early. As you know, normal fasting blood glucose ranges from 80 to 99 mg/dL (4.4 to 5.5 mmol/L). Although hypoglycemia is technically any blood glucose below 65 mg/dL (3.6 mmol/L), how low it must go to cause symptoms of hypoglycemia varies. For instance, if you have been running on the high side, sometimes you will get symptoms while your blood glucose is still normal but dropping rapidly, without ever technically getting low. If your blood glucose rarely is above normal, your symptoms may not start until you reach 55 mg/dL (3.1 mmol/L) or lower. Some people have hypoglycemic unawareness, which means that they either do not have or fail to recognize the usual symptoms. This condition is more common in anyone with tight blood glucose management and frequent lows (more on this later).

*Fear of hypoglycemia is the main reason why insulin-using adults with diabetes forgo regular exercise. To optimize your health with diabetes, it is infinitely better to learn how to prevent and manage lows instead of giving up on being active.*

The hormones that your body releases during exercise result in some of the same symptoms as hypoglycemia, which can sometimes make it hard to distinguish between getting low and the normal physical sensations from exercise like fatigue, especially during exercise in weather extremes. The typical symptoms of hypoglycemia include shakiness, hand trembling, tingling of your hands or tongue, sweating, mental confusion, irritability, poor physical coordination (clumsiness), and visual changes. Here is a more extensive list of hypoglycemia symptoms:

- Buzzing in ears
- Cold or clammy skin
- Dizziness or lightheadedness
- Double or blurred vision
- Elevated pulse rate
- Fatigue
- Hand tremors
- Headache
- Inability to do basic math
- Insomnia
- Irritability
- Mental confusion
- Nausea
- Nervousness
- Nightmares
- Poor physical coordination
- Restlessness
- Shakiness
- Slurred speech
- Sweating
- Tingling of hands or tongue
- Tiredness
- Visual spots
- Weakness

The symptoms may also vary among people and by type of activity. By way of example, one athlete with diabetes sees a spot develop in one eye while running every time he gets low; another starts kicking the back of one heel with the toe of his other foot during runs when low. Your symptoms can also change over time when your fitness levels improve or worsen, so you should learn to recognize your own unique set. Be aware that your symptoms can also differ from workout to workout depending on your exercise type, rate of glucose decline, time you last exercised, any recent lows, and environmental conditions.

## Treating Hypoglycemia

Make certain that you carry something with you to treat your lows, such as glucose tablets or gels, or hard candy. You may possibly step out of your house and forget to bring something with you, only to have a bad low with nothing to treat it. One hard-training triathlete who always carries tablets with her during her long, strenuous workouts said she often would go out to walk her dog without bringing anything along and her blood glucose would plummet. It is better to always be prepared to treat a low.

Treat your lows—at least to start—with carbohydrates. Eat something with a higher glycemic index (GI), meaning it will be digested and raise your blood glucose quickly. But do not eat things that also have a high fat content—such as chocolate candy, donuts, or potato chips—because the fat will slow down absorption. Also, your whole body normally only has about 5 grams of glucose total in your bloodstream, so do not overtreat it and end up with elevated glucose levels later. Unless your insulin levels are high, you may only need anywhere from 4 to 15 grams of glucose to raise your blood glucose to normal.

> *Treat low blood glucose with small amounts (4 to 15 grams) of rapidly digested carbohydrates, wait 5 to 10 minutes, and then recheck your glucose levels or monitor your symptoms. Consume the same amount again only if your hypoglycemia has not resolved.*

Choose the carbohydrates that work the fastest, which are the ones that contain straight glucose (also called dextrose). You can find straight glucose/dextrose in glucose tablets, glucose gels, GU energy gel, most sports drinks, candies like Smarties and SweeTARTS, and other forms. Because glucose is the simple sugar that is normally in the blood, it gets there most rapidly after you eat or drink it. These products come in measured amounts—usually 4 grams per tablet or 15 grams per gel or liquid container—which makes it easy to know how much you are getting. With some trial and error, you can determine how much each tablet, gel, or liquid is likely to raise your blood glucose. Dale, an insulin user with type 2 diabetes from Monterey, California, agrees that glucose works best. He says, "I only treat my lows with pure glucose. I used to use food, but it almost always raised my blood glucose levels higher than desired."

If you do not have any glucose tablets handy to treat hypoglycemia, you can use other foods and drinks as well, such as

- One to two rolls of Smarties (6 grams of glucose each)
- One to two pieces of hard or sugary candy (but not chocolate)
- Four ounces of regular soda
- Eight ounces of juice diluted to be half water (to speed up digestion)
- Eight ounces of sports drink (6 to 9 grams of carbohydrate)
- Eight ounces of skim milk
- Two to three graham crackers or six saltine crackers

The white sugar (*sucrose*) in regular sodas and candy also works because it is half glucose, but the other half (*fructose*, or fruit sugar) is absorbed more slowly. You can also eat bagels, bread, cornflakes, white potatoes, or marshmallows in a pinch.

Although many athletes report using fruit juice as their first choice to treat lows, you need to understand that its only sugar is fructose, which has a relatively low rate of being converted into glucose. Juice has traditionally been used for treatment for lows, but it can cause you to overtreat a low while you are waiting for its effects to kick in. Some juices (like "fruit drinks") also have added glucose, so they may work faster than 100 percent juice.

You usually should not use chocolate or other high-fat sugary foods to treat hypoglycemia because of their slow absorption rate, but what and how much you use to treat hypoglycemia with may vary by the situation. If you are likely to keep dropping from the insulin in your system, you may need to consume additional food or drinks with greater staying power—that is, containing some fat or protein to go with the carbohydrate, such as peanut butter crackers or energy bars. Milk is a good treatment option because it contains 7 to 8 grams of protein along with some fat, depending on the type. For prevention of the lows that come on later after exercise, whole milk is much more effective than skim milk or even sports drinks because it contains extra fat that takes longer to fully digest and affect blood glucose. (Chapter 4 has more on how carbohydrate, fat, and protein are broken down, along with how they affect your blood glucose.)

> *Chocolate milk is a balanced, effective recovery drink for prevention of lows and for recovery from exercise. If you cannot drink milk, try soymilk or other variations on any food or drink with a mostly equal mix of carbohydrate, protein, and fat.*

Having glucagon on hand may also be beneficial if you experience a bad low that lasts a long time or that you cannot treat by yourself. Of course, your family and friends will need to learn how to use it on you, and these kits are not easy to use. Some companies are working on creating mini-doses that you can take via a glucagon pen (similar to an insulin pen) to raise blood glucose without calories. These mini-injections work better than simply lowering insulin basal rates, and they are just as effective as glucose tablets when they are injected to treat or prevent lows during moderate exercise, without the potential for causing too much of a rise in blood glucose. Glucagon could previously only be given as a full (and usually nauseating) injection, so mini-doses are a step in the right direction. In addition, a nasal glucagon spray is in the works that may end up being much easier to use.

## Avoiding Weight Gain From Overtreating Lows

Although you cannot avoid treating a low, everything you use contains calories (at least until mini and nasal doses of glucagon are available) and those extra (albeit medically necessary) calories can still end up as excess body fat. Some heavily training athletes have reported gaining fat rather than getting leaner from all their workouts because of chasing a lot of exercise lows. To avoid gaining extra body fat, give each low a precise treatment to limit the calories. That is, if you have a minimal amount of insulin on board, do not just grab the nearest candy bar when it may only take one glucose tablet to bring your blood glucose back to normal.

Start with 4 to 15 grams of a rapid-acting sugar (preferably glucose), and only take in more glucose or follow it with a balanced food or drink if your low does not resolve itself within 10 to 15 minutes or if you anticipate needing more protein or fat in your system to prevent later lows, such as after a long workout or if you took too much insulin. Overtreating your lows just leads to rebound hyperglycemia, which will need more insulin to bring it back down, and another potential low later—followed by more calories and potential weight gain.

## Monitoring for Hypoglycemia

It is not always easy to tell right away whether your blood glucose level is too high or low right when you start feeling weird, especially during activities. When your blood glucose is changing rapidly—going either up or down—you often cannot tell which direction it is going until your symptoms progress. If it has been on the high side for a while or you are exercising hard when your blood glucose starts to decrease rapidly, you may feel hypoglycemic even when it is still elevated.

Regardless of your type of diabetes, checking your blood glucose at varying times, more often than just before meals and at bedtime, can help reveal trends that might not be apparent

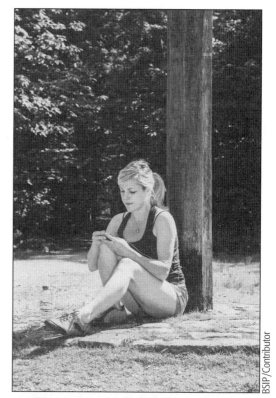

BSIP/Contributor

Checking frequently, sometimes even during exercise, may reveal blood glucose trends that might not be apparent otherwise and help you anticipate hypoglycemia.

otherwise. Continuous glucose monitors (discussed in chapter 5) can detect your glucose trends over time. You want to understand your responses because glucose spikes after meals may be as likely to lead to complications as your overall blood glucose management. Thus, checking not just before meals but also occasionally 1 hour and 2 hours afterward can show how your various meals and prior exercise may be affecting your blood glucose and how much variability you have.

Although it is recommended that you check 2 hours after your first bite of a meal, the actual peak may be closer to 72 minutes after eating and can have a variation of 23 minutes either way, based on continuous glucose monitoring. It also varies with how many carbohydrates you ate and how rapidly they were digested (for instance, beans digest differently than rice). It helps to vary the times you check your blood glucose—not just before meals and at bedtime—especially when you add in exercise. The more you check, the easier it is to figure out your patterns and when you are likely to drop during or after exercise.

## Preventing Hypoglycemia During and After Exercise

After exercise, your main concern will be prevention of later-onset lows, which can occur both because your glycogen levels are low and being replenished (making insulin sensitivity higher) and because hormonal responses to low blood glucose may be blunted after exercise. It helps if you start to restore your muscle glycogen right after exercise at the fastest rate possible by taking in adequate carbohydrate, making you less likely to get as low later. The first 30 to 120 minutes after exercise are the most critical time, when your muscles take up glucose without much need for insulin.

Also, be aware that you may have more than one time after a workout when it feels as though your body is rapidly depleting your blood glucose. At least one study has shown a biphasic increase in carbohydrate requirements to prevent lows, both right after exercise and again from 7 to 11 hours afterward. Be on the alert for this second wave of potential lows and prevent them with adequate food intake and medication changes. Here are some keys to preventing lows anytime, not just during and after exercise:

- Learn your unique patterns and trends—including your reactions to specific foods, activities, and stress—with frequent glucose monitoring.
- Test your blood glucose more frequently whenever you are performing new activities, traveling, ill, or not following your usual routines.
- If you dose with rapid-acting insulin for food intake, experiment and monitor to find the right timing of the insulin and dose.
- Keep "insulin on board" in mind. It takes 1 to 2 hours for the majority of a dose of rapid-acting insulin to clear your bloodstream; if chasing a high with more insulin that time, avoid insulin stacking.
- Never skip the meals for which you have already taken insulin.
- If you are not sure when you will eat, do not take all your insulin beforehand— wait until you have it in front of you.

- Keep track of your blood glucose for several hours to a day after exercise to catch and prevent delayed-onset lows.

- Eat a carbohydrate snack (at least 15 grams) within 30 minutes to 2 hours after doing strenuous or prolonged exercise to help restore your muscle glycogen more rapidly.

- Consume protein and fat that will stick around longer and help prevent lows 2 to 6 hours after exercise.

Refer to the additional troubleshooting and prevention tips in chapter 6 for lows, highs, and early fatigue related to exercise, all part of thinking and acting like the athlete you are.

What you consume afterward may also impact your risk of lows. Volunteers with type 1 diabetes in one study consumed water, whole milk, skim milk, sports drink A (with carbohydrates and electrolytes), or sports drink B (with carbohydrates, fat, and protein) before, during, and after 1 hour of moderate cycling in the late afternoon. The number of calories in the drinks averaged around 450, and the bike riders made no insulin adjustments. All the drinks except for whole milk and water spiked blood glucose levels above 200 mg/dL (11.1 mmol/L) between the end of exercise and dinner. Sports drink B (with the extra protein and fat) caused persistently elevated levels. Glucose declines after dinner were lowest in the people who drank the whole milk. This study shows that balanced foods or drinks (with carbohydrate, protein, and fat) may be most effective at stabilizing blood glucose over time compared with carbohydrate-only items.

> *Although carbohydrates are the most important to replace immediately after exercise to prevent hypoglycemia, extra protein and fat intake also help for longer prevention of lows because they take longer for your body to metabolize and add to your blood glucose later on.*

# Preventing Lows During Exercise With Exercise Itself

You may also be able to prevent, treat, or reverse your impending hypoglycemia during exercise by some novel means. All of these involve using the exaggerated release of glucose-raising hormones that you can get by doing an intense, near maximal, or maximal bout of activity. We will discuss these options next, which are based on research and athlete experiences.

## *Ten-Second Maximal Sprint*

A short, maximal sprint may counter a fall in blood glucose levels. This has been studied by having exercisers with type 1 diabetes perform a 10-second cycling sprint either before or after 20 minutes of easy cycling. Done before, sprinting may keep blood glucose levels from falling for the 45 minutes after exercise; done afterward, it may prevent a decline for at least 2 hours. This technique may also help anytime during exercise. Although sprinting will have a limited effect if you have extremely high levels of insulin or a blunted hormonal response, it is still beneficial as a short-term means of raising your glucose levels or preventing them from falling as quickly. As Martin Berkeley of Cardiff, Wales, said, "I always do a 10-second sprint at the end of a run. This definitely helps prevent hypos by releasing adrenaline. I can clearly see the effect on my continuous glucose monitor."

> *If you are going low and cannot stop exercising, sprint as hard as you can for 10 to 30 seconds to induce a greater release of glucose-raising hormones. But if you have a lot of insulin on board, this strategy will be less effective.*

## Intermittent Sprints (or Interval Training)

You can even keep your blood glucose higher during exercise by interspersing 4-second sprints into an easier workout, which comes closer to replicating what happens when you do sports like soccer or tennis. Doing a 4-second sprint once every 2 minutes during 30 minutes of otherwise moderate cycling has been shown to keep glucose-raising hormones higher, which keeps your blood glucose from declining as much. This effect is the result of both greater glucose release (by the liver) and less glucose uptake during exercise and recovery. Exercisers also experience the same response when they do sprint training and high-intensity interval workouts. Watch out, though, because when the hormonal effects wear off, you may end up more likely to develop hypoglycemia because doing sprints uses up more muscle glycogen.

## Exercise Type and Order of Training

You may also be able to lower your risk of exercise-induced hypoglycemia (or even hyperglycemia) by varying the type or order of training that you are doing during a workout session, such as whether you choose to do aerobic or resistance training first. We know that blood glucose levels tend to fall more during moderate aerobic exercise and less afterward when compared with resistance workouts; this causes less of a decline during the activity and more overnight. If you are already planning to do both activities during the same workout, you can vary the order accordingly.

If you are on the low side with your blood glucose, do your resistance training first, then the aerobic training to keep your glucose higher throughout the first half of your workout. If you are starting out on the high side, begin with easy to moderate aerobic training first to drop your levels and follow that with the resistance work, during which your glucose will stay more stable or rise somewhat (depending on intensity). Fabian Tukacs of Austria has found this works for him, too. He usually goes to the gym and starts his workout with a blood glucose of 100 to 115 mg/dL (5.6 to 6.4 mmol/L). After his weight training, he always does 20 minutes of cardio training; he ends with his blood glucose stable at around 100 mg/dL (5.6 mmol/L).

# EXERCISE AND HYPOGLYCEMIA: WHEN HORMONES ARE LACKING

Research has uncovered the physiology behind why low blood glucose can sneak up on you sometimes. Most athletes would not be surprised to hear that exercise can have a lot to do with it, but that is certainly not the whole story.

## Understanding Hypoglycemia-Associated Autonomic Failure

Unfortunately, if you have had diabetes for longer than 10 years, you likely have a blunted release of glucose-raising hormones (e.g., glucagon and adrenaline) in response to hypoglycemia. This means your body will release less of these hormones, so your blood glucose may stay or go lower than before. How low you go and for how long also affect whether you experience a blunted hormonal response during your next episode. Short duration lows have less of a lasting effect on your ability to respond the next time compared with longer ones, so detecting and treating hypoglycemia early can help prevent this condition.

What's more, experiencing hypoglycemia if you have *hypoglycemia-associated autonomic failure* (HAAF) may blunt your body's hormonal response during any exercise you do within a day or so, even more so in men than in women. A prior bad hypoglycemic event makes your hormones less able to respond to the next exercise-related low when it comes along. Any hypoglycemia, even mild events, may blunt your next exercise session responses somewhat, but the lower you go, the worse the impact. Being hypoglycemic for a longer amount of time also amplifies the blunting.

In a similar vein, if you did not get low but you exercised, you may have an altered response to becoming hypoglycemic the next day. This exercise-induced effect appears to occur rapidly—within a couple of hours—and can increase your risk of getting low for the rest of the day after your workout and the next one. Remain vigilant to catch any impending lows, and avoid them altogether if possible.

> *Both prior exercise and a prior low can blunt your hormonal responses the next time you exercise or go low again. Being aware of this possibility may help you make informed decisions, but avoiding bad lows whenever possible is also critical.*

## Reversing Hypoglycemic Unawareness

Mild hypoglycemia is not pleasurable, but at least it is relatively easy to treat. However, if your blood glucose drops too low without symptoms or enough time for you to treat it, you may become unresponsive or unconscious. If you ever get bad lows without being aware of them, you may have *hypoglycemia unawareness*, which affects about 20 percent of insulin users. It may become worse if you have HAAF and have exercised or had a bad low recently. It can also happen at any point during your life with diabetes: I have heard of it coming on after 60 years in long-living adults with type 1 diabetes. Although being unaware of lows is less common if you have type 2 diabetes, if you do become unaware you are even more likely to experience severe hypoglycemia.

When you are hypoglycemic unaware, your milder or missing symptoms of a low are likely related to a blunted hormone release. Because low blood glucose affects your brain's cognitive abilities, you may check your blood glucose when you are low and not even realize that you need to eat; you may resist help to treat it or fight off or run from paramedics trying to assist you. Unawareness occurs more often when you are sleeping (people apparently wake up for less than half of their nighttime lows), but it also can happen during the day. After people sleep through a low during the night (from which they eventually recover without treatment), they are less likely to recognize another low the next day. Unless someone is around to recognize that you are very low and help you get treatment, you could even have a seizure or lose consciousness.

Fortunately, you may be able to reverse this condition, at least to some extent. Although people often experience diminished glucagon release (associated with HAAF), the most common reason for unawareness developing is having frequent lows. You may be able to at least partially (if not fully) restore your normal hypoglycemic symptoms if you avoid lows for a 3-week period. If you do get low, try to avoid having another episode for at least 2 days to regain better awareness of your next one, and try to limit how low you go and how long it lasts. Some diabetes educators offer hypoglycemia unawareness training, which can teach you to become more cognizant of changes in your blood glucose levels.

# DEALING WITH HYPERGLYCEMIA AND EXERCISE

Although lows are the bigger problem for most people, many people also grapple with how to deal with exercise-induced hyperglycemia. The first question to answer is, Should you start to exercise when your blood glucose is elevated? And to follow that question, How should you deal with the rise in blood glucose that some types of activities cause?

## Exercising With Incipient Hyperglycemia

If your glucose is higher than optimal when you go to exercise, should you wait and do it later instead? It really depends on how high it is, how long it has been elevated, and whether you have developed ketones (a byproduct of fat metabolism) in your blood and urine that are the direct result of insulin deficiency (rather than from a low-carbohydrate diet). As mentioned earlier in this chapter, exercising when your blood glucose is too high and you have ketones from a lack of insulin in your body can make your glucose level go even higher.

For athletes with diabetes who are using insulin, it is often tempting to maintain higher blood glucose levels to prevent hypoglycemia, but going too far in the other direction can be detrimental to your performance as well. It has been shown that once your blood glucose goes above around 200 mg/dL (11 mmol/L), your kidneys start spilling more glucose into your urine. This matters because urinary glucose pulls extra water out of your body, so you dehydrate more easily. What's more, it can mess with your electrolyte levels (including sodium, chloride, potassium, and calcium), all of which can impair your muscle function and ultimately your performance.

So when can you exercise, or when should you wait to do it? The current recommendation from the American Diabetes Association is that if your blood glucose is over 250 mg/dL (13.9 mmol/L) *and* you have moderate or higher levels of ketones in your urine or blood, you should avoid exercising until your blood glucose is in a more normal range (or you have more insulin in your body). Some hyperglycemic athletes have reported that they give themselves insulin and work out anyway. For example, Jamie Read of Perth, Australia, said that he injects 1 unit of rapid-acting insulin directly into his muscle before exercising to keep his blood glucose from rising during high-intensity interval workouts. Neil McLagan (also from Perth) often takes half a unit 10 to 15 minutes before doing heavy and intense weight-lifting, even when he starts out with normal blood glucose. In either case—taking intramuscular insulin to lower a high or prevent one—you should be extra careful because insulin is absorbed more rapidly when given intramuscularly. Taking only a very small amount is the best policy.

If your blood glucose is over 300 mg/dL (16.7 mmol/L) and you do not have ketones, you can still be active, but using caution during exercise is recommended. Your body should respond normally when you have enough insulin circulating and you lower your glucose, assuming that your workout is not too intense and you are not dehydrated. Use your meter to monitor your response, and make sure to stay hydrated because elevated glucose levels can cause you to urinate out extra water. Particularly after eating a meal if you are taking insulin or if your body can release its own insulin when you eat, your blood glucose levels are more likely to come down naturally during exercise.

## Dealing With Exercise-Induced Hyperglycemia

Your blood glucose may rise during morning exercise or intense workouts, or for other reasons. If your blood glucose is higher than you would like after you stop exercising, you can try one (or more) of these options:

- End your workout with an easy aerobic exercise (such as walking) to cool down for 10 to 15 minutes and use up some of the excess glucose.
- Wait it out to see whether your blood glucose comes down on its own during the next couple of hours due to increased insulin action after your workout.
- Take some insulin (albeit a smaller dose than normal). If you have any ketones, this is probably the best option to ensure that you are not insulin deficient.

# BEING FEMALE: SPECIAL CONSIDERATIONS FOR ATHLETIC WOMEN

Being a woman is not a health complication per se, but your female hormones most definitely affect insulin action and can make blood glucose more challenging to manage. If you are female, past puberty, and still young enough to be menstruating or even fast approaching menopause, you will want to read this section to find out more about factoring the time of the month into your insulin adjustments. Moreover, if you are pregnant, living with diabetes, and active, you will also face some special circumstances when it comes to both diabetes management and being physically active.

## How Monthly Cycles Affect Insulin Action

A woman's normal monthly cycle has two phases: (1) *follicular*, which goes from the start of menses up to midcycle ovulation (egg release), and (2) *luteal*, spanning the time from ovulation to when your next period begins. Women are more insulin resistant during the luteal phase because of the greater release and sustained higher levels of the female hormones estrogen and progesterone during that time. Female athletes must factor these changes into the equation to achieve balanced blood glucose levels while maintaining an active lifestyle.

For example, Betty Ferreira, a regular exerciser from Toronto, Ontario, has found that her blood glucose starts to increase gradually 7 to 10 days before her menses and then instantly decreases the day her period starts. To compensate, she increases her basal insulin (Levemir) by 1 unit a day starting 5 days beforehand, and she includes an occasional extra unit or two in her evening dose. Similarly, Cynthia Fritschi from Chicago, Illinois, must increase her total insulin by 150 percent on the 3 days before her menses begin and then makes varied changes for each workout she does during that time. Heather Williams from Columbus, Ohio, has said that starting her period makes her go low.

Not all women are affected equally by monthly fluctuations, and the differences may be tied to the actual increases in estrogen levels. Generally, the higher the estrogen levels go, the more they increase insulin resistance and potentially raise blood glucose (and the need for more insulin). My own experience with aging as a woman is that hormonal swings can become even more intense and erratic as you start to approach the age of menopause (typically around 51 years of age), making blood glucose management even more challenging at times.

Using oral contraceptives can alter the normal monthly hormonal changes in women as well. Currently most of these pills and treatments contain low-dose estrogen and progestin. Because they prevent ovulation, they may reduce your insulin action somewhat, but at least your female hormone levels remain more balanced over the monthly cycle. This leads to greater predictability and easier glucose management for most women who use contraceptive treatments.

# Pregnancy, Diabetes, and Staying Active: The Ultimate Challenge

Even if you are athletic and regularly active, pregnancy releases the same hormones as the luteal phase of your menstrual cycle, which ensures that your insulin needs will go up. However, at least the hormone levels stay more consistent on a day-to-day basis, albeit elevated and rising slowly throughout pregnancy. Raging hormones during the third trimester in particular can make the mother-to-be insulin resistant and spare glucose for the fetus.

Staying physically active will keep you from having to raise your insulin doses as much, even during the last few months of your pregnancy. (In my own case, during each pregnancy my total insulin requirements went up about 2.5 times my normal amount, even though I continued exercising until the day before I gave birth to all three of my sons.) Staying active will also keep you from gaining more weight than recommended (25 to 35 pounds, or 11.5 to 16 kilograms, if you start out at a normal weight, less if you start out overweight) or getting as far out of shape. If you must stop exercising during your pregnancy for any reason, expect your insulin needs to go up dramatically, both from the hormones being released and from the decrease in insulin action that you will experience from being inactive.

Pregnancy increases the energy costs of doing any activity, so you may be using more calories, particularly during weight-bearing activities. This does not mean that you need to "eat for two," as some women claim about pregnancy. Your tagalong *in utero* starts out smaller than a peanut but ends up weighing less at birth than most watermelons, so your calorie needs should only increase by about 300 a day on average over the entire 9 months, even if you are normally active while pregnant. That breaks down to no calorie increase in the first trimester, an average of 340 calories per day added in the second trimester, and about 450 calories extra on a daily basis during the third and final one.

Your total energy requirements will vary with your age during pregnancy, your body mass index, and your physical activity level. The number of calories you expend while active may not change that much, even with your added weight, because your exercise intensity will likely decrease, particularly in the last trimester of your pregnancy. Mother Nature takes care of your baby's health by making it virtually impossible for you to work out as hard as normal (even if you try to) when you are that far along.

You should avoid certain activities when pregnant, including contact sports, sports with lots of directional changes (like racquetball), water skiing, and cycling outdoors (when balance becomes an issue). But you can continue doing most other ones. During the third trimester, consider substituting non-weight-bearing activities such as water exercise and stationary cycling for running or excessive walking. Also, do not do any exercises lying flat on your back past the second trimester because these can reduce the blood flow to your developing baby. Despite all these changes, you will likely find that diabetes management may be the least of your problems when you are pregnant, especially if you are able to stay active.

Once you give birth, expect your insulin requirements to plummet within a day or two as your hormone levels drop precipitously and start to normalize. I highly recommend breastfeeding your newborn for as long as possible. (I breastfed each of my sons for at least 1 year, and over 2 years for the last one. I even breastfed the first one until I was more than 7 months pregnant with the second!) Not only can breastfeeding provide the perfect nutrition for your baby (and possibly lower his or her risk of developing type 1 diabetes), but it also helps keep your insulin needs low and makes losing your extra baby fat—anything over the first 20 to 25 pounds (9 to 11 kilograms) you gained while pregnant—so much quicker and easier. If you get back into your normal exercise routines as soon as possible, you can reverse any detraining that occurred and get yourself back into shape.

In part II of this book (chapters 8 through 12), you will be able to find many real-life examples of how athletes, male and female, younger and older, deal with prevention of both lows and highs induced by being active. Consider using some of their recommendations on how they manage their blood glucose levels in over a hundred different sports and activities, and you will surely get better at your own unique glucose balancing act during exercise.

## Athlete Profile: **Mandy Marquardt**

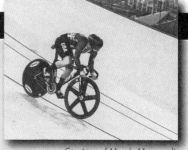

Courtesy of Mandy Marquardt.
Photographer: Richard Lyder.

**Hometown:** Allentown, Pennsylvania

**Diabetes history:** Type 1 diabetes diagnosed in 2008 (at age 16)

**Sport or activity:** Track sprint cycling

**Greatest athletic achievement:** Thirteen-time U.S. national champion; two-time U.S. national record holder, 500-meter time trial and team sprint (set in 2016); Pan American champion in 2016, Team Sprint; 2017 silver medal in Keirin, bronze in 500-meter time trial.

**Current insulin and medication regimen:** Injections, finger pricks, and a continuous glucose monitor.

**Training tips:** If I'm dealing with a high before training, I might correct it. If I have low blood glucose before training, I will eat a light snack since I want something quick and easily digestible. If it's during or after training, I communicate with my teammates and coach and take the extra time I need to feel better. It might be a rollercoaster—and calling it a day or taking extra time for a break is not a bad thing at all. I've had to do it. When that happens, after I get home I use that experience to reevaluate what I could have done differently and hopefully how to prevent it from happening again.

continued ➡

*Mandy Marquardt continued*

In my opinion, taking a break is never a bad thing. Everyone's body responds differently, and you should never be discouraged. I believe diabetes is an opportunity to learn more about your body and become an even stronger you. Listening to your body and taking recovery days are crucial because you are repairing muscle, which does the body good. Also, I think you need to figure out what makes you happy and mix it up sometimes.

*Typical daily and weekly training and diabetes regimen:* Track sprint cycling is very power based, so we spend a lot of time in the gym to build the foundation. Power off the bike converts to power on the bike, so it's important for us to continue building our strength in the gym. As a sprinter, I also focus on building and strengthening other muscle groups like my back, core, and upper body, which helps stabilize my position on the bike and prevent injury or damage. I also heavily rely on plyometric exercises for improving the explosive side of my sprint. Here is a good website that goes into detail of what track sprint training is: www.cyclingweekly.com /fitness/training/how-to-train-like-a-sprinter-334002.

► *Monday:* Morning track session, typically with an ice bath afterward. Recovery is a very important aspect of my training. I take recovery just as serious as my training.

► *Tuesday:* 2-hour gym session, then lunch and an afternoon track session.

► *Wednesday:* 1-hour road recovery ride, massage, and chiropractor appointment.

► *Thursday:* 2-hour gym session, then lunch and an afternoon track session.

► *Friday:* Morning track session. This is definitely one of the hardest days because it's coming toward the end of the week, so utilizing recovery modalities such as ice baths, compression pants, and good nutrition are all so important.

► *Saturday:* 2-hour gym session, 2-hour road ride. This is typically a "sprinter" road ride, so the pace isn't as quick compared to an endurance rider. My coach adds this in for a little maintenance, but the week workload already gives me the endurance I need. Our races are typically 10 to 30 seconds long.

► *Sunday:* Completely off, but I usually take an ice bath and try to stay off my feet as much as possible, but chores still need to get done . . .

*Other hobbies and interests:* Gardening, Netflix, getting my nails done. I graduated from Pennsylvania State at Lehigh Valley in May 2014 with a bachelor's degree in business management and marketing. When I graduated, I wanted to fully focus on my cycling career, and I took on a part-time coaching position. I also serve on the Penn State Lehigh Valley Alumni Board of Directors. I enjoy giving back to the sport and my community through mentoring and coaching student-athletes. It's fun to continue to plant roots on campus. Training, racing, and traveling take up a lot of my time, which helps me break up my routine.

*Good diabetes and exercise story:* The diabetes community is the best. I'm so honored to race for Team Novo Nordisk and the USA Cycling National Team. One of my biggest goals is to represent my country in the 2020 Olympic Games. Not only would it be the pinnacle of my athletic career, but it would also be an incredible platform to inspire, educate, and empower those affected by diabetes and to encourage them to pursue their dreams.

One of the young girls that I mentor (15-year-old McKenna McKee, who also races with type 1 diabetes) wrote me a letter that said, "I really hope you make the Olympics, because you know we will be right there to cheer you on! You are so inspiring and such a great person. If I had to choose my favorite superhero, I would say forget superheroes and meet Mandy because she's the closest you will get to meeting one." McKenna's letter is always in my backpack. It's my good-luck charm. I love the photos I have of McKenna, her mom, my mom, and me at the 2017 USA Cycling Track Nationals in Carson, California. They're very special to me! Our parents are definitely our biggest supporters.

# 3

# Ups and Downs of Insulin and Other Medications

**A**t the start of any activity, your muscles start using more glucose and your body increases the release of glucose-raising hormones (covered in the last chapter) to try to prevent a drop in your blood glucose. At the same time, your pancreas releases less insulin (if you still make any) during exercise. But if you take insulin, your body may not be able to respond normally.

You cannot stop insulin absorption from an injection or pump site after you have given it, and exercise may speed up its absorption by increasing the blood flow to your muscles and skin. As a result, instead of having less insulin in your bloodstream during exercise, you may end up with more than normal. Similarly, certain oral diabetes medications can cause a greater release of insulin or interfere with your digestion of carbohydrates taken for a low, potentially resulting in hypoglycemia. This chapter will let you know what steps you can take to prevent lows (and highs) during exercise, no matter which type of diabetes medications you use. You will also learn about other medications that may cause problems when you are active or cause you to gain weight.

## INSULIN USE

Have you ever felt like jumping on your bike and going for a ride without having to plan ahead? When you use insulin, the problem with such spontaneity is that your insulin levels during an activity can greatly affect your blood glucose (refer to figure 2.8 in chapter 2). To predict your response to working out, you must take into account the types of insulin you use, when you last took any, and how much is "on board" before, during, and after.

Different insulins have varying times to reach their peak action and unique durations, making activities (especially spontaneous ones) harder to handle. Multiple types of insulins are now on the market, and most can be taken via an insulin syringe, pen, or pump. The actions of insulins are considered ultra-rapid, rapid, short, intermediate, long, or ultra-long depending on their onset, peak, and duration. Each type potentially has a different effect on your blood glucose responses to exercise. For insulin users, exercise must often be handled with insulin changes or extra food intake to prevent hypoglycemia.

*Know when your insulin peaks and how long it lasts to anticipate your blood glucose responses to exercise and decide whether to eat more or change your insulin doses.*

# Fast-Acting Insulins

Synthetic human insulins have the same structure as actual human insulin, as well as a faster onset, quicker peak time, and shorter duration than their older animal counterparts. Human synthetic regular insulin (Humulin R and Novolin R) is still available, but few manufacturers make the beef and pork versions (which are more likely to cause allergic reactions). Regular insulin is not as widely used anymore, although it is making a comeback among people who are following a low-carbohydrate diet. I personally think (and many low-carbohydrate athletes would agree) that it is better for covering mixed meals—especially when you are eating slowly digested carbohydrates or lots of protein—because of its longer duration and slower onset compared with the newer, more rapid-acting insulin analogs. Jamie Read of Perth, Australia, apparently agrees with me that regular insulin is better to cover protein (and fat). He has used Novolin R for the last 2 years to cover his main, red-meat protein meals; he injects it about 30 minutes before the meal. He says, "I find regular matches in very well with the glucose timing of a filling red meat and vegetable meal. This way I tend to avoid those blood glucose spikes that were typical 3, 4, or 5 hours after such a meal when using NovoRapid or NovoLog."

In recent decades, even faster insulins have taken over the market from regular, including Humalog (generic name: lispro), Admelog (biosimilar to Humalog), NovoLog or NovoRapid (aspart), Apidra (insulin glulisine), and Fiasp, a faster-acting version of aspart. These products are technically insulin analogs, meaning that their structure is similar to insulin, but the order of their *amino acids* (protein building blocks) is slightly modified to make them have a faster absorption and shorter duration. The benefit of these analogs is that their action has peaked and mostly dissipated within 2 to 3 hours, lowering your risk of getting low when active after that. Most insulin pump users are now using one of these analogs for both basal and bolus insulin coverage. For a comparison of these and other insulins, refer to table 3.1. The insulin action times may vary somewhat depending on environmental conditions, activity level, injection site, and dosage taken.

Fiasp (a faster version of aspart) is now being used by some athletes, although how much faster it is remains to be seen. Professor Mike Riddell from Toronto likes to use it in his insulin pump, saying that he thinks it is more responsive to changes in basal rates and when correcting postexercise highs. By contrast, Dr. Jeremy Pettus of San Diego, California, has tried using Fiasp and did not notice much of a time difference in its peak for meals (he says you still need to prebolus with it before eating). Whether it is noticeably faster or not, it gives you one more option to try.

*For all insulins, the smaller the dose you take, the more rapidly it is absorbed. This is due to the exposed surface area of the insulin drop injected under the skin.*

**Table 3.1   Insulin Action Times**

| Insulin | Onset | Peak (hours) | Duration (hours) |
|---|---|---|---|
| Fiasp | 2–15 minutes | 0.25–2.0 | 2–5 |
| Humalog, Admelog, NovoLog/ NovoRapid, and Apidra | 10–30 minutes | 0.5–1.5 | 3–5 |
| Regular (R) | 30–60 minutes | 2–5 | 5–8 |
| NPH (N)/Isophane (I) | 1–2 hours | 2–12 | 14–24 |
| Lantus, Basaglar, Toujeo | 1.5 hours | None | 20–24 |
| Levemir | 1–3 hours | 8–10 | Up to 24 |
| Tresiba | 30–90 minutes | None | Well over 24 |

An inhaled insulin, Afrezza, is also available despite problems with its marketing (so it may or may not remain on the market). It comes as single-use 4- and 8-unit cartridges that are disposed of after using, but only about half of the dose fully hits your bloodstream; that is, a 4-unit cartridge equals about a 1- to 2-unit dose, and an 8-unit cartridge is equivalent to no more than a 4-unit dose. Its onset is similar to fast-acting insulin analogs, but its duration is reportedly much shorter.

Not many people appear to be using inhaled insulin, but those who do—like Peter Nerothin of San Diego, California—think highly of it. He says, "I use Afrezza for the rare occasions when I wake up above 300 mg/dL (16.7 mmol/L): super-fast drop and flat line stable within 45 to 60 minutes. It is like a miracle! The best part for people who are super insulin sensitive like me is that it's completely gone after about 2 hours so I can exercise. Otherwise I'd have to wait 4 to 6 hours after correction, unless I want to eat empty carbs and work out on a full stomach. I have also heard of people using it instead of a dual wave for pizza and other foods, or as a quick hit for high glycemic foods." Its main drawback is that people with certain lung conditions (like asthma or emphysema) cannot use it, and it may cause persistent coughing in others. Mike Joyce from Sarasota, Florida, uses it exclusively for meals and corrections, stating that he uses 8 units for most meals, with a 4-unit follow-up for protein. "I correct anything at 110 mg/dL (6.1 mmol/L) with a 4-unit dose, which I find works more like 1 unit of injected insulin."

# Intermediate-Acting Insulins

Some intermediate-acting insulins are still available and are more widely used in parts of the world outside the United States. NPH (trade names: Humulin N or Novolin N in the United States, and Protophane elsewhere; generic name, isophane, or I) is the most common insulin with an intermediate action. A usual regimen is NPH at breakfast along with fast-acting insulin at meals as needed during the day and a second dose of NPH at bedtime. An alternative regimen is to take fast-acting insulins for meals during the day with a single bedtime dose of NPH. If you have type 2 diabetes, you may be using NPH alone or a mixture of NPH with a faster one (e.g., a 70–30 mix or another mix).

## Basal Insulins

Long-acting basal insulins, including Lantus (generic name: glargine), Basaglar (a biosimilar version of Lantus), Toujeo (three times the usual concentration of glargine [U-300]), Levemir (detemir), and Tresiba (degludec), have replaced the use of older long-lasting insulins (like Ultralente). The main differences are their duration and how often you should dose with them. Levemir requires twice-daily dosing. Lantus, Basaglar, and Toujeo are supposed to last up to 24 hours and be taken once daily, but many athletes taking small doses (less than 20 units daily) have to split their dose and give it twice a day about 12 hours apart. (I split mine unevenly with 10 units in the morning to cover protein and fat digestion during the day and 5 units at bedtime.) The duration of all glargine insulins is quite variable and as short as 12 hours. Tresiba is the longest-acting basal insulin, lasting up to 48 hours or longer, and it can (supposedly) be given at any time of day. All basal insulins are considered peakless and cover background insulin needs, but Lantus and Basaglar have more of a peak than Levemir in the first 6 to 12 hours after each dose.

The benefit of long-lasting choices is that you will always have some basal insulin on board to cover your body's basic needs. When insulin pump sites fail, users are left with no real basal insulin coverage for hours. The main downside of basal insulins is that it is harder to make short-term corrections in basal coverage during unusual or prolonged activities unless you lower your doses in advance. Also, absorption can be inconsistent based on your injection site and activity level, as well as if you massage the injection area, go hot tubbing, or otherwise speed up how quickly it shows up in your circulation. You can end up with basal insulin levels that are at first excessive and later on deficient.

> *For many Lantus (or Basaglar) users who only need small doses of basal insulin, coverage lasts significantly less than 24 hours, so you may need to take it twice a day.*

The ultra-long-acting insulin called Tresiba is also gaining popularity among all who need constant basal insulin dosing. Not much research has been done so far on how well it works with exercise. However, Cathy DeVreeze, an athlete from Ontario, Canada, is using this basal insulin and loving it. She says it has stopped the dawn syndrome (early morning rise in blood glucose) that she has always had and could never control with other basal insulins. She usually gives a week between changes to her dosing because she finds it takes a couple of days for her body to adjust, and she has needed lower doses than she started with. You may need to supplement with extra insulin during the first few days you are switching onto it until it reaches a steady state, but take a dose that is 20 to 40 percent lower than what you needed with other basal insulins to avoid causing incessant lows from Tresiba due to its staying power.

Tresiba's long duration does make it much more difficult to lower your doses to account for extra exercise or multiple days of activity. Mike Chadwick, an athlete from Mullica Hill, New Jersey, has a unique approach to address this issue with Tresiba. He gets 50 percent of his basal insulin coverage from Tresiba and the other half from his Omnipod insulin pump (filled with Humalog). He started doing this split regimen to make sure he had some insulin on board in case his pump failed, but it allows him more basal dosing flexibility during training than Tresiba alone does. He says, "For 1-hour efforts, it's no big deal. But after 2 days of exercise on the weekends, I need to lower my basal halfway through the first day and into the second day, which I can't do with Tresiba. If Tresiba were my only basal insulin, hypoglycemia would be my only response." He finds that as his fitness increases, he requires fewer changes in his basal doses, though.

# INSULIN PUMPS

Whether you have type 1 or type 2 diabetes, if you use insulin, you may choose to use a specialized insulin pump for both your basal and bolus insulin delivery. Pumps have a small catheter placed under your skin and are programmed to cover your basal insulin needs by delivering small doses of fast-acting insulin to mimic normal insulin release by the pancreas. You give separate bolus doses with your pump to cover your food and snacks or to bring down highs. Every 3 days or so you have to change the infusion site by putting in a new catheter to avoid clogging and excessive buildup of scar tissue that can compromise your insulin delivery. (I personally have been on a "pump vacation" since 2002 because pump-induced scar tissue in my abdominal region made my insulin infusion sites go bad too frequently for my taste, although most pump users do not have such a negative experience.)

The goal of insulin pump therapy is to provide insulin just like your body would—that is, in small doses all day long, with bigger doses after meals. Although this physiological pattern can be closely mimicked using injection regimens (e.g., Levemir for basal and Apidra boluses), insulin pumps make delivery easier and offer more flexibility by allowing you to have different basal rates of insulin delivery during the day or use temporary basal settings (such as during and after exercise). Pump users have the luxury of suspending the pump or immediately reducing basal delivery of insulin for activities, which you cannot do as easily without planning ahead if you use injections.

## Insulin Pump Features

Although the number of insulin pump companies has dwindled recently, a number of pumps with various features are still available. Although you still have to be smarter than your pump, these "smart pump" features have helped take a lot of the guesswork out of it. Most pumps have options for small basal increments (0.05 unit per hour or less), temporary basal rates, insulin-on-board calculators, menu-driven programming, and various bolus patterns. Normal boluses, for instance, give the insulin dose all at once, but extended ones allow a dose to be given over a longer period to avoid peaks and valleys in coverage for foods that are more slowly absorbed; combination boluses combine these two strategies for optimal

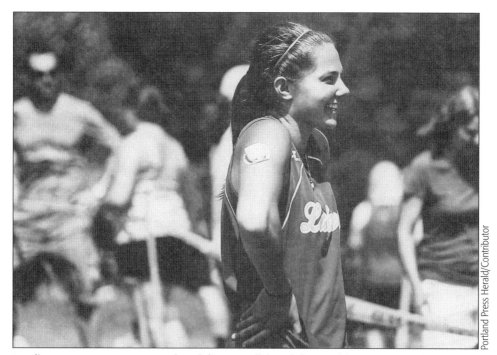

Insulin pumps are programmed to deliver small, basal doses of fast-acting insulin to mimic normal insulin release by the pancreas throughout the day. These pumps are not ideal for everyone, and the choice to use one and the one chosen should be an individual one.

coverage of foods like pizza. Some are waterproof at shallow depths. The race is on to create the best combination insulin pump therapy and continuous glucose monitoring (CGM) with algorithm-driven control systems. These "closed-loop" systems integrate features and make decisions for you, although exercise remains a sizable management hurdle to overcome (read more about these systems in chapter 5).

# Insulin Pump Exercise Strategies

Insulin pumps give users the opportunity to reduce basal insulin levels and/or bolus doses in desired amounts and for different durations. As a result, pump use may reduce your exercise-induced hypoglycemia risk compared to multiple daily injections. Some strategies using pump features may be helpful, based on the purpose and timing of insulin dosing.

## *Altered Bolus Doses Before Exercise*

You can adjust your meal and correction doses of insulin with a high degree of accuracy to accommodate for exercise. Calculate boluses as usual (entering the actual carbohydrates and blood glucose) and then adjust them using a percentage. For postmeal activity (i.e., when bolus insulin is still peaking, such as within 2 hours after eating), reduce your meal bolus by 25, 33, or 50 percent, depending on your upcoming activity.

### Lower Basal Rates During Exercise

Reducing your pump's basal rate before, during, or after exercise by programming a temporary basal rate can allow you to eat less to compensate and prevent lows, particularly when exercising for 2 hours or more. If you can plan ahead, try reducing your basal rate somewhat starting 1 to 2 hours before exercise to make sure your insulin levels are lower when you begin. Try reducing it by 50 percent, although you may need to lower it by 80 percent for prolonged exercise.

### Lower Basal Rates After Exercise

Lowering your basal insulin for a time after exercise can also keep you from getting low later when your muscle glycogen is being restored. How much you will need to reduce it will vary by person and by situation. A common starting point is to reduce your basal rate by 25 percent for 6 to 8 hours afterward if you anticipate possibly getting low later.

### Alternate Basal Insulin Profiles

You can use altered delivery patterns if you are going to be doing a full-day activity, such as during summer camp, or while engaging in intense sports conditioning, or when completing major projects around your home. Pumps allow you to switch to a basal pattern that is entirely different from your usual one, allowing for significant delivery rates during peak activity and more modest reductions when you are resting afterward. If you have a pump that allows you to alter bolus calculation formulas along with basal settings (insulin delivery profiles), such as the Tandem pump, you can also use a lesser hyperglycemia correction factor, decrease your insulin-to-carbohydrate ratios, and raise your target glucose during times when you will be more insulin sensitive.

## Challenges to and Solutions for Pump Use During Exercise

Insulin pump use does present its own set of challenges related to physical activity and sports. For instance, some athletes have issues with getting infusion sets to stay in place during certain activities or with excessive sweating. Others have complained that the pump or tubing simply gets in the way during exercise, and they may prefer to remove the pump entirely while active. Given that pumps deliver rapid-acting insulins only, removal of the pump for an excessive length of time (longer than 1 hour) can result in severe hyperglycemia and ketone formation, potentially leading to diabetic ketoacidosis (DKA). Exposing your pump to water and extreme weather conditions can also threaten its integrity and the insulin in it.

Pump use is not optimal for every sport and activity, but it can help by allowing more rapid alterations in insulin levels during activities. Some of the more common pump exercise challenges are included in table 3.2, along with potential solutions. Also refer to a list of strategies and tips used by the athletes found in chapter 12.

**Table 3.2   Insulin Pumps and Exercise: Challenges and Solutions**

| Challenge | Potential Solutions |
|---|---|
| Water damage | • Use a fully waterproof pump (e.g., Omnipod).<br>• Disconnect from the pump while you are in the water.<br>• Switch to an injection regimen for the day. |
| Extreme temperatures | • In frigid weather, keep the pump as close to your body as possible (next to the skin) to keep it warmer.<br>• In extreme heat:<br>　• Place your pump in a special cooling pouch (FRIO).<br>　• Keep your pump out of direct sunlight.<br>　• Change your insulin reservoir frequently.<br>　• Switch to an injection regimen for the day. |
| Inadequate adhesion | • Use overtape or patches on your infusion set (such as medical or waterproof tape, GrifGrips, RockaDex, or other types of patches).<br>• Place your infusion set on a less-susceptible area (e.g., buttocks or lower back).<br>• Use an adhesive aid before insertion (skin preparation like Mastisol or Skin Tac). |
| Inconvenience | • Use a tubeless patch pump (e.g., Omnipod).<br>• Disconnect from your pump during activity but reconnect hourly to replace missed basal insulin via a small bolus.<br>• Switch to an injection regimen for the day. |

# Perspectives on Insulin Pump Use and Exercise

Despite some of the benefits of pump use, they remain underused by youths and adults with type 1 diabetes for a variety of reasons. Worldwide, fewer than 20 percent of people of any age with type 1 diabetes use pumps. Pump use among youths is highest in the United States (around 47 percent), followed by Austria and Germany at around 40 percent. Among the insulin-using athletes completing the survey for this book, pump use was above 60 percent. Some studies have suggested that the top reasons why people stop using pumps include problems with insertion sites, adherence issues, cost, and interference with sporting activities. Others just feel they are uncomfortable or dislike wearing them.

If you are still having trouble making up your mind about whether a pump is right for you, consider what the active individuals with diabetes who are taking insulin consider to be benefits and drawbacks of pumps. Ultimately, it is a personal choice, but it never hurts to hear why others choose to use or not use them when making your own decision.

## Why Some Athletes Choose to Use an Insulin Pump

Probably the biggest advantage that pumping has over injections is the ability to quickly lower basal insulin levels before, during, and after activities. Almost no athletes disagree about how helpful this is for being active. Canadian Dessi Zaharieva says, "I can really fine-tune the adjustments to basal and bolus insulin pre- and postexercise with an insulin pump. It has been especially helpful in preventing nocturnal hypoglycemia!" In the mind of Vic Kinnunen, a resident of Lawrenceville, Georgia, being able to adjust his insulin as needed when exercising (and after exercise) is critical. Similarly, Emily Marrama of Lynn, Massachusetts, loves being able to reduce her basal rate before, during, or after exercising. Marialice Kern from Moraga, California, acknowledges that with a pump, it is "much easier to control the amount of insulin, and change or stop delivery when you begin/end exercising."

Many sports enthusiasts love their pumps for a variety of reasons. Conor Smith, an Ironman triathlete from Fort Washington, Pennsylvania, is particularly enamored with the Omnipod pump because it is both tubeless and waterproof. He says, "It's a huge benefit that I don't have to disconnect, especially when swimming. It's great to be able to do temporary basal rate and also great for dosing on the fly if I am running high or need to fuel." Stephen England from New York City appreciates being able to set temporary basal rates, especially when running for long periods (several hours or days). Likewise, Mike Riddell from Toronto enjoys being able to give very small amounts of variable basal insulin, along with making very small insulin corrections and setting temporary basal rates around being active. Marc Blatstein of Huntingdon Valley, Pennsylvania, simply states, "I totally enjoy the pump and don't find any drawbacks."

Judith Jones-Ambrosini, a part-time resident of New York City, thinks that being able to reduce or suspend basal activity for hours comes in handy during exercise. She says, "My insulin pump does not interfere with the types of exercise I do, so I am quite comfortable wearing my pump 24/7. In fact I would probably have a hard time feeling comfortable without it since I have been wearing an insulin pump since 1995." Saul Zuckman from Columbia, Maryland, will not leave home without his pump either. He wears a bicycle jersey with the large rear pockets and pouches to store his pump during exercise, and he tapes the infusion set to his abdomen to keep it from getting dislodged.

Emily Tiberio, of Beaver, Pennsylvania, has worked out most of the issues she has with pumps: "The Omnipod has been excellent for my running and cycling for marathon training. I have had a little trouble with rowing because I usually keep my pump on my abdomen, but it's manageable. There is some chafing during long runs (over 10 miles) around the pump adhesive, but that is also manageable. On race days, I plan it out so that my pump is on the back of my arm where I have much less chafing."

Not everyone is having a pump love fest all the time, although most pumpers keep using them anyway. Sarah McManus, a resident of Pittsburgh, Pennsylvania, does not find pumping to be necessarily less work than using injections. She says, "With the pump (compared to 35+ years on multiple daily injections), I have to manipulate my settings *a lot* to not go low while working out at my desired intensity. This is more labor intensive and takes greater decision making. But the benefit is I consume less food in order to get my blood glucose high enough to work out." Canadian Sarah McGaugh of Brampton, Ontario, complains that hers "gets in the way and bounces around during running exercises and it's painful when you land on it during physical sports." Mason Klahn of Colorado acknowledges both the good and the bad of pumping: "The benefits of the insulin pump have been lower A1Cs, faster reaction to insulin, and fewer injections. The drawbacks have been my site falling out due to a combination of sweat, different movements, and accidental cord snags." Many others cited issues with occasional infusion site failures leading to too little insulin on board during activities.

## *Why Some Athletes Choose Multiple Daily Injections*

Athletes have a variety of reasons for not pumping, including cost, lack of access, pumping issues, and even inertia ("If it ain't broken, don't fix it," says Aaron Gretz from Apple Valley, Minnesota). Some people just feel less stressed by giving themselves multiple daily injections instead. A resident of Burlingame, Vermont, Ginger Vieira wore a pump for 7 years, but after getting DKA from a pump failure, she took a break. She tried going back to pumping before pregnancy, but the "occlusions and skin irritation and insane cost of pump supplies just made it so stressful and tedious." As she says, "Syringes always get the insulin where it is supposed to go!"

It is entirely possible to do just as well with managing diabetes on multiple daily injections, and some even feel it works better for them. For instance, Del Mar, California, exerciser Blair Ryan feels like she has more control over her basal insulin delivery with Levemir injections. She says, "I used a pump for 12 years. I see the benefits for many, but I prefer long-acting insulin for basal. I've found I have reduced exercise-related hypoglycemia this way." Michael Horgan from Northborough, Massachusetts, had been on a pump for many years, and he feels it did make skiing easier for him; however, ever since his last pump died, he has been giving himself multiple daily injections and is doing just fine. Similarly, Lisa La Nasa, a resident of Valencia, Spain, used a pump for 13 years but is now on multiple daily injections, using a split dose of Tresiba, a small premeal Humalog bolus, and regular insulin to cover her low-carbohydrate eating. About being off a pump she says, "I switched to MDI (multiple daily injections) 6 months ago, and I love it!"

Sometimes pumping is viewed as an impediment to being active. According to Molly McDermott, a resident of Ottawa in Canada, she does not mind the insulin injections and is totally not interested in a pump, given all the sports she plays and the size of a pump. Multisport athlete Bec Johnson from Perth in Western Australia similarly says, "I swim, dive, mountain bike, kitesurf, and sail and couldn't make those sports work with a pump attached." Sarah Richard, a resident of Fort Walton Beach, Florida, feels similarly: "I live on the Gulf of Mexico and enjoy an active and beach-inclusive lifestyle. Giving multiple daily injections has worked well for me so far, and I plan to continue this treatment until it no longer works."

Blocked insulin cannulas or failed infusion sites were a concern brought up by quite a few athletes. Personally, I have had issues with scar tissue building up and causing infusion site failures; in my case, trying to chase my blood glucose levels back down all day after discovering that yet another site had failed was causing my A1Cs to go up. Although I can appreciate all the benefits of pumping, I can manage my blood glucose for my activities just as well or better using injections, and I do not see my extended "pump vacation" of close to 2 decades ending anytime soon.

For others, not pumping gives them more peace of mind. Melbourne, Australia, native Warwick Sickling does not want to worry about a blocked cannula leaving him with no insulin on board and skyrocketing blood glucose levels. Likewise, Cathy DeVreeze from Ontario, Canada, just started a pump vacation and is loving not having to deal with all the tubing or worries about her pump sites failing. She exclaims, "I feel free now. I don't mind the injections. I struggled for a long time with my pump." Even though Jonah Howe from Montoursville, Pennsylvania, liked his pump, he experienced issues that forced him to give it up: "I previously used an

Omnipod pump and even though it allowed me to do more physically and overall improved my insulin management, I was not able to maintain the blood glucose control that I experience on injections. In my case. absorption issues and continuous mechanical failures led to stress and high blood glucose levels."

Others are only enjoying some of the benefits, or they are waiting for other options down the road. For example, Chelsea Brown from Berkeley, California, wears a pump but only overnight, not during the day. Ruth Sproull from Newport, Vermont, does not want to get a pump until it is fully automated with CGM readings as well (see more on closed-loop systems in chapter 5). The bottom line is that there is no right or wrong here—you should use whatever works best for you.

## An Athlete's Experience Switching From a Pump to Basal Insulin Injections

This is the story of Blair Ryan, a former competitive runner from Del Mar, California, who made the switch from a pump to Levemir to cover her basal insulin needs.

"For 12 years, I ran competitively using an insulin pump without finding an insulin-to-carbohydrate ratio that would both sustain my blood glucose and give me enough insulin on board to fuel my muscles. Like many people with diabetes, when I thought about how to fuel for optimal athletic performance, I made the mistake of focusing solely on which types of carbs to consume while cutting back insulin to prevent lows. Before my high school and collegiate running practices, I was ingesting hundreds of calories I didn't want and ran with a sloshing stomach. I didn't explore insulin as fuel.

Those frustrating routines continued until 2012 when I was training for an Ironman triathlon with some friends with diabetes, Peter Nerothin and Brennan Cassidy. They received good results from injecting basal insulin, and encouraged me to try Levemir for basal. It changed my life.

Now there is a growing group of endurance athletes with diabetes, including me, who've found that by investing a little time to explore new basal insulin strategies we've made huge progress in eliminating exercise-induced low blood glucose, improved athletic performance, and reduced the emotional burden of diabetes during our training and racing. I discovered that when I am using Levemir (taken by injection twice a day) instead of Humalog insulin dripped from a pump, I don't struggle to keep my blood glucose from plummeting during exercise at any time of day like I did with a basal rate of rapid-acting insulin from the pump. With only a portion of my daily total units coming from rapid-acting insulin via injection (boluses for meals and corrections), the amount of rapid-acting insulin I have on board at any point in time is less. I can take my full morning Levemir basal injection and immediately go for a run, with little to no drop in blood glucose. I can eat lunch at work, cover the meal 100 percent with a bolus injection (still Humalog, but injected), head home for a run in the evening, start that run at 160 mg/dL (8.9 mmol/L) and end at 140 md/dL (7.8 mmol/L). I don't have to fill my tummy with carbs before the start to prevent an exercise-induced low. I have become leaner and faster, and my muscles don't feel stiff. I believe this is because the Levemir on board is putting glucose into my muscles, but not being absorbed in a way that lowers blood glucose fast."

# OTHER DIABETES MEDICATIONS

If you use any of the oral or noninsulin injectable diabetes medications, knowing their potential glucose-lowering effects is important. In general, these medications work on one or more of the metabolic targets associated with diabetes: insulin production by the pancreas, glucose release by the liver, insulin resistance in muscle and fat tissues, gut hormones, and glucose loss through the kidneys. Their classes, actions, and names are listed in table 3.3. If you change your exercise routine (or are just starting one), consult with your health care team about adjusting the doses of diabetes medications that you take.

**Table 3.3   Diabetes Medications and How They Work**

| Class | What They Are Called | How They Work |
|---|---|---|
| **Oral Agents (Pills Taken by Mouth)** | | |
| Sulfonylureas | Amaryl, DiaBeta, Diabinese, Glucotrol, Glynase, Micronase | Promote insulin secretion from the beta cells of the pancreas; some increase insulin sensitivity |
| Biguanides | Metformin, Glucophage, Glucophage XR | Decrease your liver glucose output; increase liver and muscle insulin sensitivity; have no direct effect on beta cells |
| Thiazolidinediones (glitazones) | Avandia, Actos | Increase insulin sensitivity of muscles |
| DPP-4 inhibitors (gliptins) | Januvia, Onglyza, Nesina/Galvus, Tradjenta | Inhibit DPP-4, an enzyme that breaks down glucagon-like peptide-1 (GLP-1) in the gut; delayed GLP-1 degradation extends insulin action and suppresses glucagon release |
| Meglitinides | Prandin, Starlix | Stimulate beta cells to increase insulin secretion but only enough to cover meals |
| Alpha-glucosidase inhibitors | Precose, Glyset | Slow digestion of some carbohydrates and lower postmeal blood glucose peaks |
| SGLT-2 inhibitors | Invokana, Farxiga, Jardiance, Steglatro<br><br>Zynquista (combination SGLT-1/SGLT-2 inhibitor) | Prevent kidneys from reabsorbing glucose; lose more glucose in urine when blood glucose is above a certain level |
| **Injected (Noninsulin) Medications** | | |
| Amylin | Symlin | Works in combination with insulin to control glycemic spikes for 3 hours after meals |
| GLP-1 agonists (incretins and incretin mimetics) | Byetta, Victoza, Bydureon, Trulicity, Ozempic, Eperzan, Adlyxin/Lyxumia | Stimulate insulin release; inhibit the liver's release of glucose by glucagon; delay the emptying of food from the stomach |

*If you increase your activity level, you may need to lower your doses of other diabetes medications, even ones that do not usually cause lows with exercise. Consult with your health care team about how to do this safely and effectively.*

## Oral Diabetes Medications

The oldest class of oral diabetes medications, *sulfonylureas*, was first used to treat type 2 diabetes and was the only option for many years. These drugs stimulate insulin release from the pancreas and decrease insulin resistance. The only first-generation one still on the market is Diabinese (chlorpropamide), which can last for up to 72 hours and can cause hypoglycemia during or after exercise, especially if you have kidney problems. The more commonly used, later-generation sulfonylureas are effective at smaller doses and include Amaryl, Glucotrol, DiaBeta, Micronase, and Glynase. Of these, only the latter three (all brand names for glyburide) carry a greater risk of causing exercise lows because of their action (24 hours versus only 12 to 16 for Amaryl and Glucotrol), although all can cause you to gain weight.

*Oral sulfonylureas with the longest duration, such as Diabinese, DiaBeta, Micronase, and Glynase, have the greatest potential to cause hypoglycemia during and after exercise, especially when you do any unusual or prolonged activity.*

Metformin (marketed both in its generic form and as brands like Glucophage) is in a separate class of drugs called *biguanides*. It reduces your liver's output of glucose (often elevated in the early morning in diabetes), but it can lower glucose absorption from the gut and enhance insulin action. Metformin is, by far, the most prescribed of all oral diabetes medications. Unlike sulfonylureas, it does not contribute to weight gain and is unlikely to cause hypoglycemia. Some insulin-resistant and overweight adults with type 1 diabetes take metformin, even though this drug is normally prescribed to treat type 2 diabetes, prediabetes, and other insulin-resistant conditions.

Another class of drugs called *thiazolidinediones*, or glitazones for short (including Avandia and Actos), directly enhance peripheral insulin sensitivity without affecting insulin secretion from the pancreas. Although these drugs do not usually cause low blood glucose, they can cause weight gain and have been associated with a greater risk of bone fractures and swelling of the feet and ankles. But their ability to increase insulin action, much like exercise, does makes them an attractive treatment option for type 2 diabetes.

Some medications are now available that work with gut hormones, natural enzymes, and the body's own insulin to lower blood glucose. *DPP-4 inhibitors* are oral medications that work by inhibiting DPP-4, an enzyme that breaks down glucagon-like peptide-1 (GLP-1); delayed GLP-1 degradation extends the action of insulin while suppressing glucagon release.

Prandin and Starlix are two drugs in the *meglitinides* class, which may work well for you if you eat sporadically. Taken when you eat, they cause your pancreas to release enough insulin to reduce blood glucose spikes after meals. If your exercise occurs soon after a meal at which you take either of these medications, you may have a higher risk of developing a low during the activity. They are one of the oral medications sometimes prescribed for women who have gestational diabetes.

*Alpha-glucosidase inhibitors*, marketed as Precose and Glyset, can prevent increases in blood glucose after meals by delaying carbohydrate digestion in the small intestine. Taking these medications directly before exercise if you eat extra carbohydrate during the activity would slow your absorption of them as well. These drugs also can cause undesirable side effects like flatulence and diarrhea. Exercise itself usually slows the digestion of foods, so if you are exercising after eating you may need to lower your dose of these medications or skip them.

A more recent class of medications, *SGLT-2 inhibitors,* treats diabetes by making you lose glucose through your urine. Normally you will start to lose glucose when your blood levels get to around 180 mg/dL (10.0 mmol/L), but these drugs cause release at a lower level. Because they result in more urinary glucose, taking these medications raises your risk of yeast infections slightly (especially in women), urinary tract (bladder) infections in both women and men, and dehydration. These medications have been associated with DKA in people with both type 1 and type 2 diabetes even with only moderate elevations in blood glucose, so be careful about cutting your insulin too much when using these medications. At least five athletes with type 1 diabetes surveyed for this book take a medication from this class, and one believes this medication (Jardiance, in his case) helps prevent hypoglycemia during exercise (perhaps due to a higher glucagon-to-insulin ratio), but research is needed to confirm this observation.

One medication under consideration (Zynquista) for approval by the FDA for people with type 1 diabetes combines SGLT-1 and SGLT-2 inhibitors for the first time. Although most glucose in the urine is due to the impact of the latter inhibitor, the former adds a small amount by causing loss of glucose in urine via a different part of the kidneys. If approved, it will be the first oral medication specifically approved for treatment of type 1 diabetes in conjunction with insulin therapy.

Your doctor may put you on a combination therapy that requires you to take two or more different drugs. Often you can now get combination medications that have two of these classes of drugs together, which can make taking multiple ones easier. Such combinations, however, can make the prediction of an exercise response more difficult if you do not know which classes of medications they contain. Also, starting people on insulin sooner may better preserve the remaining beta cell function, so this approach is worth considering. Similarly, if you get type 1 diabetes later in life, its full onset may be delayed enough that taking oral medications prescribed for type 2 diabetes may effectively control your blood glucose for a while, but usually you will have to start taking insulin at some point for adequate management.

## Noninsulin Injected Diabetes Medications

The turn of the millennium brought the first new drug to treat type 1 diabetes in more than 80 years since the discovery of insulin in 1921. This injected medication, Symlin (generic name: pramlintide), is a synthetic form of the body's natural hormone *amylin*, which is normally released along with insulin from pancreatic beta cells. Its main action is to improve the action of insulin after meals by slowing down how quickly the glucose coming from the food that you ate shows up in your circulation. This can reduce blood glucose spikes, make you feel full sooner, and potentially cause weight loss. As an added benefit, Symlin may also reduce oxidative stress and prevent you from developing complications, although this potential effect needs further study. Its potential side effects are severe hypoglycemia, nausea, vomiting, abdominal pain, headache, fatigue, and dizziness.

Only one of the hundreds of athletes responding to the survey for this book was using Symlin currently, and she only exercised before dinner when no Symlin was in her system. Some type 1 exercisers have tried using this medication in the past. Bill King, a runner hailing from Philadelphia, Pennsylvania, found that using Symlin with insulin boluses helped him correct his blood glucose more rapidly when spiking after a big meal. However, be careful about taking Symlin before exercise, because having Symlin on board may make it harder to raise your blood glucose if it drops. Athletes have complained about getting Symlin-induced lows that they cannot easily treat during and after exercise. In fact, one master athlete who used to use Symlin, Guy Hornsby from West Virginia, reported that he stopped using it for exactly that reason: he had too many problems getting his blood glucose to come up if he was hypoglycemic.

In addition, if you have *gastroparesis* (delayed emptying of your stomach because of damage to the central nerves by diabetes), you may not want to use Symlin at all. It can cause more frequent and severe hypoglycemia by further slowing your already delayed absorption of food (and any glucose or other carbohydrates taken to treat a low).

Other injectable medications (*GLP-1 agonists*) have mainly been intended for the treatment of type 2 diabetes, although some people with type 1 have tried using them to stimulate regeneration of their beta cells (with limited success) or to help them lose weight. Like Symlin, these medications cause food to empty from the stomach more slowly and blood glucose levels to stay more stable after meals. Some also stimulate the pancreas to make more insulin (which will obviously not work in most individuals with type 1), keep the liver from overproducing glucose, and result in weight loss. These effectively replace natural hormones released by the digestive tract (gut hormones) after meals to spur insulin release. Some (like Byetta) have to be injected twice a day, but

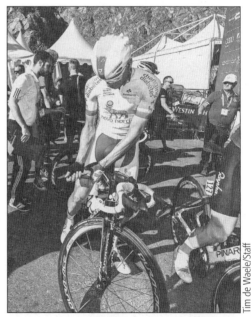

Expect to do some trial and error to figure out how best to manage your medications if they are affected by exercise, but you can do it successfully.

others are taken once a week and may be as effective as insulin while also leading to weight loss. Some pharmaceutical companies are working on getting approval for oral versions of these medications as well.

Another potential drawback of Byetta and other incretins is that they may affect your ability to exercise. Janis Eggleston, an athlete with type 2 diabetes from Berkeley, California, has reported that "I could never cycle with Byetta on board without throwing up, feeling weak, losing steam, and having 'no legs' to pedal with. I learned to drop that med early in my training season." She never took Byetta when cycling over 65 miles (105 kilometers) in 1 day because she got major lows if she did and only took her evening dose of metformin those days. Similarly, Tom Seabourne from Mount Pleasant, Texas, used to take Byetta as well, but warned, "I had extreme lows with Byetta, so I dropped to a single dose of 10 units before dinner. I tried Byetta before breakfast for a while, but it turned me into a vegetable until lunchtime. I never take Byetta before a workout!"

## Resources for Active People With Diabetes

# Diabetes Training Camp

Diabetes Training Camp (DTC) is a unique clinical resource devoted entirely to diabetes, fitness, and sport funded by the Diabetes Training Camp Foundation, a nonprofit organization. DTC offers fitness and multisport training camps for adults with type 1 diabetes, as well as boot camps for teenagers with diabetes and their parents, and other camps for adults with type 2 diabetes. These various week-long camps reach adults and teens at every level of athletic ability. What makes this organization unique is that it focuses on the exercise and athletic part of having diabetes, whether you simply want to become fitter or want to take your triathlon and marathon training to a new level. Its comprehensive, onsite staff consists of an experienced and talented crew of medical and diabetes specialists, exercise scientists, athletic trainers, dietitians, elite coaches, fitness specialists, and sport psychologists. The integrated approach of all these specialists creates a supportive and educational experience.

Founded in 2006 by Dr. Matthew Corcoran, who serves as medical director, DTC is expanding each year to offer more week-long camps and programs to fulfill the Foundation's mission of empowering the community of people with diabetes to thrive. For more information, visit www.diabetestrainingcamp.com.

There are some key points to remember about using diabetes medications and being physically active that will make managing your blood glucose easier. Without diabetes, insulin levels go down but glucose-raising hormones rise during exercise, even more so when working out hard. How much insulin you have in your bloodstream during exercise (whether it is injected, pumped, inhaled, or your own) affects whether your blood glucose stays normal, goes down too much, or rises. Finally, certain other diabetes medications besides insulin, such as select oral sulfonylureas, Symlin, and Byetta, may increase your risk for hypoglycemia during exercise, so they will need to be adjusted for activities.

# NONDIABETES MEDICATIONS AND EXERCISE EFFECTS

If you take any other medications to help lower your blood cholesterol, manage your blood pressure, or control other health problems, be aware that some of them can potentially impact your ability to be physically active. Although most drugs do not affect exercise, several common nondiabetes medications with such potential effects are statins, beta-blockers, diuretics, vasodilators, and blood thinners.

## Statins

Statins are a class of medications prescribed to lower cholesterol levels or abnormal levels of blood fats to reduce your risk of having a heart attack or stroke. Brand names include Altoprev, Crestor, Lescol, Lipitor, Livalo, Mevacor, Pravachol, and Zocor. If you are someone who is unwilling or unable to change your diet and lifestyle sufficiently to lower your cholesterol enough or you have genetically high levels of cholesterol or triglycerides (another blood fat), then the benefit of statins on lowering your cardiovascular risk may exceed its risks. Given that cardiovascular disease (leading to heart attack and stroke) is the leading cause of death in adults with diabetes of any type, doctors often prescribe statins to people with perfectly normal cholesterol levels.

Although undesirable muscular effects are not that common, statins potentially can cause unexplained muscle pain and weakness with exercise, likely related to these medications compromising the ability of the muscles to generate energy. Other muscular conditions like myalgia, mild or severe myositis, and rhabdomyolysis, although relatively rare, are doubled in people with diabetes, along with an increased susceptibility to exercise-induced muscle injury. Other symptoms, such as muscle cramps during or after exercise, nocturnal cramping, and general fatigue, generally resolve when you stop taking statins. If you experience any of these symptoms, talk with your doctor about potentially switching to another statin or a different cholesterol-lowering medication.

About one-third of the athletes surveyed (of all ages) reported taking or having taken a statin. Many take the lowest possible dose of a statin as a heart disease preventative. Some reported getting side effects such as more frequent and severe leg cramps, muscle pain, and weakness, and others have complained of dizziness and foggy memories. Although people in the survey did not report any negative side effects, a few had to either stop taking statins or switch to another drug.

For instance, Michael Krupar of Silver Spring, Maryland, found that Lipitor was awful for him. He says, "I ached constantly. There were days when I couldn't get out of bed." Sean Busby of Whitefish, Montana, found a balance in taking a statin only once a week to avoid cramping issues while also keeping his cholesterol in a normal range. Sarah from the United Kingdom started on Zocor but suffered from extreme fatigue and muscle cramps until she switched to Lipitor, which did not give her any noticeable side effects. Don Muchow from Plano, Texas, takes a low dose of Crestor because it is one of the few that does not give him exercise side effects. Mary Alice of San Diego, California, found that statins not only kept her from exercising, they just made her feel bad: "Statins very much weakened me. When I'm taking them, I cannot seem to gain muscle no matter how hard I work at strength training. When I finally went off them, I was able to make significant progress in weight training. I feel better all the time since I stopped taking any statins."

Long-term statin use may also negatively impact collagen and decrease the strength of your tendons (which connect muscles to bones) and ligaments, making them more predisposed to ruptures. In fact, statin users experience more spontaneous ruptures of both their biceps and Achilles tendons. You may want to talk to your doctor about whether you can manage your cardiovascular risk and lipid levels without taking long-term statins for this reason. The potential impact of other cholesterol medications such as Repatha (which is injected and expensive) on muscles and joints is presently unknown.

## Beta-Blockers

Another class of medications called beta-blockers (e.g., Corgard, Inderal, Levatol, Lopressor, Tenormin, and Zebeta) are used to treat heart disease and *hypertension* (high blood pressure). They lower both your resting and your exercise heart rate. If you are taking one, your heart rate will not reach an age-expected value at any intensity of exercise, and you may not be able to work out as hard as you would like to. Be aware that your exercise responses may differ from normal when taking one of these drugs, that they can blunt your hormone response to hypoglycemia, and that they can increase your risk of more severe lows during activities.

## Diuretics

Diuretics—or "water pills"—such as Lasix, Microzide, Enduron, and Lozol reduce the amount of water in your body and thereby lower your blood pressure. They can also lead to dehydration if you lose too much fluid. They are unlikely to affect your blood glucose, but using diuretics can cause dehydration with associated low blood pressure and dizziness during exercise.

## Vasodilators

Taking a vasodilator like nitroglycerin allows more blood to flow to your heart during exercise, which can keep you from having to treat chest pain (*angina*) both at rest and during exercise. Be forewarned that vasodilators can also induce a drop in your blood pressure (hypotension), which can cause you to faint or feel lightheaded during or after an activity.

## Blood Thinners

If you have a high stroke risk, your doctor may put you on a blood thinner to keep clots from forming. However, aspirin and other blood thinners like Coumadin have the potential to make you bruise more easily or extensively in response to athletic injuries or to bleed longer before clotting if you get a cut or scrape while working out. If you take aspirin chronically to reduce your risk of stroke, you may only need a dose equivalent to a baby aspirin a day to limit these possible side effects. Luckily, none of these blood thinners usually have any direct impact on your ability to exercise.

## Medications Without Exercise Effects

You may be prescribed a number of medications to treat a variety of health conditions. Luckily, many of these have no impact on your ability to exercise. For example, if you take an angiotensin-converting enzyme (ACE) inhibitor (e.g., Capoten, Accupril, Vasotec, Lotensin, or Zestril) or angiotensin II–receptor blocker (such as Cozaar, Benicar, or Avapro) to reduce your blood pressure or protect your kidneys from possible damage, you should not expect it to have any impact on your being physically active. In fact, certain ACE inhibitors may lower your risk of a heart attack during exercise if you have heart disease. Other medications that treat heart disease and high blood pressure (calcium-channel blockers like Procardia, Sular, Cardene, Cardizem, and Norvasc), depression (such as Wellbutrin and Prozac), or chronic pain (Celebrex) also have no known effect on exercise.

## Nondiabetes Medications Affecting Blood Glucose

Very few nondiabetes medications will directly impact your blood glucose levels. The main exception is any type of corticosteroids—like Prednisone or cortisone (pills or injections into inflamed joints)—which make you much more insulin resistant and cause your blood glucose to rise, sometimes dramatically. Certain statins also raise the overall risk of developing type 2 diabetes.

# LOSING WEIGHT WITH DIABETES AND MEDICATION USE

It is a well-known fact that insulin promotes fat storage; if you often end up taking too much, it can make you gain extra fat weight. You can adopt some strategies to keep the weight gain from happening from insulin or other diabetes medications, regardless of what type of diabetes you have.

Why is using insulin often associated with weight gain? On insulin, your blood glucose is (usually) in a tighter range, so you stop losing some calories in the form of glucose in your urine, as you do when your blood glucose is running on the high side. You can also gain weight from having to eat extra to treat any lows caused by insulin or other medications. I know of a heavily training Olympic handball athlete with type 1 diabetes who was gaining weight despite doing heavy training—and it was not just muscle. When asked, she admitted that she was having a lot of lows (and treating them with excess calories), which explained most of her weight gain. (Remember, even if you have no other choice than to treat hypoglycemia, calories are still calories.) You may find that cutting back on refined carbohydrates that require more insulin to cover them, exercising regularly, and checking your blood glucose to avoid taking too much of any weight-inducing medications will help you avoid gaining fat weight.

Most people with type 1 diabetes gain some weight as soon as they start using insulin. Many of them lost weight before the diagnosis—some of it muscle—so not all the weight regain is necessarily bad (some is from muscle mass). However, you can gain excess weight from taking too much daily insulin and treating lows, or even from taking the right amount of insulin but eating too many calories. Warwick Sickling from Melbourne, Australia, agrees, saying, "I'm quite a bit heavier than I was prior to being diagnosed with diabetes, and part of that is due to having to treat lows with extra carbs. However, exercise is a factor in that, but I would not give it up because the health benefits and increased satisfaction with life that comes from exercising are too valuable to me." Helen Cotton, a resident of the United Kingdom, has had similar experiences with treating exercise-related lows: "One of my biggest challenges related to being active with diabetes is weight gain due to treating increased hypos when I exercise more. I have gotten better at not overtreating them, but hypo munchies can be hard to ignore."

It is advisable to not give up exercise, but you should still avoid gaining extra fat if you can—it is often associated with being more insulin resistant and may result in you requiring even larger doses of insulin. You can lower your insulin needs by staying regularly active. Readjusting your ratio of basal-to-bolus insulin—specifically, lowering your basal doses and raising your premeal insulin—without increasing your total daily insulin dose may also prevent weight gain with type 1 diabetes.

Also, try to keep your insulin needs as low as possible—the more you take, the greater your potential for causing lows that lead to weight gain. During any physical activity, your muscles can take up blood glucose and use it as a fuel without insulin. After exercise, your insulin action is heightened for several hours (up to 72 hours). During that time, you need smaller doses of insulin to have the same effect. With that in mind, adjust your insulin doses downward to prevent lows after exercise that cause you to take in extra calories to treat them.

You may be able to avoid weight gain by looking at the type of insulins you are using. For example, once-daily Levemir used by people with type 2 diabetes causes less weight gain and less frequent hypoglycemia than NPH insulin, even combined with the use of rapid-acting insulin injections for meals. The same is likely true when using Lantus, Basaglar, Toujeo, and Tresiba. In type 1 diabetes, individuals end up eating less when using Levemir compared to Lantus, leading them to gain less weight. It also helps to dose with fast-acting insulins for the amount of food you actually eat rather than eating to match your premeal insulin doses.

*Both the type of insulins you use and the doses you take are important to consider in the overall management of your diabetes and your body weight. Make sure that your doses are regulated effectively to prevent the blood glucose lows that make you eat more.*

**Table 3.4 Diabetes Medication Effects on Body Weight**

| Cause Weight Gain | Lead to Weight Loss or Have No Effect |
|---|---|
| *Sulfonylureas*<br>Amaryl, DiaBeta, Diabinese, Glynase, Glucotrol, Micronase | *Metformin*<br>Metformin, Glucophage, Glucophage XR, Riomet, Glumetza |
| *Meglitinides*<br>Starlix, Prandin | *DPP-4 inhibitors*<br>Januvia, Onglyza, Nesina/Galvus, Tradjenta |
| *Thiazolidinediones*<br>Actos, Avandia | *GLP-1 receptor agonists*<br>Byetta, Victoza, Lyxumia, Bydureon, Trulicity, Ozempic, Eperzan, Adlyxin |
| *Insulin*<br>All types of insulin (especially taken before meals instead of dosed afterward based on actual food eaten) | *SGLT-2 inhibitors*<br>Invokana, Farxiga, Jardiance, Steglatro Zynquista (*SGLT-1/SGLT-2 inhibitor*) |
| | *Amylin analog*<br>Symlin |
| | *Alpha-glucosidase inhibitors*<br>Precose, Glyset |

Even when you exercise more, some noninsulin medications may be working against your ability to lose weight. Focus on reducing the diabetes medications that contribute to weight gain and replacing them (if needed) with ones that do not affect body weight or help with weight loss, and avoid using too much of those that contribute to weight gain. Table 3.4 shows which medications fall into each category.

As you can see by the topics covered in this chapter, the more you know about your diabetes and other medications, their actions, and how they may (or may not) be affected by exercise, the easier it will be for you to adjust and have as normal a response as possible to being active. You will have to go through some trial and error to figure out how best to manage all these medication variables for yourself, but many athletes with diabetes do it successfully, and so can you.

## Athlete Profile: **Charlie Kimball**

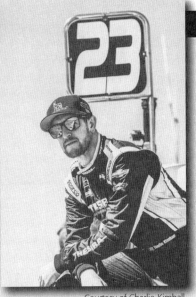

*Courtesy of Charlie Kimball.
Photographer: Chris Bucher.*

***Hometown:*** Camarillo, California (Residence: Indianapolis, Indiana)

***Diabetes history:*** Type 1 diabetes diagnosed in 2007 (at age 22)

***Sport or activity:*** IndyCar series racing (motorsports)

***Greatest athletic achievement:*** First licensed driver with diabetes in the history of IndyCar; first licensed driver with diabetes to qualify for and compete in the Indianapolis 500 (2011); first driver with diabetes to win an IndyCar series race (Mid-Ohio, 2013).

***Current insulin and medication regimen:*** Multiple daily injections with continuous glucose monitoring and traditional fingerstick blood glucose testing; Tresiba once daily, Fiasp for meals and corrections; and multivitamins daily.

***Training tips:*** I adjust my insulin doses and nutrition based on the type of training planned for that day, as well as how many days I have trained in that week. Multiple training sessions in a week seem to "stack" for me, and I become more sensitive to insulin doses.

***Typical daily and weekly training regimen:*** I follow this schedule during the week leading up to a race weekend.

► ***Monday:*** Travel/rest day. I'm more insulin sensitive after a race weekend, so I adjust my carb ratios accordingly (i.e., the carbs I eat need less insulin to cover them).

► ***Tuesday:*** Morning training session: typically I do a higher weight session, so I need some more insulin for strength training.

► ***Wednesday:*** Morning training session: usually a lighter, longer reaction circuit, so I need some more preworkout carbs.

► ***Thursday:*** Travel/setup day: focus on refueling from the training days so that I am well-prepared for the race weekend.

► ***Friday:*** Practice day: I typically don't change my basal dose, just adjust my carb ratios so that my blood glucose hits a target of 150 to 175 mg/dL (8.3 to 9.7 mmol/L) for every on-track session.

► ***Saturday:*** Qualifying day: each day I'm on track driving I eat a very similar breakfast and a measured/weighed lunch of pasta, grilled chicken, and salad.

► ***Sunday:*** Race day: depending on the time of the race, I typically eat my pre-race meal (the same as practice and qualifying days) about 1.5 to 2.0 hours before the green flag.

***Other hobbies and interests:*** Boating, mountain biking, surfing, snowboarding, home improvement, grilling. My wife Kathleen and I have two dogs: Taj, a husky, and Lilah, a black Labrador (Lilah has been trained as a diabetes alert service dog).

continued ➡

*Charlie Kimball continued*

> **Good diabetes and exercise story:** After my diagnosis, I spent some time away from the race track, refocusing and learning about my diabetes management. As I was getting closer to being back in a car, I kept asking myself the same questions: Am I the same athlete as I was before my diagnosis? Would I still be competitive? There is a mountain trail near my parents' home I had biked countless times—before my diagnosis. A few months after my diagnosis, I got the courage to try it again, and I beat my previous best time. That helped me prove to myself that I can be just as competitive and successful as I was before. I backed that up with a podium finish at my first race driving with diabetes!

# 4

# Eating Right and Supplementing for Activity

**A**s a physically active person, you are likely to be bombarded with claims about the superiority of certain diets and guarantees that specific nutritional supplements will enhance your athletic performance. With the fierce competition that exists in sports nowadays, athletes look for any edge to improve their athletic ability. They will try almost any supplement or technique to get it—caffeine, amino acids, sports drinks, carbohydrate loading, and hydrolysates, to name just a few. In reality few of these advertised *ergogenic aids* (i.e., anything that enhances performance) for athletes are scientifically proven to boost your physical prowess. Moreover, as an athlete with diabetes, you may have special concerns about the effects of various diets and supplements on your blood glucose, as well as what to consume to perform optimally during exercise.

## EFFECTIVE DIETARY PRACTICES OF ACTIVE PEOPLE

Active people can eat more than one way and perform effectively in sports, and the "best" way may be different for everyone. The diets and nutritional practices of athletes with diabetes are as varied as the sports and activities that they do. No one likes to have to stop exercising because of low blood glucose, so preventing hypoglycemia during and after any activity is a high priority for everyone. Becoming low unexpectedly can be especially inconvenient if you are on a run or a long bike ride and still a good distance from your destination. Prevention of lows has a lot to do with your food intake both before and during the activity, but supplementing during exercise may also be performance enhancing. In general, rapidly absorbed carbohydrate is most effective to take during exercise to keep your blood glucose and performance up, but protein and fat may be helpful in preventing lows as well. The following sections include some basic points to remember about the different classes of nutrients and dietary patterns, along with some nutritional supplements.

# Carbohydrate: Critical to Making It to the Finish Line (Fast)

Despite claims and beliefs to the contrary by Paleo, keto, carnivore, and other "low-carb" diet advocates, carbohydrate is the body's most important energy source for many types of exercise. Muscle *glycogen* (the main storage form of carbohydrate) is the only fuel used by the lactic acid system (discussed in chapter 2) for many power activities, as well as being the primary energy provider during most moderate and vigorous aerobic exercise. Whenever you eat carbohydrate, it is broken down by enzymes in your digestive tract, absorbed through the wall of your small intestine, and released primarily as glucose into your blood, making it the most important simple sugar found there. Your muscles can take up and use blood glucose, but they generally use more of the glycogen already stored there during exercise as long as it is available.

The more intensely you exercise, the greater the rate of muscle glycogen depletion in the muscle fibers you are using. Your liver also releases its more limited glycogen stores as glucose into the bloodstream to help maintain your levels during exercise. Glycogen is critical to most harder activities, so if you deplete your muscle and liver stores during exercise, you will become fatigued and either have to stop exercising or slow down considerably. You have heard of athletes "hitting the wall" or "bonking," often around the 20-mile (32-kilometer) mark of a marathon. When that happens, it means they have run out of glycogen and either must drop out of the race or walk/jog the rest of the way. Your body cannot use fat as effectively either once your carbohydrate stores are severely depleted.

> *Fat "burns" in a carbohydrate flame, so you cannot use fat as effectively as an alternative fuel during exercise once you have depleted most or all your body's carbohydrate (glycogen and blood glucose) supply.*

In general, most exercisers (even without diabetes) can benefit from taking in some carbohydrate before and during prolonged exercise to help maintain their blood glucose levels. Supplementing with carbohydrate does not slow down your use of muscle glycogen much because the rate at which glycogen is broken down is primarily determined by the intensity of your workout. However, any carbohydrate that you take in during exercise is rapidly metabolized and begins to be available for use as an alternate fuel within about 5 minutes. The type of carbohydrate that you should consume (if any) depends on factors such as how long you will be exercising, how hard your workout is, and what your blood glucose and insulin levels are before and during the activity, as you will see in the sport-specific examples offered in part II of this book.

## Carbohydrate Intake and Its Glycemic Effects

The current dietary recommendations for all adults suggest that 45 to 65 percent of daily calories should come from carbohydrate intake. This is the equivalent of 225 to 325 grams of carbohydrate if you eat 2,000 calories daily (each gram of carbohydrate contains 4 calories, but subtract out any fiber). Most people with diabetes find that amount to be on the high side if they are serious about keeping their blood glucose levels stable and as close to normal as possible. Whether you eat that amount or less, it likely matters more which types of carbohydrate you consume when it comes to treating or preventing hypoglycemia, restoring muscle glycogen, keeping your insulin action high, and optimizing your sports performance.

Carbohydrates with a higher *glycemic index* (GI), by definition, are absorbed more rapidly and have a more immediate impact on your blood glucose. It then follows that if you want to treat hypoglycemia quickly, you should use higher-GI carbohydrates, such as those found in glucose tablets or gels (which have a GI of 100 on a scale of 0 to 100), regular soda, sports drinks, skim milk, hard candies, jelly beans, bagels, bread, crackers, pretzels, cornflakes, white potatoes, and more. If you develop a low during exercise, one of these sources will treat it most rapidly, and you can use any of them to raise your blood glucose quickly before exercising.

By way of comparison, foods with a low GI include high-fiber carbohydrate sources such as apples, cherries, beans and legumes (e.g., black, kidney, and chickpeas), dates, figs, peaches, and plums, along with whole milk, kefir, and yogurt, none of which raise blood glucose quickly during hypoglycemia. Likewise, you probably should not rely on medium-GI foods like bananas, grapes, oatmeal, orange juice, pasta, rice, yams, corn, and baked beans to raise your blood glucose rapidly. Carbohydrate foods with a high fat content also have slower absorption rates than those with less fat. Potato chips and doughnuts are examples of high-carbohydrate, high-fat foods; if eaten for the treatment of lows, they would definitely not work as rapidly or be as effective.

Almost all recommended exercise carbohydrate intake in this book refers to higher-GI carbohydrates for optimal treatment and prevention of hypoglycemia, at least during the first hour of exercise. During prolonged physical activities, it is also possible to supplement with carbohydrates that have a different absorption rate—and, in some cases, with both protein and fat. Although people differ in their GI responses, certain foods generally elicit lesser blood glucose peaks and may not be as effective during exercise. When optimizing your blood glucose after workouts to restore glycogen as quickly as possible, however, you can use carbohydrate-rich foods with varying GI values and even protein to a lesser extent. Just be aware that if you take in most of your calories as protein and fat after exercising, it will take longer to restore your muscle glycogen than if you take in some carbohydrate as well.

## Using Glucose (and More) to Treat and Prevent Lows

Glucose tablets, gels, and liquids have some benefits for rapidly treating lows that other substances do not have. Glucose is the simple sugar that ends up in your bloodstream most rapidly and abundantly, and it is the primary fuel for your brain and nerves under normal circumstances. By way of comparison, other simple sugars, such as the fructose found in fruit, must be converted into glucose in your body, so they have a lower GI value and a slower effect on raising blood glucose. Traditionally, people have used orange juice and other fruit juices to treat lows, but they really are not the fastest to use because most juices have only a low or moderate glycemic effect.

Another benefit of using glucose to treat lows is that it usually comes in precisely measured amounts—4 grams per tablet or 15 grams per gel—so you can consume a specific amount of this quick carbohydrate without overdoing it. With a little practice, you can easily determine how much each 4-gram glucose tablet or 15-gram gel or liquid is likely to raise your blood glucose level under different insulin or exercise conditions.

What you treat hypoglycemia with may need to vary somewhat by situation, however. If you are only slightly low, you may just need a glucose tablet or two. If you are low and likely to keep dropping from whatever insulin you have on board, then you may need to take in glucose plus additional food or drink with greater staying power, such as peanut butter crackers or a Balance bar that have a balance of carbohydrate, protein, and fat. Milk can also be a reasonable option because it contains protein along with some fat, depending on the type (e.g., whole, 1 percent, 2 percent, or skim). Skim milk works quickly for treatment of lows, but at least one study has shown that for prevention of hypoglycemia after exercise whole milk is more effective than skim milk or sports drinks, likely because of the extra fat in it that takes longer to digest and boosts blood glucose hours later.

## Supplementing With Carbohydrate Before, During, and After Exercise

Carbohydrate supplementation may enhance your athletic performance whether or not you have diabetes. In general, taking in extra carbohydrates is not usually needed to boost performance in events lasting an hour or less if you start with normal muscle and liver glycogen stores and moderately low levels of insulin. But you may need to take in extra carbohydrate for exercise lasting less than an hour if you have too much insulin on board.

If your blood glucose is normal or slightly low before exercise, you may also need 10 to 15 grams of a moderate- or high-GI carbohydrate without any insulin coverage when you start certain activities, especially if your glucose typically drops during the first 30 minutes and you are starting out in a normal range. Also, if you are running low on glycogen for any reason, your muscles will use more blood glucose than normal, and you will likely have to supplement. During marathons or triathlons, extra carbohydrate (30 to 60 grams per hour, or sometimes more) can help maintain your blood glucose and provide an alternate fuel for muscles, enabling you to keep going at a faster pace for longer without having to slow down or stop. Consuming extra carbohydrates even helps during intermittent, high-intensity sports like soccer, field hockey, basketball, tennis, and ice hockey.

If you train hard on a regular basis, your workouts will feel easier if you take in enough carbohydrate every day to restore your muscle and liver glycogen levels between them. When you have diabetes, you must be especially careful to manage your blood glucose before and after exercise so that your glycogen repletion takes place as normally as possible. Your body needs adequate insulin, especially starting more than an hour after exercise when the glucose uptake into your cells becomes more dependent on insulin availability. Taking in at least some carbohydrate immediately after you finish a workout or event (within the first 30 minutes to 2 hours) will speed up your initial glycogen replacement and help lower your risk of developing lows later, all with minimal need for insulin during that period.

> *Carbohydrate intake after exercise helps ensure that your glycogen stores are adequately reloaded by the time your next workout rolls around. Full glycogen repletion can take 24 to 48 hours (with adequate carbohydrate intake, possibly longer with limited intake), but manage your blood glucose to optimize its replacement.*

## What Happens to Glycogen Stores If You Limit Carbohydrates?

The time it takes for full muscle glycogen reloading after exercise depends on how much you used up while active and whether you are taking in a diet with adequate carbohydrate and calories. If you eat a low-carbohydrate diet, while you likely have adapted to using a greater relative amount of fat during moderate-intensity or easier workouts and endurance activities, fully restoring your glycogen may take longer than usual and negatively affect your ability to do activities at a higher intensity on a regular basis. You may want to consider taking in more carbohydrate of any GI than your normal intake to promote glycogen storage after you have largely depleted it through activity. Also, make sure you take enough insulin (if you use it) to get those carbohydrates properly replaced in the least amount of time. (See the further discussion on the impact of keto and other low-carbohydrate diets on exercise later in this chapter.)

> *Your body restores glycogen most rapidly during the first 30 to 120 minutes after exercise. To minimize your risk of lows, take in some carbohydrate (and possibly protein) and tightly manage your blood glucose during this "window of opportunity" for carbohydrate storage.*

## Consuming Fluids and Carbohydrates in Sports Drinks

Gatorade, Powerade, All-Sport, GU energy gels, Power Bars, Clif Bars—with so many sport drinks, gels, and other sport-related supplements to choose from, how can you choose which ones to use, if any? Take a closer look at sports drinks and other fluids, including some trendy ones like coconut water. You probably should not be drinking any of these during rest if you have diabetes because of their high GI, but during activity may be another story.

Most sports drinks have been formulated for optimal digestion when active. During exercise, a fluid that is a 5 to 10 percent carbohydrate solution (meaning that it contains 5 to 10 grams of carbohydrate per 100 milliliters, or about 3.4 ounces) will empty from your stomach as rapidly as plain water, can hydrate you effectively, and will provide you with carbohydrate. If you are more worried about your blood glucose dropping than getting dehydrated, choose one with a slightly higher carbohydrate content. Not surprisingly, drinking one with 10 percent carbohydrates has been shown to keep your blood glucose higher than consuming a similar quantity of a sports drink with only 8 percent.

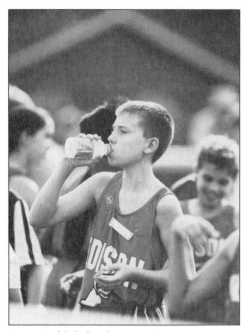

A sports drink that has 5 to 10 grams of carbohydrates per 100 milliliters (3.4 ounces) is easily absorbed, can hydrate you, and provides you with carbohydrate.

Only consume more concentrated drinks (above 10 percent) before or after exercise because their emptying from your stomach is somewhat delayed. Fruit juices are usually more concentrated than 10 percent and should be diluted for faster absorption during exercise, but remember that their GI is usually lower than many other choices. You may also want to avoid straight juice because drinks with high amounts of fructose (fruit sugar) may cause abdominal cramps or diarrhea, likely because fructose is absorbed more slowly than glucose and it pulls water into your stomach and small intestines. Because fructose is transported from your gut into your bloodstream differently than glucose, many sports drinks are now formulated to contain some of both types of simple sugars (albeit with less fructose than glucose) to optimize the availability of various sugars during exercise.

How do you know if you need fluids and electrolytes when you work out or compete in an athletic event? Whether you use sports drinks or just plain water depends on how long your activity is going to last. During an exercise session of an hour or less, you can effectively maintain hydration with either nothing or water alone (see the more general hydration tips summarized in chapter 5), although athletes with diabetes may need the extra carbohydrates in sport drinks for blood glucose reasons at times. Do not worry about replacing electrolytes (like sodium, potassium, and chloride) during shorter events (an hour or less) because sweating does not immediately unbalance them—sweat is more dilute than blood, and it contains less sodium and other electrolytes, so you are sweating out less than you are leaving in your blood.

For medium-length workouts and events (lasting an hour or two), water alone will keep you hydrated, but taking in sports drinks or other substances with carbohydrates may prolong your endurance by preventing drops in your blood glucose and providing your muscles with an alternative source of carbohydrates (besides muscle glycogen). See table 4.1 for the carbohydrate and electrolyte contents of some popular sports and energy drinks to help you choose which one you may want to use.

During prolonged activities lasting more than a couple of hours, such as a full Ironman triathlon, you will need to replace the electrolytes lost during the event, especially when you are consuming lots of fluids. Otherwise, you may end up with a dilution of sodium in your blood that causes *hyponatremia* (low sodium levels), otherwise known as *water intoxication*. Its symptoms include light-headedness, hcadaches,

### Table 4.1    Sports and Energy Drinks

| Product | Carbohydrate Content | Other Ingredients |
|---|---|---|
| Accelerade | 14 g per 8 oz (240 mL): 6% carbohydrate solution, plus protein; sucrose, whey protein, and soy protein | Sodium, 125 mg; potassium, 45 mg; protein, 3.3 g; 67% daily vitamins C and E; 20% daily magnesium |
| All-Sport | 17 g per 8 oz (240 mL): 7% carbohydrate solution; sugar and glucose | Sodium, 55 mg; potassium, 60 mg |
| Coconut Water (Vita Coco Brand) | 11 to 17 g per 8 oz (240 mL), based on flavor: 4.6% to 7.1% carbohydrate solution | Sodium, 25 mg; potassium, 470 mg; 100% daily vitamin C |
| Gatorade | 14 g per 8 oz (240 mL): 6% carbohydrate solution; sugar and dextrose | Sodium, 107 mg; potassium, 30 mg; phosphorus, 25 mg |
| Monster Energy | 27 g per 8 oz (240 mL): 11% carbohydrate solution; sucrose and glucose | Sodium, 180 mg; caffeine, 80 mg; 100% daily vitamins $B_6$ and $B_{12}$ |
| Powerade | 14 g per 8 oz (240 mL): 6% carbohydrate solution; high-fructose corn syrup | Sodium, 100 mg; potassium, 25 mg; some niacin, vitamin $B_6$, and vitamin $B_{12}$ |

nausea, repeated vomiting, and malaise. For the most effective hydration, take in fluids before you start, during the activity, and afterward, but do not go overboard on the amount, even if it has some electrolytes. Even an excess of sports drinks can cause water intoxication, despite containing sodium and other electrolytes.

In general, fluids are absorbed fastest when drunk cold and when containing less than 10 percent carbohydrate to promote faster emptying from your stomach. Ice-cold water will get into your body relatively more rapidly than a lukewarm drink, but taking in more than 500 milliliters (17 ounces) at a time will slow its emptying and increase your risk for water intoxication. While you are exercising, start drinking before you feel thirsty because thirst is not triggered until you have already lost 1 to 2 percent of your body weight as water. Taking in a large mouthful (1 to 2 ounces, or 30 to 60 milliliters) at a time may be sufficient.

*Anything you drink during exercise should ideally be dilute (less than 10 percent carbohydrates), be cold, have a volume of less than 500 milliliters (17 ounces), and contain some electrolytes if you are exercising more than an hour.*

## Getting Carbohydrates and More via Sports Gels, Bars, Chews, and More

If you do not need extra fluids sloshing around in your stomach during activities but still need carbohydrates, protein, or fat to prevent lows, you may want to try gels, bars, chews, or other more solid sources. Carbohydrate-based gels like GU have a set quantity (e.g., 15 grams) of carbohydrate, which makes your consumption easier to track; also you do not get extra fluids along with the carbohydrates if you

**Table 4.2    Sports and Energy Gels**

| Product | Carbohydrate Content | Other Ingredients |
|---|---|---|
| Accel Gel | 20 g fructose and sucrose per 41 g (1.4 oz) gel | Protein, 5 g (whey protein from milk); fat, 0 g; sodium, 100 mg; potassium, 50 mg; vitamins E and C (100%); various flavors |
| Carb Boom! Energy Gel | 26 g maltodextrin and fruit puree in 41 g (1.4 oz) gel | Sodium, 50 mg; potassium, 45–60 mg; various fruit flavors |
| Clif Shot Energy Gel | 24 g maltodextrin and cane sugar in 34 g (1.1 oz) gel | Sodium, 60–90 mg; potassium, 55 mg; various flavors |
| Glucose Gel or Liquid (generic) | 15 g glucose per tube or container | None |
| GU Energy Gel | 21–23 g maltodextrin and fructose in 32 g (1 oz) gel | Sodium, 60–125 mg; potassium, 30–40 mg; various flavors |
| Hammer Gel | 20–22 g maltodextrin and fruit puree per 33 g (1 oz) gel packet | Sodium, 25–35 mg; potassium, 35 mg; amino acids (L-leucine, L-alanine, L-valine, L-isoleucine) |
| Honey Stinger Gel | 24–27 g honey per 32 g (1 oz) gel (some flavors with tapioca syrup as well) | Sodium, 50 mg; potassium, 50–85 mg; six B vitamins; some flavors with caffeine (from green tea concentrate) |
| PowerBar Gel | 27 g maltodextrin and fructose per 41 g gel | Sodium, 200 mg; potassium, 20 mg; chloride, 90 mg; many flavors with 25 to 50 mg of caffeine added |

already are sufficiently hydrated or at risk for hyponatremia. For glucose gels or liquids, one packet equals almost four to more than six glucose tablets, and a gel or liquid may be easier to get down while you are exercising, especially if you do not need any extra fluids. Refer to a select list of sports and energy gels and what they contain in table 4.2.

More solid sources of carbohydrates—and protein and fat as well—can be found in sports and energy bars, chews, and other items (listed in table 4.3). Many sports bars and chews allow you to take in some longer-lasting protein and fat along with the carbohydrates, which can help prevent lows later on during longer workouts or events. These may work better either before you start exercising or during longer duration events. Some people also eat them afterward to prevent lows then as well.

## Carbohydrate Loading: Effective If Done Right for Even a Day

Most athletes can benefit from taking in enough carbohydrate before long-distance events to start exercising with fully restored or even supercompensated glycogen stores. Traditionally, this loading technique consisted of 3 to 7 days of a high-carbohydrate diet combined with 1 or 2 days of rest or a reduction in exercise volume, a method known as *tapering*. For endurance athletes, loading is recommended to consist of taking in 8 to 10 grams of carbohydrate per kilogram of body weight (e.g., 560 to

**Table 4.3   Sports and Energy Bars, Chews, and More**

| Product | Carbohydrate Content | Other Ingredients |
|---|---|---|
| Clif Bar | 41–45 g carbohydrate per 68 g bar | Protein, 10–11 g; fat, 3–6 g; fiber, 4–5 g; sodium, 170 mg; potassium, 450 mg; vitamins; minerals; various flavors |
| Clif Shot Blok Chews | 24 g carbohydrate per three pieces (30 g) | Sodium, 50 mg; potassium, 20 mg; various flavors, some with more sodium and added caffeine |
| Glucose Tablets (generic) | 4 g glucose per tablet | None |
| Honey Stinger Energy Bar | 30 g carbohydrate per 50 g (1.75 oz) bar | Protein, 5 g; fat, 5 g; fiber, 1 g; sodium, 160 mg; potassium, 130 mg; various flavors |
| Honey Stinger Energy Chews | 39 g carbohydrate per 50 g (1.75 oz) packet | Protein, 1 g; fat, 0 g; fiber, 1 g; sodium, 80 mg; potassium, 40 mg; 100% daily vitamin C; various flavors |
| Honey Stinger Waffles | 21 g carbohydrate per 30 g (1 oz) waffle | Protein, 1 g; fat, 7 g; fiber, <1 g; sodium, 60 mg; various organic flavors and gluten-free options |
| Gummy Candies | 22 g carbohydrate per 34 g (1 oz, or ~10 bears) | Protein, 0 g; fat, 0 g; sodium, 10 mg |
| Jelly Belly Sport Beans | 25 g carbohydrate per 28 g (1 oz) package | Sodium, 80 mg; potassium, 40 mg; 10% daily thiamin, riboflavin, niacin, and vitamin C |
| PowerBar | 44 g carbohydrate in 57 g bar | Protein, 10 g; fat, 4 g; fiber, 2 g; sodium, 200 mg; potassium, 140 mg; vitamins; minerals; essential amino acids; various flavors |
| PowerBar Performance Energy Blasts (gel-filled chews) | 46 g carbohydrate in 57 g bar | Protein, 3 g; fat, 0 g; sodium, 30 mg |
| PowerBar Protein Plus Bar (or Bites) | 25–40 g carbohydrate in 74 g bar (or pouch) | Protein, 20–30 g; fat, 5–10 g; fiber, 1–6 g; sodium, 120–260 mg; potassium, 80–300 mg; calcium; iron; varies by flavor |

700 grams for someone who weighs 70 kg, or 154 pounds)—but that is admittedly a lot of carbohydrate to handle if you have to match it with insulin or are very resistant, and it is not necessary.

Even a single day with enough carbohydrate and food intake and rest or tapering can effectively maximize your carbohydrate stores, so you do not need to spend a week, or even 3 days, overconsuming it. Maximal glycogen storage is dictated by how much muscle mass you have, but it is typically around 300 to 400 grams total in all your skeletal muscle, along with 75 to 100 grams of liver glycogen, for the average person. As long as you consume enough calories and taper or rest for a day, taking in up to 40 percent of your calories as carbohydrates is more than adequate to fully reload your glycogen. For someone consuming 2,000 calories and resting on a pre-event day, that amounts to around 200 grams of carbohydrate—more than enough

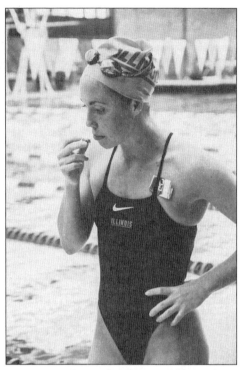

Many sports bars provide you with protein and fat along with carbohydrates, which can help prevent your blood glucose from dropping later during longer workouts or events.

if you are not starting out fully depleted. It's also likely that you can fully restore your glycogen on far less carbohydrate, especially if you have been following a low-carbohydrate diet and are fully fat-adapted.

The key for carbohydrate loading to be effective for exercisers with diabetes is to ensure that your muscles can take up any available glucose, which only happens if you have sufficient levels of insulin and enough sensitivity to it to prevent hyper-glycemia and promote glucose uptake. Consuming higher-fiber carbohydrate sources and those with a lower glycemic effect will help prevent an excessive rise in your blood glucose and be effective for loading. In fact, a study showed that participants actually end up with higher glycogen stores when they maintain more normal blood glucose levels while load-ing with less carbohydrate (50 percent of calories from carbohydrate instead of 59 percent in that study). To optimize your liver glycogen replacement, keeping your blood glucose as close to normal as possi-ble is also most effective.

*To maximize your glycogen stores, all you really need is 1 day and a combi-nation of rest, enough calories in your diet, and good blood glucose levels for that day. You do not need to do traditional carbohydrate loading to make this happen.*

## Fat: Its Use Depends Largely on Exercise Intensity and Duration

Both the fat stored in your muscles (i.e., *intramuscular triglycerides*) and circulating around in your blood (*free fatty acids*) can provide some energy for muscle con-tractions. Although carbohydrate is the main (and muscle preferred) energy source during most moderate and vigorous exercise, fat is an important contributor to your fuel needs, particularly during low-intensity or slower and prolonged activities like walking the dog, taking an all-day hike, or running a marathon.

Fatty acids are stored in your fat (*adipose*) tissue as triglycerides and released by hormones (mainly epinephrine) to circulate to your active muscles. If you have too much insulin in your bloodstream, it can inhibit or impair the release of stored fats from adipose tissues during exercise. Not much intramuscular fat (triglycerides stored in your muscles) is used during activities—unless they are extremely prolonged, lasting many hours at a moderate intensity—but later when you are resting they kick in some of the energy for recovery, which is largely fueled by fat from all sources. Fat is hardly used at all during high-intensity aerobic and anaerobic exercise (which both use the first two energy systems), which rely almost solely on carbohydrate for adenosine triphosphate (ATP) production.

> *Fat use during hard exercise is limited, contributing most during prolonged endurance and lower-intensity activities, but fat provides most of the fuel for recovery from any activity.*

## How Does Fat Affect Blood Glucose?

Calculations for giving insulin boluses to manage meal spikes in your blood glucose have previously only factored in the carbohydrate content of a meal, but recent studies have confirmed that fat (and protein) can change how much insulin you need. High-fat meals require more insulin than low-fat meals with the same amount of carbohydrates, and dietary fat can make you more insulin resistant hours later (when more fat is available and your body is using less carbohydrate). A high intake of protein can have a similar impact on your blood glucose later (within 2 to 4 hours after you consume it). You may need an extra bolus of rapid-acting insulin 2 to 5 hours after eating a lot of protein or fat to cover the rise in blood glucose that can occur.

Along those lines, your blood glucose may stay more stable overnight if you eat a high-fat or high-protein bedtime snack, such as ice cream, yogurt, soymilk, or a Balance bar on days when you have been particularly active. Fat is metabolized much more slowly than carbohydrate and will provide an alternative energy source for your muscles for up to 5 to 6 hours after you eat it, whereas protein is fully digested within 3 to 4 hours and carbohydrates in the first hour or two.

## How Much Fat Do You Need and Which Types?

The current dietary guidelines recommend a fat intake of 20 to 35 percent of daily calories. Fat calories add up quickly because each gram contains around 9.5 calories, which is more than twice what a gram of carbohydrate or protein contains. You may already consume more than 35 percent of your calories as fat, which is fine as long as you take into account the type of fat. It is prudent to minimize your intake of saturated fats (mostly solid at room temperature, found in meats, butter, cheese, and more) because these can increase insulin resistance and may raise your risk of heart disease. Also, cut out all trans fats, which are unhealthful, particularly the hydrogenated fats added to foods by manufacturers, and interesterified fats, a newer trans fat substitute. All these fats may raise the levels of the "bad" cholesterol (low-density lipoprotein [LDL]) in your blood and raise your risk for heart disease and stroke accordingly. If you have a moderate fat intake after exercise to prevent later-onset lows, pick more healthful fats such as those found in nuts and seeds, peanut butter, olives and olive oil, fish, avocados, flaxseed, and dark chocolate (70 percent or higher), and at least consider choosing the lower-fat varieties of dairy products (e.g., fat-reduced ice cream, yogurt, and cheese).

## Does Fat Loading Enhance Performance?

Eating high-fat foods while training (a practice called *fat loading*) may potentially be detrimental to your performance unless you have been adapting to a lower carbohydrate intake for several weeks already. If you do eat low amounts of carbohydrates most of the time, your body will adapt to using more fat during exercise and maintain your endurance performance once you are fully adapted, but your race times may not improve because harder intensities still require more carbohydrate use as a fuel. You may want to consider replenishing carbohydrates for a day or 2 before you attempt any moderate or higher intensity events. Also, any fat you eat right before or during exercise will not be digested and ready for use for many hours (and may raise your blood glucose afterward). Fat may slow the absorption of carbohydrates during exercise, so you may have to supplement with straight carbohydrates or protein during most activities if you need energy sooner rather than later.

## What About Following a Keto Diet?

A current dietary trend (for people with and without diabetes) is to eat a very low-carbohydrate (5 to 10 percent of calories), high-fat (60 to 80 percent) diet that leads to the formation of *ketones* in the body. This *ketogenic* (or "keto") diet can lead your body to adapt to using as much fat as possible during exercise in place of carbohydrate sources. (At rest, fat use is already higher than carbohydrate use.) The brain and nervous system require around 130 grams of glucose a day to fuel their activity. But when your carbohydrate intake is less than that, ketones can become an alternate energy source for your brain, nerves, and active muscles.

Ketones consist of three primary compounds derived by the liver directly from free fatty acids (*acetoacetate, beta-hydroxybutyrate,* and *acetone*). These then circulate throughout the body and can be measured in your blood and urine. Those of us who started out with diabetes and urine tests years ago are familiar with testing for urinary ketones (mainly acetoacetate), but these fail to tell you what your actual blood levels are. Acetone makes your breath smell "fruity" and can be measured in your breath by some devices (although it can be affected by your hydration status and alcohol consumption). Some blood glucose meters are also able to co-test for blood levels of one of the ketones (beta-hydroxybutyrate); blood levels are considered the most accurate indicator of your level of ketosis.

- Very low ketones: Less than 0.5 mmol/L
- Mild ketosis: 0.6 to 1.5 mmol/L
- Optimal ketosis: 1.6 to 3.0 mmol/L (indicative of adaptation to keto diets)
- Very high ketones: Greater than 3.0 mmol/L (as seen in diabetic ketoacidosis)

When ketones increase naturally during periods of low food intake (such as fasting or starvation) or during extended bouts of exercise, they are not necessarily harmful and can supply energy for ATP aerobically in place of carbohydrates, and your levels may not even get that high. The only problem is when they are produced due to severe insulin deficiency, as is often the case in insulin users who miss a dose or just do not take enough insulin to cover their basal needs and food intake. In their case, ketones over 3.0 mmol/L (but often as high as 10 mmol/L) plus hyperglycemia due to insulin deficiency can lead to diabetic ketoacidosis (DKA), which is a dangerous medical condition and potentially fatal.

> *Your ketone levels while on a "keto diet" are not likely to ever be as dangerously high as you might experience during DKA.*

## Are All Low-Carbohydrate Diets High in Fat?

For years, a very-low-carbohydrate diet championed by Dr. Richard K. Bernstein has been the primary one followed by some people with diabetes, until the last decade when fad weight loss plans such as the Paleo and LCHF (low-carbohydrate, high-fat, or keto) diets have been become mainstream—not just for losing weight, but also for their purported ability to boost athletic performance and improve blood glucose management.

All these eating plans are lower in carbohydrates, but they differ in the types of noncarbohydrate macronutrients or foods they recommend. Dr. Bernstein's plan advocates a higher protein intake, moderate fat, and very low carbohydrates (less than 10 percent of calories with only 30 grams of carbohydrates daily: 6 grams at breakfast and 12 grams at both lunch and dinner). The Paleo diet focuses on unprocessed foods that nomadic early humans supposedly ate (higher protein and no legumes, dairy, grains, or processed foods). But few truly Paleolithic foods are even available nowadays, and this diet varies widely in its percentages of calories coming from carbohydrates (22 to 40 percent, which is not necessarily that low), proteins (19 to 35 percent), and fat (28 to 47 percent). The LCHF (keto) diet gets 70 percent of its calories from fat and 15 percent from carbohydrates. (An even newer fad, the carnivore diet, contains no carbohydrates at all—nothing but meat intake—which would undoubtedly fail to supply you will all the essential nutrients you need from your foods.) Honestly, these diets remind me of the no-carbohydrate starvation regimen that everyone with type 1 diabetes used to survive for a few months (or years) after diagnosis back before insulin was discovered in 1921. Have we really come full circle, back to those extreme diets in mainstream eating for diabetes?

## How Does Low-Carbohydrate Eating Affect Athletic Performance?

The effect of special diets on physical performance is the question particularly relevant to athletic individuals with diabetes who are choosing to go low carbohydrate. We have often preached the importance of carbohydrate loading (think "pasta party") for endurance athletes before events. Can you still perform at the top of your game while eating very few carbohydrates? We do know that taking in carbohydrates can help: at least one study in adults with type 1 diabetes has shown that it is possible to balance blood glucose levels and prevent lows while doing long-duration endurance events and consuming 75 grams of carbohydrates per hour, the same as many endurance athletes without diabetes do. For intermittent sports like soccer and rugby, it also appears that ingesting 30 to 60 grams of carbohydrates per hour has the ability to prevent the fatigue or hypoglycemia that can occur toward the end of a game (although this has only been studied in athletes without diabetes).

That said, it appears possible to use more fat as a fuel after becoming adapted to low-carbohydrate eating. Highly trained, keto-adapted ultraendurance athletes have extraordinarily high rates of fat oxidation, even though their use of muscle glycogen is not lower. Glycogen repletion during and after a 3-hour run is also similar to athletes on higher-carbohydrate diets. Can this improve your performance in most events? It is likely that it does not—despite an enhanced ability to use fat as a fuel after adaptation—but most find their performance is at least maintained, although it is unlikely to be better.

By way of example, keto-adapted, off-road cyclists (without diabetes) experience greater fat use—but at the price of having higher heart rates at the same workload during training—after following LCHF diets with only 15 percent of daily calories from carbohydrates. Keep in mind that with their average calorie intake, they are still eating nearly 150 grams of carbohydrates daily, much more than many low-carbohydrate advocates recommend. To my knowledge, no published studies to date have been done on keto adaptation and performance in exercisers with diabetes, and we do not really know much about the long-term impact of such low-carbohydrate diets on health or blood glucose management (although at least one study on the latter is currently underway in Scandinavia).

On the other hand, if you are doing activities that rely more heavily, or even exclusively, on muscle glycogen stores for energy like many endurance–power and power sports and activities, a low-carbohydrate diet may be detrimental to how well you perform. But many athletes with diabetes have adopted a low-carbohydrate approach to diabetes management and still perform well (or well enough) during their athletic endeavors, particularly in endurance and ultraendurance sports. If you are going to try eating this way, give yourself a few weeks of adapting to a lower carbohydrate intake—whether your eating is more focused on fat or protein—before you do an athletic event, or your performance will likely suffer in that case.

### How Low-Carbohydrate Do You Really Need to Go?

I was surprised by the large number of athletes surveyed for this book who claimed to be following very-low-carbohydrate dietary regimens. Based on their responses, it appears entirely possible to undergo fat adaptation and exercise regularly—at least when engaging in endurance-type training and events. These exercisers worry less about getting hypoglycemic during events because they have lower levels of insulin on board. But keep in mind that many others have accomplished the same reduction in the risk of lows simply by not taking bolus insulin within a few hours of being active (even if they are eating more daily carbohydrates), regardless of their carbohydrate intake.

However, there are several caveats to any conclusions based on these survey results. All normal dietary patterns by these active individuals (most with type 1 diabetes) were self-reported, and I did not have any way to analyze their actual daily carbohydrate intakes. Some claimed to eat only 20 grams of carbohydrates a day, but it is possible they were not including the carbohydrates from every food they consumed, including the many avocados (12 grams of carbohydrates per medium avocado), olives (2 to 3 grams of carbohydrates per 10 olives), and nuts (which have about 10 percent of calories from carbohydrates) they were eating.

Any carbohydrates you take in during activities, even if you need them to prevent or treat lows, count toward your daily total intake. What's more, if you are an average active individual who requires about 2,000 calories per day, and 15 percent of your calories come from carbohydrates (like most LCHF keto diet advocates), that still equates to 75 daily grams, which is not nearly as low as the 20 to 30 daily grams many of these athletes claimed to be eating or that Dr. Bernstein recommends. My guess is that many people on "low-carb diets" are actually taking in more daily carbohydrates than they think they are.

So how low do low-carbohydrate athletes with diabetes really need to go? In all likelihood, it depends on the sport and the level of athlete. Without a doubt, most of us can benefit from avoiding or limiting our intake of refined carbohydrates and foods with a higher GI to better manage our diabetes, but going to the extreme of avoiding nearly all carbohydrates or severely restricting our intake may not be necessary. If you do decide to try a low-carbohydrate diet, keep in mind that adapting to training with fewer daily carbohydrates requires several weeks—do not just cut carbohydrates for a few days and expect to feel good during any type of exercise.

> *Adapting to a lower-carbohydrate diet may allow your body to become more efficient at using fat during even moderately high-intensity activities, but give yourself a few weeks to fully adapt before you try competing in an endurance event, or your performance will likely suffer.*

## How the Diets Athletes Follow Impact Their Exercise Performance

Although I personally choose to follow a more balanced diet with a moderate intake of lower-GI carbohydrates (making up less than 40 percent of my total calories, but likely closer to 30) with the rest of my calories split between protein and fat (slightly more slanted toward fat), it is mostly because I prefer plant-based foods and do not care for meat (I have not eaten mammals of any kind for nearly 4 decades). As a semi-vegetarian (which is an actual type of *vegetarianism* involving not eating beef, pork, or other meat), I do not particularly like poultry, fish, and seafood that much, but I eat some because it makes managing my blood glucose easier. I balance it by avoiding most bread and white flour products and strictly limiting how much I eat of rice, white potatoes, highly processed carbohydrate foods, and other rapidly absorbed, high-GI carbohydrates. I eat lots of fiber. I also exercise daily doing a variety of activities and experience few lows when active. My last A1C while following this dietary regimen was 5.6 percent, and that value has been within my normal range for the past 30 plus years (since I got my first blood glucose meter). I do not actively eat a low-carbohydrate diet, but I admit to being very carbohydrate-conscious and careful with my intake—and it has ended up being lower in carbohydrates than for most people without diabetes.

For the many athletes with diabetes who swear by extreme low-carbohydrate diets that are either high in fat (like a keto diet) or higher in protein (like Dr. Bernstein's diet) or who follow another dietary regimen (like me), how do our dietary choices impact both our blood glucose management and our ability to be active? Here is what some of the respondents told me.

> "I eat mostly low carb, but find that I often need to eat more carbs after sports in order to prevent overnight lows. I try to eat 30 percent of my daily calories from carbs, 30 percent protein, and 40 percent fat each day."
> —Molly McDermott (Ottawa, Canada)

> "I stick to a low-carb diet. I eat a lot of meats, salads, eggs, and nuts. I avoid bread, pasta, processed food, and any type of sugar unless my blood glucose is low. I found that a low-carb diet makes it way easier to control my blood glucose throughout the day, especially during exercise. The more Humalog I use, generally the more tired I feel, and I also gain weight much easier and faster."
> —Aaron Gretz (Apple Valley, Minnesota)

> "I normally eat a plant-based (vegetarian) nutritional lifestyle. I almost always work out fasted in the morning as I've discovered this is how I feel best and how I can maintain the best control over my blood glucose. I also practice intermittent fasting, with my first meal each day generally at about 11:00 a.m. and my last food intake around 8:00 p.m. My carb intake varies daily, and I don't particularly aim to eat low carb as I eat a lot of fruit, sweet and regular potatoes, and beans. I eat eggs almost every day and rarely eat any kind of dairy product."
> —Daniele Hargenrader (Philadelphia, Pennsylvania)

> "I eat reasonably low carb most of the time, though I do 'carb up' for race days and tests sometimes (for performance reasons)."
> —Jennie B. (United Kingdom)

> "I have been following a low-carb, high-fat diet for a couple of years. It makes it easier to keep blood glucose levels stable and keeps me full so I'm less tempted to snack between meals. Though I don't eat low enough carb to stay in ketosis. I eat 40 to 60 grams of carbohydrate per day."
> —Andrea Limbourg (Paris, France)

> "I follow the metabolic efficiency diet. I eat about 125 to 150 grams of carbs per day with a diet focused on low glycemic carbs, fiber, healthy fats, and proteins. I avoid white flour and high glycemic foods."
> —Conor Smith (Fort Washington, Pennsylvania)

> "I stick to low carb unless in an environment of heavy training (marathon training). Consuming periodic glucose during endurance exercise and events

can optimize my performance. I eat no fast food and a healthful diet full of greens and fish."

—Bill King (Philadelphia, Pennsylvania)

"Per Dr. Bernstein's protocols, I eat low carb, moderate protein. I typically exercise in the morning and do not have active bolus insulin on board. I will eat small portions of dried fruit to bring my blood glucose up to 120 mg/dL (6.7 mmol/L) if it's below that when I start. If I am going to do a race that will last more than 90 minutes, I will use UCAN 60 minutes before the race for slow-acting carbohydrate during the event."

—Jason Sperry (Mannsville, New York)

"I eat low-carbohydrate, high-protein, high-healthful fat meals. I recently cycled from Perth to Sydney, solo and unsupported in a time frame of 20 days, following low carb. As a fat-adapted athlete, this also disproved any theories that such exercise must be performed consuming a high-carbohydrate diet."

—Neil McLagan (Perth, Western Australia)

"I am, for the most part, on a Paleo diet. My carb intake is ~20 to 40 grams a day. By not needing to cover a large carb intake, my boluses are less, thus I am not partaking in an odyssey of hours of either being hugely high or low due to a miscalculation. The law of small numbers is the key here."

—Jay Handy (Madison, Wisconsin)

"Changing my diet to no starchy carbs has been magic. I dropped Lantus from more than 30 units down to 18 per day since dropping *all* starchy carbs. I eat no breads, pasta, cereal . . . The carbs I consume include veggies only. Most of my workouts now require no insulin management, and I seldom get low."

—Tom Seabourne (Mount Pleasant, Texas)

"I am carb-conscious. I do not eat low carb but make smart carb decisions. I aim to eat unprocessed, homemade food as much as possible. I love cooking in the backcountry and enjoy finding recipes that are dehydrated, light-weight, nutritious, and carb-rich for trekking days, and fueling."

—Jen Hanson (Toronto, Canada)

"I was most helped by switching my diet and way of handling my diabetes to the Dr. Richard K. Bernstein method. I spent 47 and a half years stuffing glucose in my face all day long when I was skiing, hiking, or swimming just to keep my blood sugar above 100 mg/dL (5.6 mmol/L) and then having it fly up to the 200 to 300s later. Now that I'm eating very low carb, this problem is *greatly* minimized. Eating this way has significantly flattened my blood glucose graph and prevented the precipitous, scary lows of the past. I'm so thankful to have found this way of handling type 1 diabetes."

—Mary Alice (San Diego, California)

"I tend to eat low on the glycemic index and very little gluten. I substitute bean noodles for wheat, and quinoa is a staple. I eat a lot of slow-cooked meals with beans and vegetables. Breakfast is usually full-fat Greek yogurt. During trail races, I eat hard-boiled eggs and potatoes, items that provide nutrition but don't require a bolus. I don't drink sports drinks or anything with sugars that need insulin. For low correction, I eat dried fruit which I find is kinder on the stomach than simple sugars in sports drinks. I don't eat GU or other sports gels. The less insulin in my system around exercise the better. This is not to be mistaken for low-carb or low-calorie diet; it's just low-GI."

—Blair Ryan (Del Mar, California)

## Protein: Important During Recovery for Muscle Repair

During most exercise, protein contributes less than 5 percent of the total energy, although it may rise to 10 to 15 percent during a prolonged event, such as a marathon or Ironman triathlon. Regardless, protein is never a key energy source for exercise, but it is critical for other reasons. Taking in enough protein in your diet allows your muscles to be repaired after strenuous exercise and promotes the synthesis of hormones, enzymes, and other body tissues formed from *amino acids*, the building blocks of protein.

About half of the 20 amino acids (shown in table 4.4) are considered *essential* in your diet, meaning that you must consume them or your body will suffer from protein malnutrition, which causes the breakdown of muscles and organs over time. Your body can make *nonessential* amino acids by itself, but you need to have enough of all of them—essential and nonessential—to synthesize protein during

**Table 4.4  Amino Acids**

| Essential Amino Acids | Nonessential Amino Acids |
| --- | --- |
| Histidine | Alanine |
| Isoleucine | Arginine |
| Leucine | Asparagine |
| Lysine | Aspartic acid |
| Methionine | Cysteine |
| Phenylalanine | Glutamic acid |
| Threonine | Glutamine |
| Tryptophan | Glycine |
| Valine | Proline |
| Serine | Tyrosine |

recovery from exercise. This is vital to experience any increase in the strength, aerobic capacity, or size of your muscles. Animal sources of protein (including meat, poultry, fish, dairy products, and eggs) are considered complete protein because they contain all the essential amino acids. Most plant foods—except for soy, buckwheat, quinoa, and hemp—contain proteins that are lacking in one of more of the essential amino acids and are best eaten in combination (such as beans and rice) at meals or during the day. Eating a wide variety of plant foods (of different colors) is best from a nutritional standpoint anyway.

The current recommended intake of protein is 10 to 35 percent of total daily calories, with each 1 gram of protein containing 4 usable calories (the nitrogen part of an amino acid is excreted if the protein is used for energy). Athletes who train regularly likely can consume anywhere in that range as long as they are minimally consuming at least 1.2 to 1.8 grams of protein per kilogram (or 2.2 pounds) of body weight, which works out to 84 to 126 grams of daily protein for a 70-kilogram (154-pound) exerciser. Typically, an ounce (28 grams) of chicken, cheese, or meat contains 7 to 8 grams of protein.

Protein takes 3 to 5 hours to be fully metabolized after you eat it—more time than carbohydrate but less than fat—and a portion of it is converted into glucose, which can raise (or prevent drops in) your blood glucose when it finally gets digested. Both protein and fat can increase the rise in your blood glucose long after eating, and their impact is additive, meaning that fat and protein separately contribute to the rise.

Low-carbohydrate diets can alternately be higher in protein or in fat, but some recommend taking in at least 30 to 40 grams of protein at each meal to enhance maximum protein uptake. You are likely getting this much protein or more already if you are following a low-carbohydrate, high-protein diet (like Dr. Bernstein's) to manage your diabetes. Protein requires some insulin—usually within a few hours of consuming it when a portion of it is converted into glucose—but not right away. Check your blood glucose levels a few hours after exercise taking in protein and dose then with insulin if your blood glucose starts to rise to ensure those amino acids get into your muscles and any converted into glucose do not stay in your bloodstream.

Given that protein is not a major energy source during exercise, you really do not need to worry about consuming any protein right before or during an activity. Taking in some protein along with carbohydrate right after hard or long workouts may help your body replenish its stores of muscle and liver glycogen more effectively, as digested protein can be converted into glucose as needed by your liver (mostly using the amino acid *alanine*). Although the benefits of taking in protein after workouts have not been studied in athletes with diabetes, consuming carbohydrates with a small amount of protein (in a ratio of 4:1) after an activity may help prevent lows later and speed up recovery, although others show no benefit beyond what you get with proper refueling. Protein is protective against getting low later. You may also want to have some in your bedtime snack (along with fat and carbohydrate) when you are trying to prevent nighttime lows after a day of strenuous or prolonged activity.

## Resources for Active People With Diabetes

### Riding on Insulin

The Riding on Insulin (ROI) organization empowers, activates, and connects the global diabetes community through shared experiences and action sports. In addition to establishing a comfortable environment, they strive to help families explore new passions, challenge type 1 diabetes, and celebrate each other's successes, including through a multisport racing team. They offer 1-day "shred" events for kids ages 7 to 17 who are living with type 1 diabetes and their siblings. They hold their camps across four countries—the United States, Canada, New Zealand, and Australia—and serve over 500 kids each year. Their programs include ski/snowboard camps, mountain bike camps, the ROI Race team that participates in everything from 5K to Ironman triathlons, and winter racing like cross-country ski races, and skiing and snowboard competitions. Their camps have also been used to conduct clinical trials for major universities, hospitals, researchers, and scientists to help push new medical devices to market such as the "artificial pancreas."

Founded by professional snowboarder Sean Busby in 2004, this group was born out of Sean's desire to give back to the kids who had inspired him to keep snowboarding after his own complicated type 1 diabetes diagnosis at age 19. He read stories online through the JDRF Children's Congress event of kids and teens living with the disease, and he figured if they could do it—who knew no other different life—then surely so could he. He wanted to give back to those kids for inspiring him. To find out more about what ROI does and learn how to donate and how to get involved, visit them online at www.ridingoninsulin.org.

## NUTRITIONAL SUPPLEMENTS: NECESSARY, HELPFUL, OR HYPE?

The number of advertised nutritional supplements that claim to enhance athletic ability is staggering. Most of the "proof" for these claims comes from studies done by the manufacturer of the product or from testimonials by people, often celebrities, who claim to use them. Thus, the problem for most athletes is determining which nutritional claims to believe.

Probably the best ergogenic aid for most athletes with diabetes is simply keeping your blood glucose as close to normal as possible during exercise. Your performance can suffer from early fatigue (caused by hypoglycemia) or sluggishness (a common result of elevations). You need to maintain your blood glucose in a narrow range during exercise to prevent either of these problems. (See some troubleshooting tips at the end of chapter 6 for possible solutions.) That said, some supplements may help your performance, but others are likely to make things worse. Refer to table 4.5 for nutritional supplements that may potentially benefit athletes with diabetes and table 4.6 for those with a potentially harmful impact.

Some of these supplements should rightfully appear in both tables (beneficial and harmful) depending on whether you go to extremes. For instance, when you

**Table 4.5   Potentially Beneficial Supplements for Athletes With Diabetes**

| Nutritional Supplement | Potential Beneficial Effects |
|---|---|
| Antioxidants | May reduce oxidative damage to cell membranes induced by exercise and hyperglycemia, and slow down aging |
| Caffeine | Increased release of fatty acids, better hormone response to exercise hypoglycemia, and lessened risk of getting low |
| Carbohydrate and glucose intake | Appropriate amounts of carbohydrate before, during, and after exercise may prevent exercise-induced lows |
| Chromium, vanadium, and zinc | Possible improvement in insulin sensitivity (especially in type 2 diabetes) |
| Magnesium | Improved function of over 300 metabolic pathways involved in producing ATP from various fuels, reduced risk of exercise-related muscle cramps, lower resting blood pressure |
| Sports drinks | Prevention of hypoglycemia, dehydration, and electrolyte imbalance during prolonged exercise, especially in the heat |
| Water and fluid replacement | Prevention of dehydration, especially with hyperglycemia or during exercise in the heat when you sweat more |

**Table 4.6   Potentially Harmful Supplements for Athletes With Diabetes**

| Nutritional Supplement | Potential Harmful Effects |
|---|---|
| Amino acid, whey, or other protein supplements (including hydrolysates) | Taking too much of one or several amino acids can cause an imbalance in the body; all protein can potentially stress your kidneys due to causing excess nitrogen excretion (and is not recommended if you have diabetic kidney disease) |
| Caffeine | Potential for greater water loss and dehydration due to its diuretic effect, especially in the heat; too much caffeine can lead to an abnormal heart rhythm |
| Carbohydrate loading | Potential for hyperglycemia before, during, or after exercise, as well as a reduction in insulin sensitivity; potential for hypoglycemia if consumed before exercise with too much insulin taken to cover it |
| Creatine | Potential for added stress on your kidneys, especially if you have any stage of kidney disease, due to excess urinary excretion of its breakdown product creatinine |
| Fat loading | Slower carbohydrate absorption rates during exercise if consumed before or during activity, increased insulin resistance, ketone production, and obesity in the long term |

supplement with sports drinks, avoid taking in too many carbohydrates or you can end up with high blood glucose instead. Similarly, carbohydrate loading can ensure you have enough muscle and liver glycogen levels both before and after exercise, but only if you have enough insulin on board to prevent hyperglycemia. If not, you will not get as much glucose into storage in your muscles. Antioxidants taken in mega doses may have a pro-oxidant (or the opposite) effect. Excess nitrogen from amino acids—even essential ones that you need—must be converted into a waste product called *urea*, which is then excreted by your kidneys or sweat glands, making them work overtime; too much protein can, therefore, be as harmful as too little. Also, although most studies have shown that taking creatine supplements may create some stress on your kidneys during the initial loading period (lasting 5 to 7 days), during smaller maintenance doses its impact is minimal if you have normal kidney function.

## Amino Acid or Protein Supplements: Do You Need Them?

Have you heard about people using amino acid or protein supplements to try to bulk up? As we have discussed, *amino acids* are the building blocks of proteins, and you must consume enough of the essential ones (refer back to table 4.4) to build and repair your muscles and other body proteins. You can buy almost every amino acid individually as a supplement, and many more are offered in combinations (e.g., branched-chain amino acids). Athletes have tried supplementing with practically all the amino acids to produce a performance-enhancing or strength-boosting effect.

Whey protein, derived from milk protein, has been a long-time favorite because it has a high amount of three essential branched-chain amino acids (leucine, isoleucine, and valine), considered by many bodybuilders and strength athletes to be the ultimate amino acids for muscle growth and repair. A newer trend is for athletes to supplement with protein *hydrolysates*, or smaller (partially predigested) particles of whey or other proteins. Despite costing even more than other supplements, nothing has shown that these particles promote a greater uptake of amino acids into your muscles. Likely they are a waste of good money.

The biggest myth about amino acid supplements, and protein in general, is that you have to load up on them to gain muscle mass. As I previously mentioned, the protein requirement for strength-training athletes may be about twice as high as is normal for nonathletes, but most people in the United States already consume more than the higher amount of protein recommended for athletes in their own diets. To gain 1 pound (0.45 kilogram) of muscle mass a week (a realistic amount), a strength-training athlete needs only an additional 14 grams of quality protein per day, which is easily attainable in less than two glasses of milk or 2 ounces (57 grams) of lean meat, chicken, fish, or cheese—along with an adequate intake of calories.

Taking specific supplemental amino acids may actually cause an imbalance in your body by leading to an overabundance of some amino acids and a relative deficit of others. What's more, you can still gain extra fat weight or have high blood glucose if you take in excess calories as amino acid supplements, which are stored simply as excess body fat or converted into blood glucose. The supplements are also expensive. As an exerciser with diabetes, you should also consider the potential effects of excess protein consumption on your kidneys; if you have healthy kidneys, excreting it is not an issue, but it may put a strain on kidneys with long-term damage.

> *Taking amino acid or protein supplements is generally a waste of money and can potentially put additional strain on ailing kidneys. If you want more protein in your diet, simply increase your intake of healthful foods high in protein such as egg whites, nonfat milk, beans and legumes, and lean meats, fish, and poultry.*

# Vitamins: Do You Need Supplements With a Healthful Diet?

Many athletes take supplemental vitamins and minerals; maybe you are one of them. In some cases, there may be either sports-related or diabetes-related reasons to supplement with certain vitamins and minerals. Many athletes supplement with specific vitamins, such as antioxidants and vitamin $B_{12}$, in hopes of improving performance or enhancing recovery. Diabetes itself can affect your vitamin and mineral status, but that does not always mean that you need a supplement. The ones that you may want to consider taking are discussed in this section.

## *Multivitamin and Mineral Supplements*

A wide range of vitamins and minerals affect glucose metabolism and insulin sensitivity, yet people with diabetes routinely do not get enough of them, especially when on calorie-restricted diets. If you choose to supplement, consider taking adequate amounts of the B vitamins, antioxidants (like vitamins C and E and alpha-lipoic acid), magnesium, and chromium. Also, select supplements that do not contain fillers (such as sugar and artificial colors and flavors) or common allergens (e.g., gluten, wheat, dairy, yeast, or corn). Avoid taking in excess copper or iron because these minerals can lower insulin action.

## *Antioxidants*

Exercise increases the production of oxygen free radicals like *superoxide*, a chemical substance with a lone, unpaired electron that can damage cell membranes and DNA. By exercising, you already enhance your natural antioxidant enzyme systems that squelch most of these potentially damaging compounds. The vitamins with antioxidant qualities are C, E, and beta-carotene (a precursor to vitamin A). Other potential antioxidants are $CoQ_{10}$ (ubiquinone) and the mineral selenium. Another powerful antioxidant found in foods is alpha-lipoic acid, which may help prevent and treat nerve-related problems (common to diabetes) and protect against other oxidative damage.

Antioxidant supplements are believed to help limit the cellular damage that may occur from free radicals produced during exercise, or in the case of diabetes from

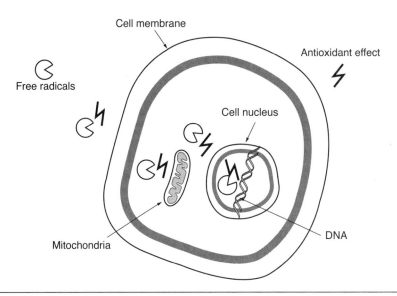

**Figure 4.1** Antioxidant vitamins may help your body prevent some damage from free radical formation resulting from exercise and high blood glucose.

higher blood glucose levels, as depicted in figure 4.1. Although these supplements do not enhance sport performance, they may play a role in protecting your muscles from cellular damage during strenuous training and protecting the rest of your body from free-radical–generated complications.

**Vitamin C.**   Besides having an antioxidant effect, vitamin C (*ascorbate*) helps form the collagen that makes up connective tissues, ligaments, and tendons. It also aids in the absorption of iron from the gut and in the formation of adrenaline. Some people take large doses of vitamin C to prevent the common cold and other viral infections. Although doses up to 1,000 milligrams of this vitamin appear to be safe, 200 milligrams per day is likely enough, which you can easily get through a diet with plenty of citrus fruits, green leafy vegetables, broccoli, peppers, strawberries, and potatoes.

**Vitamin E.**   This vitamin helps maintain the fluidity of red blood cells and protects cell membranes from oxidative damage. Supplementing with 400 to 800 IU (international units) does not appear to be harmful and may prevent damage. In people with diabetes, vitamin E supplementation may improve blood flow to the back of the eye (retina) and creatinine clearance (an indicator of normal kidney function), but it does not improve blood glucose levels. This vitamin is recommended for athletes who are training at high altitude or in smoggy areas where oxidative stress may be greater. A fat-soluble vitamin, it is found naturally in vegetable oils, margarine, egg yolks, green leafy vegetables, wheat germ, and whole-grain products.

**Vitamin A and Beta-Carotene.**   Supplements high in beta-carotene but low in vitamin A may also be beneficial. Both beta-carotene and vitamin A help maintain skin and mucous membranes, night vision, and proper bone development. Diets rich in vitamin

A or polyphenols (found in grapes and other foods) have protective effects against autoimmune attacks of beta cells and, therefore, have the potential to prevent type 1 diabetes (at least in diabetes-prone mice). Vitamin A is found in animal products like liver, milk, and cheese, whereas beta-carotene (its precursor) is higher in plant sources, particularly carrots, sweet potatoes, and other yellow or orange vegetables. Because your body can synthesize vitamin A as needed from beta-carotene, supplement with the latter and avoid taking large doses of vitamin A, which can be toxic.

**CoQ$_{10}$.** Found in the mitochondria (the powerhouses of the cells) and also known as *ubiquinone*, CoQ$_{10}$ is not an official antioxidant vitamin but rather a lipid, or form of fat. It plays an important role in your cellular ability to use oxygen to make ATP. Although it has been used as a supplemental antioxidant to potentially protect the heart muscle from tissue damage, its potential benefits remain unproven. Taking it is not advised although it is often pushed on endurance athletes.

**Selenium.** A deficiency in selenium, the main antioxidant mineral, can affect exercise performance, mainly by causing unchecked muscle or mitochondrial damage. Selenium has not been proven to be an effective ergogenic or a way to prevent diabetes-related health problems. You can easily obtain adequate amounts by eating grains grown in selenium-rich soil (as found in the United States and Canada) or eating seafood and organ meats. If you do take it as a supplement, do not exceed 200 micrograms daily.

**Alpha-Lipoic Acid.** Alpha-lipoic acid is a strong antioxidant with beneficial effects on diabetic peripheral neuropathy, as well as potentially memory-enhancing functions in people with Alzheimer's disease. If you would rather get it naturally (albeit in a lower dose), consume more spinach, broccoli, tomatoes, potatoes, green peas, and Brussels sprouts.

## Vitamin D

The only vitamin that works as a hormone is vitamin D. Its active form, *calcitriol*, helps your body absorb calcium and deposit it in your bones, but is also involved in a whole host of other cell activities around the body. A lack of vitamin D is associated with conditions like cancer, asthma, high blood pressure, depression, dementia and Alzheimer's disease, and autoimmune diseases (e.g., type 1 diabetes, multiple sclerosis, and Crohn's). Its deficiency has been linked to both of the main types of diabetes: to the onset of type 1 diabetes through autoimmune mechanisms and to type 2 through increased insulin resistance, especially when combined with low calcium intake. People commonly become more deficient in this vitamin as they age.

Close to 90 percent of active vitamin D is formed through exposure to sunlight, but deficiencies today are far more widespread due to a combination of more time spent indoors, lavish use of sunscreens (to prevent skin cancer and wrinkles), and consumption of nutrient-poor foods and drinks. You do not need much sun exposure to make enough vitamin D in your skin—maybe about 15 minutes on 3 days each week on your face and hands—but living in a high-latitude region and aging both reduce how much of this vitamin your skin can make from ultraviolet light exposure. Consider supplementing with up to 800 IU per day (particularly if you are older) and eating more foods rich in vitamin D like fortified dairy products, nuts and seeds, and vegetable oils.

## Vitamin B₁

Vitamin $B_1$, also known as *thiamin*, is often deficient in people with both type 1 and type 2 diabetes. It is essential for the metabolism of glucose, the normal function of your nerves, and muscle glycogen use during exercise. Both exercise and a high-carbohydrate intake increase the need for this vitamin, and a deficiency can lead to muscle weakness, pain in your calves, and damage to your nervous system and heart. Drinking too much alcohol can strip this vitamin from your body. Vitamin $B_1$ is a water-soluble vitamin widely distributed in plant and animal foods, such as whole grains, legumes, and pork, so you can take in enough by eating a balanced, healthful diet. If your blood glucose is frequently higher than desired, a daily supplement of up to 100 milligrams cannot hurt. Other B vitamins such as riboflavin and biotin may also be important for people with diabetes.

## Vitamin B₁₂

Athletes use and abuse vitamin $B_{12}$ (also called *cobalamin*) because they believe that it enhances red blood cell production, improves oxygen-carrying capacity during endurance events, and may even increase muscle mass. Although a deficiency of this vitamin can potentially impair your performance, it does not help you if you already get enough in your diet. Vitamin $B_{12}$ is found only in animal products (meat, dairy products, and eggs); therefore, vegetarians, especially vegans who do not eat any meat or animal byproducts, likely need $B_{12}$ supplements to prevent *pernicious anemia*, a form of anemia that causes weakness, fatigue, and malaise. Taking supplements of this vitamin is otherwise generally not necessary or recommended, although large doses are considered harmless.

# Minerals: Check Your Intake of Iron, Calcium, and Magnesium

Minerals exert their effects on many energy-producing pathways in the body because of their involvement with metabolism and the enzymes involved in ATP production. Deficiencies in a mineral like iron could certainly have a negative effect on your exercise capacity, and diabetes itself can potentially cause certain mineral deficiencies. Among the minerals that athletes with diabetes may consider supplementing with are iron, calcium, magnesium, zinc, and chromium.

## Iron

An iron deficiency can affect your endurance capacity because this mineral is part of the *hemoglobin* molecule that carries oxygen in your red blood cells. Any reduction in hemoglobin reduces your oxygen-carrying capacity and may make your muscles feel unusually fatigued during aerobic activities. Iron deficiency is a common problem, especially in endurance athletes and premenopausal women. Dietary iron is found in both animal and plant sources, but the iron in plants (e.g., spinach, which contains the *ferric* form) is not absorbed as well as that found in meat, poultry, and fish (i.e., *ferrous* iron). You may benefit from iron supplements if you do not get enough in your diet or receive it mainly from plant sources. Premenopausal women need about 15 milligrams daily, whereas men require only about 10 milligrams. However, taking iron if you are not deficient will not improve your exercise capacity and can reduce your insulin action, so do not supplement with iron unless you are deficient.

## Calcium

Although calcium intake does not directly affect sport performance, adequate amounts are crucial to the long-term health of your bones and other bodily systems. Many older people experience *osteoporosis* (thinning of the bones), which greatly increases the risk for bone fractures. Both weight-bearing exercises and resistance training can stimulate the retention of calcium in bones, but your diet also needs to contain enough calcium. Sources of dietary calcium are dairy products, egg yolks, legumes, broccoli, cauliflower, and dark green leafy vegetables, to name a few. Supplementing with calcium (as well as foods rich in vitamin D to increase calcium absorption) is recommended for anyone taking in less than 1,000 to 1,200 milligrams daily (up to 1,500 milligrams when you are older). With diabetes, be diligent about getting adequate amounts of this mineral because diabetes itself can cause greater loss of bone minerals.

In addition, limit your intake of phosphorus, found in colas and widely distributed in foods, because it can leech calcium from your bones. Also do not take in excess amounts of sodium, protein, or caffeine because they all can reduce calcium in bones.

## Magnesium

A component of more than 300 enzymes that control metabolism in your muscles, magnesium affects the use of ATP, oxygen, and glucose during muscle contractions as well as the health of your bones. It is believed to have an anti-inflammatory effect (and most chronic diseases like heart disease have chronic inflammation as an underlying cause). Deficiency has been associated with conditions like high blood pressure, abnormal heart rhythms, asthma, premenstrual syndrome, and many others. Although supplementing is not likely to improve your sport performance if you are not deficient in this mineral, having enough magnesium in your body may prevent muscle cramping and general muscle weakness. Deficiencies are more common in athletes and people with diabetes. Strenuous exercise apparently increases urinary and sweat losses, which may increase your magnesium requirements by up to 20 percent.

A significant number of athletes have magnesium intakes that may result in a deficient status, such as those participating in sports requiring weight control (e.g., wrestling and gymnastics). In their case, an increased intake of magnesium will have beneficial effects on exercise performance, and taking in less than 420 milligrams per day for male athletes and 320 milligrams for female athletes may result in a deficiency. In addition, low intake of magnesium has been linked to a higher risk for developing type 2 diabetes. In people with diabetes, low magnesium levels have been linked to a higher incidence of retinopathy (diabetic eye disease) and depression, as well as higher overall blood glucose levels. To get enough magnesium, consume foods like nuts, seafood, green leafy vegetables, dairy, whole-grain products, and even dark chocolate. You may also benefit from taking a magnesium supplement (not to exceed 350 milligrams daily), particularly if you are physically active with diabetes and female.

### Zinc

Zinc is a mineral involved in wound healing, growth, protein synthesis, and immune function. Like magnesium, it is also an activator of more than 300 enzymes, some of which involve ATP production using the lactic acid system. Low-calorie diets or excessive sweating may contribute to its loss, and having diabetes may make you more prone to deficiencies from losing more through urine when you have hyperglycemia.

In adults with type 2 diabetes, zinc supplements may reduce insulin resistance. However, zinc supplements have not conclusively been found to enhance muscular strength or athletic performance, and the intake of large doses may interfere with absorption of iron and copper, impair immune function (instead of improving it), and raise levels of low-density lipoprotein cholesterol while decreasing the "good" high-density lipoprotein. Thus, it is best not to supplement with doses above what is recommended, which is 8 milligrams (women) or 11 milligrams (men) per day. Better yet, simply consume an adequate amount by eating organ meats, poultry, seafood (especially oysters), dairy products, asparagus, spinach, or whole-grain products.

### Chromium

Believed to enhance insulin sensitivity, chromium may improve your blood glucose, storage of glycogen, and performance during endurance exercise. People with type 2 diabetes have taken it to try to improve insulin sensitivity, and athletes have hoped it increases lean body mass and reduces body fat. Chromium supplements will not affect muscle or fat mass, muscular strength, or muscular endurance, or make you lose weight. In fact, taken in excess, this mineral may accumulate in the cells and cause damage to your DNA. Only take chromium if you consume a high-carbohydrate diet, exercise strenuously, or have inadequate intake. Better yet, get chromium through food sources, including organ meats, oysters, cheese, whole-grain products, nuts, asparagus, and beer. Limit any supplements to 200 micrograms a day.

# Caffeine: Going Beyond That Morning Cup of Coffee

Do you need to have that cup of steaming java in the morning to start your day off right? If so, you are probably drinking it more for the caffeine than any other reason. Caffeine is a stimulant found naturally in coffee, tea, cocoa, and chocolate that works directly on the central nervous system and increases arousal. At the same time, it increases your body's release of adrenaline, which can mobilize fat and provide an alternative fuel for muscles.

Caffeine also stimulates calcium release in contracting muscles, allowing greater force production and muscular strength—which is probably its most important effect as far as athletes are concerned. It potentially increases performance in almost any event or physical activity that you choose to do, long or short, intense or easy. Most athletes use caffeine in an attempt to improve how well they perform and feel. Table 4.7 lists the main sources of caffeine.

Currently, all doses of caffeine are legal in sports, although it has a history of being banned and limited by the International Olympic Committee. Its turbulent status may stem from the fact that it is one of the few supplements that can improve your performance, even in running times for various distances from 1 mile (1.6 kilometers) up to marathons and in power events. You may be able to increase the effectiveness of caffeine by abstaining from it for 2 or 3 days before your event and then consuming it right before you start. A short period of withdrawal causes you to be less habituated to its effects, although you may suffer through withdrawal symptoms like headaches and irritability.

A more recently discovered effect of caffeine is that it may enhance your body's release of hormones in response to hypoglycemia and your brain's ability

### Table 4.7 Main Caffeine Sources

| Caffeine Source | Amount of Caffeine (mg) |
|---|---|
| Coffee | |
| Brewed, 8 oz (240 mL) | 95–165 |
| Instant, 8 oz (240 mL) | 63 |
| Espresso, 1 oz (30 mL) | 47–64 |
| Decaffeinated, 8 oz (240 mL) | 2–5 |
| Tea | |
| Green, 8 oz (240 mL) | 25–29 |
| Black, 8 oz (240 mL) | 25–48 |
| Bottled, 8 oz (240 mL) | 5–40 |
| Cocoa, hot, 8 oz (240 mL) | 5 |
| Soda, caffeinated, 12 oz (360 mL) | 40–55 |
| Monster Energy, 8 oz (240 mL) | 86 |
| Red Bull, 8.4 oz (250 mL) | 80 |
| 5-Hour Energy shot, 2 oz (60 mL) | 200 |
| Chocolate, dark, 1 oz (30 mg) | 12 |
| Tablet (No Doz or Vivarin) | 100–200 |

to respond to adrenaline with improved function during lows. It has also been shown that taking in 5 to 6 milligrams per kilogram of body mass of caffeine (typically around 300 to 400 milligrams) before exercise may keep your blood glucose from falling as much during exercise. Bec Johnson, a resident of Perth, Australia, will use caffeine if she anticipates that she will drop during training; she has a coffee beforehand, and it keeps her levels steady. Beware of later onset lows, though, because you likely did not consume many calories along with your coffee that have any staying power.

Caffeine has a diuretic effect, meaning that it can make you lose more body water as urine. This effect is largely overridden during exercise, but be cautious about maintaining proper hydration when ingesting caffeine, especially if you exercise in a hot environment where you sweat more or when your blood glucose is elevated. Another concern is that caffeine increases insulin resistance, although this effect will be minimized while you are active. When caffeine comes naturally in coffee, it appears to have a lesser effect on insulin action than straight caffeine (perhaps because of the other compounds found in coffee), but drinking coffee may still raise your blood glucose at rest. For instance, Jorden Rieke of Cleveland, Ohio, reports that she boluses about 1 unit to cover each small cup of coffee she drinks.

## Creatine: The Power Supplement, but for Diabetes?

Creatine is an amine present in animal products but also formed in your liver and kidneys from other amino acids. Normally, your daily dietary intake of creatine is 1 gram, and another gram is synthesized by your body. Creatine is present in all muscle cells both in its free form and as creatine phosphate (CP), a main component of the phosphagen energy system (refer to chapter 2). Many athletes have tried creatine supplements to increase their performance in power sports. The supplements do increase free creatine and CP stores in muscles, but you gain water weight retained in muscles with the extra creatine.

Loading up with 20 to 30 grams of creatine monohydrate in four equal doses over the course of a day for 5 to 7 days may improve your performance in explosive sports like power lifting and field events. After taking it, you may be able to train at a higher level, which could lead to an increase in your muscle mass and gains in strength and power, but it will not help you in endurance activities and may work against you due to weight gain. The initial creatine-loading phase is typically followed by a maintenance dose of 2 to 5 grams per day. Other athletes have tried supplementing with 3 grams per day for 4 weeks without a loading phase, and doing so works equally well. Most athletes then cycle off creatine for a while before starting again. Drink plenty of fluids because supplements can have a dehydrating effect. Also, if you have any evidence of kidney disease, you are best advised not to load up on creatine because of the stress it can place on your kidneys.

# Athlete Profile: **Jen Hanson**

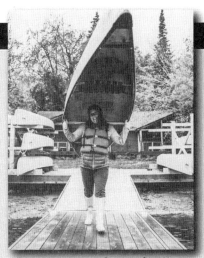

Courtesy of Jen Hanson.
Photographer: Mike Last.

***Hometown:*** Sunderland, Ontario, Canada

***Diabetes history:*** Type 1 diabetes diagnosed in 1987 (at age 3)

***Sport or activity:*** Backpacking, backcountry travel

***Greatest athletic achievement:*** My greatest formal athletic achievement was competing as a member of the championship varsity women's wrestling team at Brock University. But if we're talking about backpacking/ backcountry travel, it involves coming to a point in my relationship with my diabetes where I don't feel limited when doing backcountry travel. I have spent weeks off the grid, several days' travel away from emergency medical services. Although diabetes has always been along for the ride, it is just another factor to take into consideration when planning for an adventure. In 2016 and 2017 I completed two multiday treks as a guide of a group of adventurers with type 1 diabetes, and each was its own accomplishment for its own reason.

In 2016, I completed the challenging 36-kilometer (22.4-mile) trek of the Long Range Traverse in Gros Morne National Park in Newfoundland, Canada. This remote trek involved map and compass work to guide us over mountain passes and through valleys. The weather was incredibly varied, swinging from sweltering heat to near-hypothermic conditions. The diabetes challenges were exacerbated by the unknown in what lay ahead. Similarly, in 2017 I trekked the 58-kilometer (36-mile) North Coast Trail on the northernmost tip of Vancouver Island in British Columbia (Canada). Although the paths were marked well enough that we were not concerned about getting lost, the terrain was rugged and incredibly varied. On any given day, we were challenged with navigating river crossings, scaling steep wave-beaten cliff faces using dangling ropes, and traversing cobblestone beaches (that is, ankle-rolling, bowling ball–shaped stones, often covered in a slimy, slippery green algae).

***Current insulin and medication regimen:*** I use an insulin pump (Tandem t:slim X2) and a CGM (Dexcom G5) and take about 60 units daily split between basal and bolus doses, along with taking Jardiance, an SGLT-2 inhibitor.

***Training tips:*** My biggest tip while traveling in the backcountry would be to learn to live on less. When traveling in the backcountry, everything I need I carry on my back. I typically travel with a group and assume that half my backpack will be used for group gear and food. I typically travel with a 60-liter pack, meaning that I have only 30-liters to house my personal items for a trip. For someone without diabetes, packing all personal items into 30-liters (including a sleeping bag, sleeping pad, rain gear, cold-weather gear, water bottle, headlamp, camp shoes, clothing, etc.) is a stretch, but I typically use half of my 30-liter personal space for diabetes and emergency supplies. Figure out what you absolutely need and what you don't. Invest in

continued ➡

*Jen Hanson continued*

high-quality, lightweight gear and odor-repelling clothing like merino wool, which can be a lifesaver for both you and your trek mates! (And don't forget, you don't have to buy new. Check out your local thrift shop for some great deals!)

Also, get to know your body the best you can. Typically, on a backcountry trip, I'll be trekking for 8 to 10 hours, with a brief lunch/rest stop. All of that moving, especially with a weighted backpack, can wreak havoc on your blood glucose if you're not used to it and, let's be honest, it's hard to get used to day after day of 10 hours of travel. It's not something that is easy to train for. Over the years, I have gotten to know my body by doing shorter hikes both with and without a weighted backpack, and I've learned how my body reacts to long, flat walks versus short spurts of intense uphill work. I've been mindful of how my body recovers from consistent activity and become comfortable with resetting temporary basal rates when getting close to camp for the night.

***Typical trekking day routing and diabetes regimen:*** On a multiday trek where I expect to be active for 6 hours a day or longer, I will use a preprogrammed basal pattern in my insulin pump that assumes a 24-hour, 60 percent basal rate. Any adjustments below assume that already reduced (from my normal) basal rate.

- ► *Sunrise:* Wake up, put on coffee, begin prepping breakfast and packing up camp, look over maps, and go over activity expectations for the day. I am specifically looking for whether we'll be doing lots of climbing and descending, or whether we can expect a flatter route. I make best guesses at the terrain that is ahead (inland paths, which can often be easier on the legs, versus cobblestone beaches). I look for total mileage for the day and make best guesses at where and when we'll land for lunch. Whenever possible, I consider guidebooks and previous hiker logs (brought from home). If I am expecting a particularly challenging morning, I set a temporary basal rate of 50 percent below my already reduced rate during this activity. I try to drink 1 liter of water before leaving camp each morning and carry another 2 liters with me for the morning.

- ► *7:00 a.m.:* Breakfast of oatmeal or quinoa with freeze-dried fruit, nuts, peanut butter, chia seed, and coffee/tea, along with a regular bolus. (If not overly hungry, or if my blood glucose is already higher than I'd like, I'll often put my oatmeal or quinoa in a baggy and snack on this during the first hour of hiking by cutting a small hole into the corner of the bag).

- ► *8:00 a.m.:* Begin trekking. Check in with blood glucose levels consistently in the first 30 minutes while breakfast is kicking in and blood begins to get pumping with the activity.

- ► *10:30 a.m.:* Depending on how my blood glucose is trending, I will typically consume 1 Clif Bar (45 grams of carbs) without insulin throughout the morning.

- ► *12:00 noon:* Aim for lunch, which typically consists of pita bread/crackers, salami meat, cheese, peanut butter, and trail mix, taken with a normal lunch bolus. If water is easily accessible, finish 2 liters of water and refill.

- ► *12:30 p.m.:* Consider the afternoon trail. If expecting a challenging afternoon, maintain a 50 percent reduced basal. If the afternoon is looking less challenging, I don't set a temporary basal (but remember, I'm already using a basal rate pattern that is at 60 percent of normal).

- ► *2:00 p.m.:* Depending on how my blood glucose is trending, I will typically consume 1 Clif Bar (45 grams of carbs) without insulin throughout the afternoon.

▶ **3:30 p.m.:** If nearing camp within the next hour, I will ensure my basal rates are back to my already lowest levels during this activity with no temporary rate set.

▶ **4:00 p.m.:** Arrive at evening camp, set up, relax, swim/bathe, and begin dinner prep. Finish 2-liter bottle of water and refill.

▶ **6:00 p.m.:** Dinner: typically, a high-carb meal with a rice or pasta base and freeze-dried protein and vegetables. Bolus as normal. Drink 1 liter of water.

▶ **Sunset:** Prepare for bed. If the day has been challenging or if I have had more than two lows, I will set an overnight temporary basal of 60 percent. I ensure that I have plenty of snack stores in smell-proof containers *in* my tent. (That's another whole story, but we weigh the risks of low-snacks in tents before heading out on the trail.)

I will often leave my temporary trek basal set for 2 or 3 days post-trek. I find that my body becomes incredibly efficient and my insulin needs stay very low, even when I'm off trail.

*Other hobbies and interests:* I have recently started learning to kiteboard/kitesurf, and I'm loving it. I've run into some challenges related to my diabetes devices and the ocean: do I stay connected or disconnect? You can be in and out of the water a lot when using a kite, especially when learning, and I worry about my pump being ripped off. I haven't found a solution to see my Dexcom data while out in the water. So far, I've been kiting in places where it is not safe to leave valuables on the beach (Nicaragua and Cuba). Still figuring this one out! I love music. I play guitar and enjoy seeing live music whenever possible. I also enjoy watching sports, and in Toronto we have a wonderful sport culture.

*Good diabetes and exercise story:* I will always remember the lessons learned from a good friend of mine who was prepping for her first overseas adventure with diabetes. She spent time learning how her body reacted to different exercises, temperatures, and foods. She researched the area she was traveling to, found out where she'd go if she were to have a diabetes emergency while in the new country, and made sure she had twice the supplies she'd need for a successful trip. She felt totally prepared for anything diabetes could throw her way and set off. On the plane ride to Kenya, she boarded the plane and promptly fell asleep. Part way through the plane ride she got up to use the restroom and stepped on her glasses, breaking them in half. It was at that point she realized that although she had meticulously planned for every diabetes emergency that could come her way, she forgot that it's not all about the diabetes. For her month abroad, she wore a pair of glasses with a healthy dose of duct tape on the bridge across her nose. It has always reminded me, no matter how much I prepare for my diabetes, not to forget all of the other factors that make for a great backpacking or trekking experience.

One of the best tools I have given myself as an athlete with type 1 diabetes is the ability to flip back and forth between multiple daily injections and pumping. I have learned how my body reacts to long-acting insulin and rapid-acting boluses and am just as familiar with that routine as I am with my preset basal on my pump. I know how to convert my basals into long-acting insulin doses. I always trek with long-acting insulin as a backup; and knowing that, should an emergency occur, I know exactly what to do has relieved much anxiety.

# 5

# Using Technology and Monitoring to Enhance Performance

In the earlier days of diabetes treatment, before blood glucose meters existed, physicians often advised their patients who were using insulin not to engage in any physical activity. Without a doubt, being active can increase your risk for low blood glucose both during and after an activity, especially if you are an insulin user, and being active can even cause hyperglycemia. But you can take advantage of some of the latest technologies to help you exercise more safely and effectively, along with general activity recommendations and some precautions—particularly if you have any diabetes-related health issues. This chapter addresses all these topics in one place.

## AIMING FOR AN IDEAL EXERCISE BLOOD GLUCOSE

There is no official ideal blood glucose range to start with and maintain during physical activity, but we do know that being too low negatively impacts performance, as does being too high. As for what blood glucose target or range most athletes aim for, it depends on a number of factors, including the type, intensity, and duration of their activity. A consensus statement about exercise and type 1 diabetes published in *The Lancet* in 2017 suggested that a reasonable target for most people doing aerobic exercise lasting up to an hour is 126 to 180 mg/dL (7.0 to 10.0 mmol/L), only aiming higher for added protection against lows in some situations. For anaerobic (power) exercise or high-intensity interval training session, you may want to start with your glucose lower—around 90 to 126 mg/dL (5.0 to 7.0 mmol/L) simply because the intensity of the activity may cause your blood glucose to stay more stable, fall less than during aerobic workouts, or possibly even rise slightly.

> *An ideal or optimal blood glucose target during most physical activities may be in the range of 108 to 144 mg/dL (6.0 to 8.0 mmol/L).*

Most of the athletes surveyed for this book said the range of 80 to 180 mg/dL (4.5 to 10.0 mmol/L) was their stated target during exercise. Only a few of them aim for lower or higher than that range, although most admittedly have a narrower target. Canadian Scott Lahrs from West Kelowna, British Columbia, agrees with recommended ranges for performance reasons, saying, "My aim is to be 6.0 to 8.0 mmol/L (108 to 144 mg/dL). I feel the strongest at 6.0 mmol/L (108 mg/dL), but it gives me less opportunity to catch lows. Above 10.0 mmol/L (180 mg/dL), I start to feel a little sluggish—and above 15.0 mmol/L (270 mg/dL) very sluggish!"

But the blood glucose target depends on the activity and other factors. Just to give you a few examples, Chris Creelman, a resident of Lumberton, New Jersey, tries to keep her blood glucose as close to 100 mg/dL (5.6 mmol/L) as she can, saying, "With high-intensity interval training my glucose will jump here and there throughout the workout with the intensity of the exercises. As soon as I am done, though, my glucose usually starts to drop." Brooklyn, New York, resident Riva Greenberg uses a similar range of 80 to 150 mg/dL (4.5 to 8.3 mmol/L) for all her activities, but she likes to start on the higher end for walking. Jason O'Toole of Ireland also varies his target based on his activity: 126 to 180 mg/dL (7.0 to 10.0 mmol/L) for cycling, just to make sure he has some leeway if he needs to make a big effort, and a tighter range of 90 to 144 mg/dL (5.0 to 8.0 mmol/L) for walking. For surfing, he aims for 5.5 to 9.0 mmol/L (100 to 162 mg/dL) in the water, but uses a different target range of 4.5 to 7.5 mmol/L (80 to 135 mg/dL) for all other sports. Likewise, Ginger Vieira from Burlington, Vermont, sets the lower end of her range at 80 mg/dL (4.5 mmol/L) for all her activities, but she varies the higher end depending on whether she is doing fasted (120 mg/dL [6.7 mmol/L]) or nonfasted (150 mg/dL [8.3 mmol/L]) exercise.

# GETTING THE MOST FROM DIABETES TECHNOLOGIES

Technology and software related to diabetes and health management are advancing faster than most people can keep up with. Every day a new app seems to come out to keep track of something, be it your blood glucose levels, insulin on board, and carbohydrate counting or your calories, daily steps, and fitness goals. In the diabetes world, the latest management technologies guide people in making more informed and effective regimen change decisions—the most important of which are integrated systems that can take charge of the decision making by combining delivery of insulin via pumps, continuous glucose monitoring (CGM), and a control system with potential *artificial intelligence* (AI) capabilities. Next down the pike is integration of wearable technologies, which can add information related to heart rate and more. More improvements will make AI even more capable of "learning" and updating algorithms to match the changes and patterns in your metabolic state.

Given the challenges of exercising with diabetes, the latest technologies can be beneficial for managing your blood glucose and maximizing the benefits of physical activity. Insulin pumps (covered fully in chapter 3) offer a more fine-tuned ability to regulate basal insulin levels and bolus doses. Blood glucose meters give immediate feedback on where your glucose is starting and how you are responding to an activity. The CGM devices provide an added level of safety by offering the opportunity for improved decision making in real-time and retrospectively. Closed-loop systems that integrate a pump and CGM manage the decision making for you; they can potentially improve your blood glucose management before and during exercise and allow you to avoid any unwanted rises and falls in your blood glucose after workouts. All forms of technology have inherent drawbacks and limitations, but you can overcome most of their issues with planning and knowledge.

## Blood Glucose Meters (and Their Precursors)

If you began your journey with diabetes after the advent of home blood glucose meters, consider yourself lucky. Back in 1968 when I began my life with diabetes, no one had blood glucose meters to use for self-monitoring, much less target blood glucose ranges for exercise. All we had were urine tests, which measured the excess glucose and ketones in urine. You would pee in a cup, then put 5 drops of urine with 10 drops of water into a test tube with a tablet. The test tube mixture changed color in a range from cool blue (no glucose) to flaming orange (4+ glucose). It did not give you the foggiest idea of what your blood glucose was doing right then; it only told you whether you had been higher than optimal a few hours before. In other words, you could be shaking with the symptoms of a low while watching your urine turn bright orange, the indication of being very high. The ketone test strips merely confirmed what you already knew: you had some ketones in your urine (and therefore your blood) most of the time because the diabetes management tools were lacking.

The next generation of urine test strips eliminated the precise drops and test tubes, but they were not necessarily an improvement. After dipping the test strip in your urine, you had to match the color of the strip to a chart on the side of a bottle. Your six choices ranged from light blue to dark brown, corresponding to negative (0), 100, 250, 500, 1,000, and 2,000 mg/dL or more. This still did not give you a clue about the level of your blood glucose.

The blood glucose test strips of the early 1980s would only estimate your blood glucose within maybe 40 mg/dL (2.2 mmol/L), assuming your glucose was under 200 mg/dL (11.1 mmol/L). Over that range, from one color block to the next, the number jumped up by 100 to 200 mg/dL or more. In other words, blood glucose strips still were not remotely precise enough to allow anyone to safely make regimen changes.

Relatively small and affordable blood glucose meters did not become widely available to individuals until the mid-1980s. I got my first one in 1986 after I had already been living with type 1 diabetes for 18 years. My first meter still had significant potential for user error because you had to blot the blood off the strip halfway through the 2-minute testing period. Even with access to reasonably accurate blood glucose measurements for the first time, we all experienced a steep learning curve while figuring out what to do with our food or insulin in response to the readings.

The moral of this story is that we have come a long way with diabetes technology, even if all you use currently is a blood glucose meter that gives you feedback in only 5 seconds. Appreciate having the ability to check what your blood glucose is doing at any given moment and learn to use that vital information to expertly manipulate your medication doses and diet.

> *With access to a blood glucose meter, you have the primary tool you need to manage your diabetes effectively, especially with exercise as an added variable. Check as frequently as you need to, with the goal of avoiding both lows and highs.*

Even if you do not normally get low during exercise, checking frequently is still advisable, especially before you start and after you finish working out. Once you learn your usual responses to activities, you can usually anticipate how to react to keep your blood glucose in an optimal range to perform well.

## Continuous Glucose Monitors

In the past decade or so, a number of continuous glucose monitoring (CGM) devices have received approval from the U.S. Food and Drug Administration (FDA), the European Commission, and across the world. To date, all of them are still invasive: they require that you place and keep a probe of some sort under your skin to get readings. While many innovators are working on noninvasive CGM devices, none have been approved or are available yet for use. At least one company (Senseonics) has FDA approval for an implantable CGM device called Eversense, which lasts for 3 months at a time, and they are seeking approval for up to 180 days. (I have heard that their sensors go in easily during an office visit, but they are more difficult to remove after 90 or 180 days. That is not surprising: that time span is more than sufficient for your body to develop an inflammation and grow new tissue around a foreign object embedded in your skin.)

These monitors by themselves only give you information—much like a blood glucose meter does—but you still have to check the readings and make regimen adjustments yourself. However, getting feedback in real-time or at least every 1 to 5 minutes, 24 hours a day, can be extremely useful when you are trying to learn your patterns, see the trends, or keep your blood glucose in a tighter range with less hypoglycemia. The accuracy of these meters has been improving over time, but they are all still limited by their physiological methods: there is a lag of at least 6 to 20 minutes between the glucose they measure (in *interstitial* spaces between cells in the skin) and your actual blood glucose. This lag can be even greater during times when your blood glucose levels are often changing rapidly, such as after a meal or during exercise.

The CGM devices and models approved and available in the United States as of the publication of this book are shown in table 5.1. "Flash" glucose monitoring (as offered by the FreeStyle Libre device) is a recent innovation, possessing some but not all features of traditional CGM. Flash monitors can provide instantaneous glucose values and recent trends, but they lack the alerts for lows and highs.

Insurance reimbursement also has become more reasonable since CGM devices were first introduced over a decade ago. (I paid $35 out of pocket for each 3-day sensor for the first-generation Dexcom CGM I tried.) Currently, at least one model is covered by Medicare for anyone with type 1 diabetes age 65 and over. Studies

**Table 5.1    Available Continuous Glucose Monitoring Systems and Features in 2019**

| System | Features | Connections/Display Options |
|---|---|---|
| Dexcom G5 and G6 | • Glucose values every 5 minutes<br>• Rise and fall trending information<br>• High and low glucose alerts<br>• Data and alerts can be shared via phone app in real-time<br>• Integrated into open APS hybrid closed-loop system for automated basal insulin delivery (using Medtronic paradigm pump)<br>• Sensors last 7 to 10 days<br>• G5 requires calibration every 12 hours; G6 model requires no calibration<br>• Downloadable to multiple software options and web-based platforms | • Handheld receiver<br>• Android and iOS smartphones<br>• iPads<br>• iWatch<br>• Tandem X2 insulin pump<br>• Animas Vibe insulin pump (older G4 model only) |
| Medtronic Guardian Connect | • Glucose values every 5 minutes<br>• Rise and fall trending information<br>• High and low alerts<br>• Integrated into hybrid closed-loop system for automated basal insulin delivery (using Medtronic 670G pump)<br>• Sensors last up to 7 days<br>• Requires calibration every 12 hours<br>• Downloadable to Carelink software<br>• Sugar IQ program provides pattern recognition and feedback | • Guardian Connect smartphone app<br>• Medtronic 670G insulin pump<br>• Medtronic 630, 530, Revel pumps (Enlite sensor only) |
| FreeStyle Libre | • Glucose values every minute<br>• Rise and fall trending information, but no real-time alerts available<br>• 10-hour warmup period<br>• Sensors last for 10 days<br>• Requires no calibration<br>• Downloadable to LibreView software | • Handheld scanner<br>• "Flash" monitoring by passing scanner over monitor<br>• Readings on phone every 5 minutes using Ambrosia BluCon device with app<br>• LibreLink app for all smartphones to scan for reading and trend arrows |
| Senseonics Eversense | • Real-time glucose readings<br>• Implanted fluorescence-based sensor (the size of a headphone connector)<br>• Sensors used for 90 days (XL version approved for 180 days in Europe already)<br>• Sensor insertion and removal done by a physician<br>• Rise and fall trending information<br>• High and low alerts<br>• Day-long initial warmup period<br>• Requires calibration every 12 hours<br>• Data easily transmittable to medical team via mobile app | • Smart transmitter worn on skin over implanted sensor<br>• Mobile app (iOS or Android) for displaying glucose values, trends, and alerts on phone or other mobile device<br>• App charts by day, week, 2 weeks, month, or quarter<br>• Ability to enter events (food, insulin, activity, etc.) via app<br>• On-body vibratory alerts as well as on-screen alerts<br>• Bluetooth transmitter can be removed and recharged without discarding the sensor |

have shown that people with type 2 diabetes—especially those using insulin—can also benefit from using CGM, but coverage for them has been an even harder sell to insurance companies so far. In any case, the number of model choices has declined recently, and their cost is still prohibitive for people who lack the insurance coverage.

What's more, CGM technology is not infallible. As I have noted, a major drawback of CGM devices used during exercise is that their glucose readings are not fully real-time because they measure glucose levels in your skin rather than in your blood, and it takes some time for glucose to move between these two parts of your body. Also, CGM users may have problems getting the device to stay put, similar to the issues experienced by pump users with their infusion sites. (Refer back to table 3.2 for solutions on resolving adhesion issues and to the list of strategies used by athletes in chapter 12; most of the tactics used to secure a pump infusion site will also work for CGM devices.) Other reported challenges include variable sensor accuracy, variable performance between sensors, breakage of sensor filaments, transportation of the sensor display, and inability to calibrate CGM during exercise. (If you have the option, you may want to use an integrated watch to display your values.) Although technical failures during exercise are possible even with the newer versions of these monitors, CGM is still the wave of the future when it comes to monitoring and managing blood glucose.

*Exercisers have reported a compression effect when wearing the CGM sensor in areas underneath compression shorts, resulting in a greater lag time in readings due to reduced blood flow to areas with compressed skin. This can also happen when you lie directly on the sensors.*

If you have access to CGM, you may be able to use either traditional CGM or Flash monitors to enhance your exercise experience in a variety of ways.

- Seeing your glucose values before exercise tells you whether you are likely to need extra carbohydrates, insulin reductions, or an insulin bolus.
- Knowing your glucose trends before you start to work out can also help you make more informed decisions about any necessary changes in your food or medications.
- High and low alerts during and after exercise can help you avoid dangerous glucose extremes, particularly if you set your alerts at preemptive or conservative levels.
- Reviewing your trend graph reports after working out can show you the patterns of your exercise highs and lows, particularly if you use event markers or workout logs.

Many exercisers swear by their CGM devices and do not want to have to live without them (and hopefully they will not ever have to). But if you do not have access to CGM due to lack of insurance coverage, availability in your country, or other reasons, do not despair—you can still learn your glucose patterns by using frequent checks with a blood glucose meter, as most of us have done. In general, most athletes using CGM have found that observing their glucose trends (shown by up, steady, or down arrows) can be helpful during exercise, even when the readings lag behind actual blood glucose or are sometimes inaccurate.

## Athletes' Views on CGM Use and Exercise

It is worth considering what other active individuals with diabetes view as the benefits and drawbacks of using CGM devices. According to the *T1D Exchange* (which collects data on type 1 diabetes), despite evidence that CGM use may lead to lower A1C values, over a quarter of those who had started using CGM in one study stopped within a year. The reasons they gave for quitting included devices not working properly or not being accurate enough (71 percent), problems with the sensor insertion or adhesive (61 percent), and too expensive or not covered by insurance (58 percent)—all similar to the responses from the athletes surveyed for this book who were not using CGM. Others simply do not want to wear a second device along with their insulin pump or find CGMs uncomfortable or too big.

Among the nearly 300 additional athletes surveyed for this edition, CGM use was close to 75 percent, which is a greater percentage than for insulin pumps. CGM use was far more widespread among the athletic population than in the general population with type 1 diabetes. So why do more of these athletes choose to use a CGM device?

Personally, I do not find CGM that useful during exercise itself because interstitial glucose values lag behind actual blood glucose; I also do not find them accurate enough during rest when I am in a tight blood glucose range. For instance, CGM often reports I am at 60 mg/dL (3.3 mmol/L) when I am actually closer to 90 mg/dL (5.0 mmol/L) and vice versa, which leads to a lot of frustration on my part (and lack of sleep when this happens at night). Kerry White from Avon, Colorado, agrees: "It can assist with rapidly dropping and rising blood glucose levels, but it is often too delayed to really be useful." Despite the accuracy issues, Bill King of Pennsylvania still finds CGM useful and has a fallback plan for exercise: "Access to glucose level and forward predictions is priceless for me. Accuracy can be an issue, so I carry a backup glucose meter when racing or riding long distances."

The CGM lag time can be annoying, but it is not reason enough to choose against wearing one for most athletes. Sarah from the United Kingdom likes being able to quickly scan the Libre sensor on her arm to see trend arrows and to head off lows. The only downside she sees is its measurement of glucose in interstitial fluids, which can cause up to a 20-minute delay in the glucose values changing during exercise. Jeanette Styles of Eugene, Oregon, agrees, saying, "The CGM lets me see trends, which is very helpful. But oftentimes it is too slow to let me see real time changes."

Molly McDermott from Ottawa, Canada, says, "CGM is the best thing to happen to me. It has made controlling and preventing my lows and highs much easier because I know it before it happens." John Boyer, an athlete from Mount Airy, Maryland, agrees that seeing blood glucose trends is CGM's greatest advantage. He also likes the high and low alerts and the fact that he can share his values virtually with exercise partners. The only drawback he sees is when he is not looking at the trend and gets too focused on the exact number, which can easily lead to overcompensation. Massachusetts resident Fatima Shahzad concurs "The best advice I have is to practice patience with the CGM trend arrow. Sometimes it is pointing up or down for a while, but in the next 5 minutes it flattens out, right after you have made a treatment decision to either take insulin or ingest glucose. In times like that, I often just use my glucometer and do not trust my CGM because I end up with another issue to treat." Dan Stone of Middletown, Pennsylvania, agrees that the only drawback of CGM is when it is inaccurate or occasionally can be misleading in making overcorrections, but he says, "I would give up my pump before my CGM." Jeanette Styles also finds herself getting obsessed and stressed out watching the numbers so closely that it can get in the way of her enjoying a simple run.

Others, like Emily Tiberio from Beaver, Pennsylvania, use the CGM to warn them about impending lows during exercise. She loves using her CGM for long runs and cycling because otherwise she can confuse exhaustion with feeling low. It also makes it easier for her to fuel throughout training by watching her trends. Likewise, Neil McLagan, a native of Australia, likes that CGM provides him with greater and more frequent insight into his glucose, gives him the ability to predict trends, and permits fewer disruptions to his exercise routine. Hailing from Raymond Terrace, Australia, Declan Irvine simply states, "Before, I was running blind, and my performances were sometimes let down by my blood glucose." Tristan Rice from Chico, California, sees only benefits: "I've run marathons both with and without a CGM, and having the visibility into current trending (rapid dropping, for example) is an absolute must-have for me." He feels that having a CGM has allowed him to overcome his biggest challenge while running with diabetes.

Athletes do acknowledge some of the other drawbacks of CGM use. California resident Blair Ryan notes, "CGM use has been key for me during training and racing for visibility into my trends and current blood glucose without having to stop and test. The downside is that the CGM is often a little slow to catch lows, and by the time my alert sounds I'm already low. I've adjusted up the low alert threshold, which helps in all but the steep declines." For her, this is not that big of a deal because she usually only exercises with basal insulin (via injection) in her system and rarely has her blood glucose plummet rapidly. Estelle Grey, an athlete from Cape Town, South Africa, admits it does not always work for her for other reasons: "I am an endurance swimmer, and although the CGM and pump are waterproof, the connection fails." Bec Johnson from Australia, on the other hand, uses flash monitoring with her FreeStyle Libre, and she finds she can use it in the water by putting the receiver in a waterproof phone bag. The main drawback she sees is that the sensors are sometimes inaccurate.

To deal with its adhesion issues, Molly McDermott just covers her CGM with a sleeve or medical tape to protect it, while some people use waterproof tape (and reapply it often). Others put GrifGrips (grifgrips.com), RockaDex patches (rockadex .net), or similar products over their CGM devices to hold them in place. You can also use skin preparations like Skin Tac wipes to increase stickiness before putting them on, although many athletes say that they still have trouble with adherence when they sweat a lot during exercise.

Don Muchow of Plano, Texas, finds that Skin Tac keeps him from sweating most of his sensors off, but he also likes using waterproof dressings, which keep his sites fairly dry during normal circumstances. On super-long runs, he admits to wearing two CGMs in case one is not accurate or the sensor is failing, which allows him to run until a planned stop, during which he can change sensors and calibrate to avoid running blind. His advice is to check frequently and compare the numbers on the CGM to get a good sense of what your actual race will be like.

Klara Pickova from the Czech Republic admits that sweating makes the sensor itchy sometimes. But she still appreciates its benefits, such as seeing glucose levels and trends and using it with some automatic pump features (e.g., predictive suspension or hybrid closed-loop—see more on this topic in the next section).

Finally, although weather conditions may also affect the functionality of CGM devices, their users have found some workarounds. Sarah Davies of Melbourne, Australia, shares that getting her FreeStyle Libre was life changing, but she adds that getting the Ambrosia BluCon device, which sends readings every 5 minutes to her phone via an app, improved her life even more because she no longer had to pass a scanner over the Libre to get each reading. However, she has needed to figure out ways to keep it working in extreme weather. "I wrap the BluCon in cling wrap in extreme weather, and it still seems to work. Be mindful of cold when FreeStyle sensors do not work, and add arm warmers over them as needed."

## Closed-Loop and Hybrid Systems

The march toward creating effective, failure-proof *closed-loop* systems for insulin users is ongoing, but the drive to be the first company to market one reached a fever pitch during the second decade of the new millennium. Such a system can determine dosing and deliver insulin based on CGM feedback without your intervention, or with limited input from you about meals or exercise (making it more like semiautomated).

CGM devices are currently being paired with insulin pumps to create these closed-loop systems run by algorithms. They work most effectively when metabolic conditions are relatively stable, such as overnight during sleep. Effective use of hybrid (semiautomated) closed-loop systems has the potential to produce more stable glucose control leading up to exercise than can be achieved by traditional means. However, the technological issues with CGM during exercise (such as the time lag and rapid changes in blood glucose) make these systems less helpful for managing glycemia during physical activities. These systems have limited ability to prevent hypoglycemia during exercise because they only make minute adjustments to basal insulin; users must continue to make their own food and bolus insulin adjustments before and during exercise. It is also necessary to wear the pump, without disconnecting, during exercise for the algorithm to work, and not everyone can do this easily—including participants in aquatic or contact sports.

Many *hybrid closed-loop* systems have already implemented an automatic suspend (insulin) mode to be used overnight whenever your CGM data indicate a low coming on—but users must watch out for potential rebound hyperglycemia later after having gone for a while without any basal insulin delivery. Although the hybrid systems are not perfect, some users are already benefiting from them. For instance, Betty Murdock of Australia uses a CGM with a "low suspend" option on her pump, making it semiautomated as a closed-loop system. She says, "I can exercise confidently knowing my pump and CGM will alert me if I'm heading low and will auto-suspend until my blood glucose is heading up again." San Francisco, California, native Mary Alessandra Lucas also enjoys having the low-glucose suspend auto-mode keeping her from getting low during exercise (despite her complaints that her pump can get in the way, get sweaty, and fall off—and sometimes she gets tangled in the cord).

At least one person, Mark Rosenbaum from New Bern, North Carolina, is not quite as sold on this hybrid technology as others, though. He listed the benefits and drawbacks of his current Medtronic MiniMed 670G system: "The benefits are that in manual mode I can use a temporary basal rate during exercise or temporarily suspend. There is no drawback in manual mode. In auto mode, the major benefit is there is less chance of having a severe low blood glucose during intensive exercise. The drawback is that the pump will deliver little to no insulin for 1 to 2 hours if the CGM senses blood glucose is going down. This has resulted in subsequent elevated glucose levels for me. Overall, I have better results in manual mode."

You may be able to adopt or adapt some of these strategies to enhance your use of these hybrid systems during physical activity:

- Apply the temporary rise in your blood glucose target at least 1 hour before the time you plan to start exercising, if possible (because it takes at least this long for a change in basal delivery to effectively lower insulin and raise your blood glucose).

- Switch the system to "manual" mode (that is, turn off the self-adjustment algorithm) before and during exercise to allow you to fully use temporary basal rates and manual bolus overrides.

- Override your pump's bolus recommendation before exercise and enter smaller (or no) boluses for the carbohydrate you are eating.

- If your pump will not let you manually adjust the recommended bolus doses, enter less carbohydrate into the bolus calculator than what you are really eating before exercise, and do not enter the carbohydrates you snack on while you are active.

- Let the closed-loop algorithm take over after exercise to help prevent later-onset lows.

You may have heard that, in lieu of waiting for FDA-approved systems, some insulin users have come up with their own workaround called *looping*. This is not really an official term or practice but rather refers to a homemade hybrid system that uses (1) an old Medtronic pump (like the Paradigm 522), (2) an iPhone, (3) your CGM device (Dexcom or Medtronic), and (4) a "Riley Link" device to connect them all together. This jerry-rigged system uses an app to determine the basal rate adjustments you need on your pump based on CGM data, and then it uses the Riley Link (carried separately) to essentially hack the pump and make those changes (which is why an older, hackable pump is necessary). You still have to bolus for meals and give corrections for highs, but looping can be pretty efficient for managing your basal rates to prevent lows. Your pump can be completely controlled from your phone using the app, and you can adjust your glucose goals as desired, including putting in an exercise target. It can also give you a predicted glucose curve when you enter carbohydrates or bolus insulin doses. Alternatively, you may consider upgrading to a pump like the Medtronic 670G, which already has an integrated Medtronic Guardian CGM (refer back to table 5.1) that works like a hybrid system with its "auto mode" and "suspend before low" modes.

What if you do not or cannot wear a pump but want to use a hybrid system in the future? Hope is on the horizon. The truly critical element in semiautomated systems is an accurate and reliable CGM on which the algorithms rely. Recently, the integrated algorithms have become so much more efficient and capable of learning over time that the insulin delivery system is fast becoming less relevant—you may not even need to use an insulin pump. In fact, a "smart" insulin pen, combined with a CGM and app system, is being developed, and it will cost far less than integrating an insulin pump in such systems. (Personally, I am looking forward to using a hybrid insulin pen system because I build up too much scar tissue to use insulin pumps in the long term.)

## Technology-Driven Spontaneity

What do you do when someone asks you to participate in a physical activity on the spur of the moment, but you just took some insulin? You may be stuck trying to compensate for this activity entirely with food, but you may have some newer options that come from technology. For starters, if you wear a pump you can choose to lower your basal insulin delivery, and you can use its insulin-on-board calculator to see how much insulin you need to offset with either insulin reductions or food intake. However, just using your blood glucose meter can help you stay on top of your glucose levels, so check often during the activity. If you use a CGM, you can continue to monitor throughout to detect downward trends and treat yourself early enough to prevent lows (but just remember that there is a lag time). If you use the other wearable devices we will be discussing next, feedback on your heart rate, steps, or other variables can help you figure out how many extra calories you may need to take in to match your activity and prevent a drop in your blood glucose. With these newer technologies, at least you have options that you may not have had otherwise.

## Exercise Technologies and Wearable Devices

You may benefit from exercise-related technologies that allow you to monitor your heart rate, blood pressure, steps, sedentary time, exercise intensity, calorie use, and other variables in real time. For instance, heart rate monitors are good for achieving and maintaining appropriate exercise intensity, particularly if you are a data-driven person and are motivated by such feedback. However, keep in mind that you need to use individualized target heart rates (refer to chapter 1) based on your health status. Any medications that you are taking that may limit your heart rate also need to be considered. Many apps can track your heart rate in real time and allow you to train more effectively.

Tracking steps and other physical activity can also be useful. Step counters can motivate you to be more active throughout the day, not just during your planned workout times. Keeping a daily log of step counts can allow you to determine correlations between your activity and blood glucose responses. Apps for tracking workout progress and analyzing glucose patterns related to different forms of exercise can supply the feedback, allowing you to make regimen adjustments in real time to avoid glucose lows and highs. Many smartphones now also have integrated accelerometers that can give you data on all daily movement including your steps, along with your sleep patterns and other useful information. It is likely in the future that some of the issues surrounding exercise with fully closed-loop systems may be addressed with wearable devices that provide input about changes in activity and heart rate that can impact your blood glucose.

# GETTING READY TO BE ACTIVE

Whether you choose to partake of the latest technologies or not, it helps to keep some general principles in mind whether you are already regularly active or getting ready to be. These vary somewhat by your diabetes type, but are largely based on whether you have to manage your insulin levels during exercise because you use insulin. Read through these general recommendations as well as the precautions for any complicating health issues and keep these points in mind to get the most out of your workouts.

## Making Regimen Changes for Type 1 Diabetes

The responses to physical activity are so individualized and variable that making uniform recommendations for regimen changes is nearly impossible. However, a limited number of studies have attempted to do that, and their recommendations are listed here. Most of this information was covered in detail in earlier chapters, but the recommendations are summarized here with a reminder that almost none of these adjustments would be possible without the advent of glucose monitoring that allows you to make informed decisions based on immediate feedback about your levels.

- In general, you will need to increase your carbohydrate or other food intake and/or reduce your circulating insulin levels for aerobic activities.
- For low- to moderate-intensity aerobic activities lasting 30 to 60 minutes during fasting or with only basal insulin on board, you may need only 10 to 15 grams of carbohydrate (or nothing at all) to prevent hypoglycemia.
- When active soon after taking a bolus insulin dose, you may need more in the range of 30 to 60 grams of carbohydrate per hour.
- In some cases, you may be able to lower your insulin doses by 25 to 75 percent and either reduce or completely eliminate your need for extra food or carbohydrate to prevent lows during exercise.
- Avoid exercising if your blood glucose is >250 mg/dL (13.9 mmol/L) and moderate or high ketones are present, and use caution if your glucose levels are >300 mg/dL (16.7 mmol/L) without ketones.

# Being Active With Type 2 Diabetes

Exercise recommendations for people with type 2 diabetes who do not have to take insulin differ somewhat from anyone who uses insulin (with type 1 or type 2 diabetes) simply because they rely on a combination of diet, exercise, and noninsulin medications to manage blood glucose and overcome insulin resistance. Anyone with type 2 diabetes who is starting to exercise after being sedentary may need an evaluation by a physician to ensure that being more active will not worsen any existing health problems (see later in this chapter for determining who needs a checkup first). Even if you do not use insulin, you can benefit from blood glucose monitoring to determine the effects of exercise, although you are less likely to have lows or develop diabetic ketoacidosis (DKA).

Even if you do not get low blood glucose during exercise, checking your level frequently is still advisable, especially beforehand and afterward. Doing so can be motivational, especially when you see your blood glucose go down from an activity. Depending on your medications, you may have to make some changes to keep your blood glucose optimal. For instance, if you use certain oral medications (discussed in chapter 3), you may have a higher risk for developing hypoglycemia. Luckily, although you are not likely to develop DKA even if your blood glucose is on the high side, knowing your starting level is still important so that you can prevent lows and dehydration from physical activity.

If you are able to manage your blood glucose well most of the time and do not have any serious diabetes complications, then exercise away to your heart's content. Keep certain precautions in mind, though, particularly ones related to staying properly hydrated. If you have any complications, you may also need to take extra care to avoid problems. The following sections will teach you more about which precautionary measures to take.

# Preventing Dehydration and Overhydration

If your blood glucose has been running high, you may be prone to dehydration because of extra water loss through your urine (*polyuria*). Likewise, if you have central nerve damage (more on this later) that makes you dizzy when you stand up or change positions rapidly, you may be more likely to become dehydrated during exercise and not realize it. Normally, thirst centers in the brain are not activated until you have already lost 1 to 2 percent of your body water, and central nerve damage can make you even less likely to realize that you need more fluids until it is too late. A resident of hot and humid Homestead, Florida, Archie Jones has his own strategy: "Hydrate often. If I do not feel a slight urge to pee during exercise, I drink more."

What can you do to stay safe? Make certain that you hydrate adequately before exercise and drink fluids early and frequently to compensate for sweat losses during exercise, especially when it is hot outside. Drinking cool, plain water works for moderate exercise lasting up to an hour. For longer workouts, consider using sports drinks or diluted fruit juices to replace both water and carbohydrates. Keep drinking afterward because it may take up to a day to restore fluids lost through sweat and ventilation. As Mark Robbins, an exerciser from Victor, New York, warns, "During extreme weather (i.e., hot and humid) try to remain hydrated. Dehydration seems to cause the body to react as if it is under severe stress, and my blood glucose levels go way up." Here are some additional hydration tips.

- Drink cool, plain water during and after exercise, especially during warmer weather, and take frequent breaks to have a chance to cool down, preferably out of the heat and direct sunlight.
- Do not force yourself to drink more than the amount of fluid that satisfies your thirst. Otherwise, water intoxication may result.
- To know how much fluid to replace after exercise, weigh yourself before and after a prolonged activity and replace only as much weight as you have lost (1 liter of water weighs 1 kilogram, or 2.2 pounds).
- If you prefer fluids with some flavor, try flavored waters, sports drinks that have no added carbohydrate or calories (such as Champion Lyte), or Crystal Light (with a pinch of salt if you want it to taste more like a sports drink).
- Drink regular sports drinks (containing glucose) only when you need some carbohydrate to prevent or treat hypoglycemia during physical activities.

An equally valid concern is *overhydration*, or drinking too much fluid. In some cases, taking in too much fluid is worse than dehydrating, as discussed in the last chapter. One rule of thumb is that you should not weigh more after exercise than you did when you started; if you do, you probably consumed too much fluid. Whenever you start to feel thirsty, swig a mouthful (about 1 ounce, or 30 milliliters), and drink that amount every 10 to 15 minutes or so. If you do not sense when you are getting thirsty, just start drinking about 15 minutes into your exercise session. If you have already had plenty to drink and need to raise your blood glucose, try glucose tablets or a gel instead.

## Resources for Active People With Diabetes

# Diabetes DESTINY

The mission of Diabetes DESTINY (Diabetes Exercise and Strategies—Together in Network with You) is to empower youth to be active, stay healthy, and achieve their optimum performance through proven type 1 management strategies. Each year in the spring, their camps have a full medical team on site (with an endocrinologist, registered nurses, certified diabetes educators, and dietitians), along with a variety of successful athletes with type 1 diabetes who meet with the kids. The purpose of the camps is to provide a safe environment for kids to learn and experience the strategies that others have used to exceed their expectations. Over camp weekends, the attendees engage in very fun activities and get exposed to a lot of teaching moments as well.

Founded by runner Bill King with help from fellow person with type 1 diabetes, the late Ron Denunzio, this organization and its camps fill a void by connecting active athletes and kids with type 1 diabetes. Get more information at www.diabetesdestiny.org.

## Deciding When to Have a Checkup First

Using technologies to enhance your fitness and your health still require that you use some common sense to avoid issues before they arise. For instance, do you know whether you need to see your doctor before you start to exercise? Basically, you probably do not need a checkup before engaging in easy workouts or moderate activities like brisk walking, but having one before you begin more vigorous workouts is a good idea if you are older and have not been regularly active. If your blood glucose has been pretty good overall, you have already been physically active, and you do not have any serious diabetes complications, then exercise away.

If you are very active, getting an extra checkup before you replace your current exercise regimen with another workout routine is unnecessary. However, having regular visits to your doctor or other health care provider is a good idea for anyone with diabetes. If you have a checkup, get your blood pressure, heart rate, and body weight measured, and ask whether you need to do an exercise stress test, which usually involves walking on a treadmill or riding a stationary bike for around 10 minutes. The American Diabetes Association recommends an exercise stress test only if you are over 40 and have diabetes or if you are over 30 and have had diabetes for 10 or more years, smoke, have high blood pressure, have high cholesterol, or have eye or kidney problems related to diabetes. Above all, this recommendation applies only to people planning to do vigorous training that gets their heart rates up high. If you will just be doing mild or moderate aerobic activity or resistance training, such extensive (and often expensive) testing is usually not needed.

If you have a checkup, it should likely include a urinalysis, kidney function testing, serum lipid evaluation, and electrolyte analysis, along with screening for any diabetes-related complications, including heart, nerve, eye, and kidney disease. Although such health problems do not usually keep you from exercising, doing so safely and effectively with them may require special accommodations or precautions. Doing regular, moderate to vigorous activity can reduce your risk of having a heart attack, even if you have already had one before. Just realize and respect your limitations. Take extra care to prevent problems during exercise if you have any preexisting health issues and take certain precautions, particularly related to keeping your blood glucose in balance and staying hydrated. If you have any concerns, check with your health care provider at your next visit to discuss any measures that may be important for you while exercising.

## Determining Your Readiness for Physical Activity

If you think you are ready to start exercising and do not fall into any categories that really require you to get medical clearance or have a checkup first, you can still determine your own readiness to be physically active by using self-tests like the Physical Activity Readiness Questionnaire for Everyone (PAR-Q+). An online version of this questionnaire can be accessed online at http://eparmedx.com, where you can also find downloadable print versions. This website also links to the online electronic Physical Activity Readiness Medical Examination (ePARmed-X+), which you may be prompted to take if you answer yes to any of the questions on the PAR-Q+ that indicate that you may need additional assessment.

The PAR-Q+ is simple to take and will recommend whether you should seek further medical advice before becoming more physically active or need to engage in a fitness appraisal. It asks you questions that assess your risk for having a cardiovascular or other event during physical activity.

# EXERCISING SAFELY WITH HEALTH COMPLICATIONS

If you have any diabetes-related or other health problems, it is likely you can still exercise safely, but you may need special precautions. *Microvascular* (small blood vessel) complications include nerve damage, eye problems, or failing kidneys, and the large vessel (*macrovascular*) complications involve heart or peripheral artery diseases and high blood pressure.

## Peripheral Neuropathy

If you have some peripheral loss of sensation from nerve damage (i.e., *neuropathy*), you have a greater risk of injuring your feet due to blunted signals of pain or discomfort from high impact, friction, or pressure from your shoes and socks. Exercise may improve circulation in your lower legs and feet and help prevent the ulcers that can be associated with loss of feeling in these areas. Being active cannot fully reverse peripheral neuropathy, but it can slow its progression and prevent you from becoming less fit from being inactive. Even if you are not aware of having lost any sensation, if you develop an ulcer on the *plantar* (bottom) surface or sides of your feet you probably have this condition. Have a doctor look at any changes on the skin of your feet right away to avoid the possibility of gangrene and amputation of your toes or part of your foot.

The American Diabetes Association recommends using silicone gel or air midsoles in shoes, as well as socks made of polyester or a cotton and polyester blend (most moisture-wicking athletic socks nowadays are not straight cotton) to prevent blisters and keep your feet dry and minimize exercise-related trauma. Having appropriate footwear is vitally important to the health of your feet and lower leg joints, especially when exercising. Your shoes should fit snugly without excessively squeezing or constricting your feet. You can find tips for picking appropriate shoes in chapter 7.

If you have limited or no sensation in your feet, consider switching to non-weight-bearing exercises, which can improve tone, balance, and awareness of your lower extremities. The recommended exercises include swimming, pool walking, water aerobics and other pool-based exercise, stationary bicycling, rowing, arm ergometer work, upper-body exercises, tai chi, qigong, yoga, seated aerobic and resistance exercises, and other non-weight-bearing activities. Moving your joints through their full range of motion can also help prevent contractures, particularly of your lower limbs. For example, Connie Hanham-Cain from Albany, New York, has some neuropathy in her feet and joint changes related to that, making certain types of exercise harder for her to do at this point in her life. To compensate, she has turned to other activities that she can do more successfully, such as tai chi, qigong, in-place or chair movement stretching, and belly dancing exercise.

To prevent injury, avoid activities like prolonged walking, jogging, treadmill exercise, and step exercises that can cause blisters or foot trauma that you may not be able to detect. You do not have to avoid all activities done on your feet, but mixing up your activities by cross-training and not doing any daily activity on your feet may help. Combined resistance and interval exercise training are both good to do occasionally. All these activities—both the ones that make you carry your weight and those that do not—can improve your fitness, muscle tone, balance, and awareness of your lower extremities. You will also want to work on improving your flexibility and balance to prevent falls, which are more common if you lose sensation in your feet.

Daily foot monitoring before and after exercise is critical to catching and treating problems early. Check your feet for sores, blisters, irritation, cuts, or other injuries that can develop into ulcers. If you cannot easily pull each foot up to look at the bottom, place a mirror on the floor and hold your foot over it to inspect them yourself or ask someone else to look for you. If you have unhealed ulcers, minimize walking or weight-bearing activities until they are fully healed. While they are healing, keep your feet clean and dry, avoid swimming, stay off your feet, and inspect them daily.

> *Despite some potential health issues associated with exercise, the benefits to people with diabetes generally far outweigh the risks. Use diabetes as your excuse to be more active, not as a reason to become or remain inactive.*

## Autonomic Neuropathy

Long-term damage to your central nervous system (*autonomic neuropathy*) can manifest in a variety of ways, almost all of which may impact your ability to be active. It may affect your ability to respond with a normal heart rate to exercise, to change your body position without getting faint during activities, to manage your body temperature, or to digest your food normally. You may be more likely to experience *silent ischemia* (reduced blood flow to your heart muscle that does not have symptoms), leading to an undetected, "silent" heart attack.

Your chances of dying suddenly during exercise are higher if your heart has become unresponsive to nerve impulses (a condition known as *cardiac autonomic neuropathy,* or CAN), particularly if you have some underlying heart disease. With CAN, you may experience an elevated heart rate at rest (100 beats per minute or higher rather than the normal 72 beats), and how much your heart rate goes up during exercise may be blunted.

What should you do if you have CAN? Take a conservative approach to exercise and physical activities. Have your doctor test your heart's responses before starting an exercise program so you know how exercise affects your heart rate. Warm up for at least 10 minutes and cool down longer than normal, particularly when you are doing strenuous activity. Your exercise heart rate will likely be lower than expected, so use a subjective rating (such as "somewhat hard" for moderate activity) or the "talk test" (refer back to chapter 1). If you ever suddenly feel extremely fatigued or have other unexplained symptoms, stop exercising and get checked out by a doctor if the symptoms persist more than a couple of minutes.

For other manifestations of autonomic neuropathy, when you change your body position rapidly during an activity your blood pressure may drop (a condition called *orthostatic hypotension*) and make you feel lightheaded or dizzy, or you may faint. Avoid activities with rapid postural changes (like racquetball) because your blood pressure may not respond fast enough and you can faint. Keep yourself fully hydrated during exercise to remove the potential for dehydration to add to these symptoms. Barry Toothman, a type 2 exerciser from Lake Charles, Louisiana, knows this all too well: "I have generally low blood pressure (due to my fitness level) and orthostatic hypotension (likely a complication of diabetes), which causes dizziness when I rise from a seated or reclining position. It can be quite severe. If I'm not careful and allow myself to become significantly dehydrated from exercise, the result can be basically a sick day."

Autonomic neuropathy can also impair your ability to regulate your body temperature effectively. Your body is less able to move blood around to help you cool down, making you more likely to overheat and get dehydrated during exercise. Avoid exercising in extreme hot or cold environments because you may not be able to regulate your body temperature well at either end of the spectrum, and stay fully hydrated by drinking fluids during exercise, especially when you are exercising in hot and humid conditions.

Finally, this condition can also affect how quickly you digest your food. With *gastroparesis* (a delayed emptying from your stomach), if you try to treat a low by eating carbohydrate during exercise, raising your blood glucose may take longer. You may also experience lows followed by highs during and after exercise due to this delayed digestion. Eat only small portions and avoid eating a large meal before exercise, which can delay the emptying of food from your stomach. During exercise, monitor your blood glucose closely, but also check it before and afterward because you are more likely to develop lows. To treat a low, take glucose tablets before your blood glucose goes down to 100 mg/dL (5.5 mmol/L) to prevent severe hypoglycemia.

## Diabetic Eye Disease

Having diabetes can lead to any of eight different eye issues over time, including cataracts, macular edema, and retinopathy. The good news is that you can lower your risk of getting any of these by managing your blood glucose and limiting your postmeal spikes. All eye diseases have the potential to obscure vision and make participation in certain activities (such as outdoor cycling) more dangerous. But they are not usually a complete barrier to exercise.

One of the more common eye diseases and a leading cause of blindness related to diabetes, *proliferative diabetic retinopathy* results from the formation of weak, abnormal blood vessels in the back of your eyes (*retina*) that can break, tear, or bleed into the *vitreous fluid*. When retinal hemorrhages happen, blood fills the inside of your eye and obscures your vision (albeit sometimes only temporarily because it will often clear out later on its own over time). Exercising does not make the proliferative process faster or worse, but you may need to take certain precautions depending on whether you just have background retinopathy or a more advanced and active stage of retinopathy.

For instance, if you have retinopathy that is only mild or moderate, with no active bleeds (*retinal hemorrhages*), simply avoid activities that dramatically increase the blood pressure inside your eyes, such as heavy resistance training, breath-holding during exercise, or doing activities with your head lower than your heart. However, if you have severe, or *proliferative*, retinopathy (that is, with active or ongoing growth of the abnormal retinal vessels that can hemorrhage or detach your retina), stick with exercises like swimming, walking, low-impact aerobics, stationary cycling, and other endurance exercises done at a low to moderate level, but only do them if your eyes are not actively bleeding internally. (You should be able to see when such hemorrhages occur so long as your vision is not already totally blocked by prior bleeds that have yet to fully clear.)

*If you notice sudden, dramatic changes in your sight while exercising, stop all activity immediately and check with your eye doctor for further guidance.*

With severe proliferation that seems to be stable, avoid all activities that dramatically increase your blood pressure, such as heavy weightlifting, power lifting, or Valsalva (breath-holding) maneuvers. For severe retinopathy that is unstable (with occasional active hemorrhaging), avoid activities that cause a large increase in your blood pressure and involve pounding, jumping, jarring, or putting your head down lower than your heart (which increases the pressure inside your eyes). This means no boxing, competitive contact sports like basketball or football, weightlifting, running or jogging, high-impact aerobics, most racket sports, or strenuous trumpet playing. The last thing you want to do is cause your eyes to experience a retinal tear, retinal detachment, or vitreous hemorrhage. Exercising while you are experiencing a retinal hemorrhage will likely cause the release of extra blood into your eye and further block your vision, so wait until the hemorrhage has stopped and then see your eye doctor before doing any exercise more intense than normal walking.

Given that some people with stable retinopathy may have some permanent vision loss, it is essential to factor that into your strategy when picking which exercises to do. Take the example of Judith Jones-Ambrosini, a New York resident with a long history of living well with type 1 diabetes. She says, "I have poor vision due to proliferative retinopathy that goes way back to the mid-1970s. As a result of extensive early laser therapy done at that time (the only treatment available then, one that destroyed peripheral areas of the retina to save central vision), I have very poor depth perception and night vision and limited peripheral vision." She further explains how she considers this in choosing her activities: "So I always place myself in strategic spots in exercise or dance or tai chi classes so I do not bump into my neighbors. I'm also cautious when I ride my bicycle in local run/walk races (due to my lack of peripheral vision)." Nowadays, treatment options are more advanced and usually more of the peripheral retina is salvaged as well.

## Diabetic Kidney Disease

It is entirely possible to be active no matter what level of diabetes-induced kidney damage you may be experiencing. If you are in the early stages of kidney disease, exercise may increase the rates of albumin (protein) excretion in urine. But there is no evidence that regular endurance activity speeds progression of this disease. In fact, it is well known that exercise increases protein excretion in people without kidney disease (through *exercise-induced proteinuria*); to get accurate results on your kidney function tests, do not do hard exercise right before getting the levels of microalbumin and protein in your urine checked. If you are in the later stages of kidney disease, your exercise capacity may be limited by fatigue, but doing light to moderate exercise as you are able is still good for your endurance and will not damage your kidneys. If you are on dialysis, you can even exercise on a stationary cycle during your treatments with no ill effects. Do not exercise, however, if your hematocrit, calcium, or blood phosphorus levels are unstable because of the need for dialysis. If you have had renal transplant surgery, wait 6 to 8 weeks until your new kidneys are stable and free of rejection before restarting your exercise.

## Heart Disease

Heart disease—which is caused by plaque formation in the coronary arteries and reduced blood flow to the heart muscle—has been associated with insulin resistance and inflammation. But it may not be as directly related to how well your blood glucose is managed. Exercise itself lowers your risk of heart disease by favorably altering elevated blood lipids and clotting defects and lowering your insulin needs. It also leads to a decrease in your circulating blood fats (specifically your *triglycerides*). If you have central nerve damage, be especially vigilant for any unusual sensations during exercise that may indicate you are not getting enough blood to your heart (such as unexpected, extreme fatigue) because you may not get the usual symptoms like chest pain and discomfort.

Your risk of a heart attack or stroke is greater if you have had diabetes longer than 10 years and if you have any other cardiovascular risk factors (like being overweight, sedentary, older, or a smoker), evidence of microvascular vessel damage, peripheral artery disease, or central nervous system damage. In such cases, you may need a medical checkup and possibly a graded exercise test done under a doctor's supervision before you embark on a moderate- or high-intensity exercise program (see the earlier section on when to have a checkup first). An exercise stress test may be able to detect any significant coronary artery blockage or abnormal heart rhythms that can make some types of exercise unsafe for you to do.

One of the best ways to prevent a second heart attack is to exercise regularly, but take precautions and choose your activities wisely. If you know you have cardiovascular problems, at least initially exercise in a supervised environment like an outpatient or a community-based cardiac rehabilitation exercise program where you can be monitored easily. Start with easy aerobic exercise, progress slowly, and include some resistance training. Lifting a heavier weight 10 to 12 times may increase your blood pressure more than aerobic exercise does, but it does not raise your heart rate as much. Your blood pressure rises more and sends more blood to your heart muscle during resistance training, making it easier for your heart.

> *If you experience chest pain due to reduced blood flow to your heart muscle from clogged arteries during walking, choose a different activity such as resistance training.*

If you have some coronary artery blockage from plaque buildup, moderate weight training may be a safer activity for you than most higher intensity aerobic ones, and resistance training is recommended nowadays for almost everyone to increase strength and preserve muscle mass. If you prefer walking or another aerobic activity but experience *angina* (chest pain) when active, keep your heart rate about 10 beats per minute lower than the point at which you start to experience chest pain or tightness. For example, work no harder than 120 beats per minute if you have symptoms that start at a pulse of 130 beats.

Exercising only slightly increases your risk of having a cardiovascular event like a heart attack (*myocardial infarction*) while you are doing it. But training regularly lowers your chances, so being active is still always better for you. If you experience a sudden, unexplained change in your ability to exercise (such as extreme fatigue that comes on quickly), without any other symptoms, immediately stop exercising and consult with your physician as soon as you can to rule out *silent ischemia* (a reduction in blood flow to your heart that does not give you the usual pain due to autonomic neuropathy). Do not delay in calling 911 or seeking other immediate medical attention if you are experiencing any signs or symptoms of a heart attack. Treatment in the first few minutes is critical for surviving a major cardiac event with minimal lasting problems. Be on the lookout for:

- Chest discomfort, which can feel like indigestion, uncomfortable pressure, squeezing, fullness, or acute and stabbing pain that lasts or is intermittent.
- Discomfort somewhere other than your chest, showing up as pain radiating down one or both arms or the back, neck, jaw, or stomach, which is known as *referred pain* because it originates in your heart due to lack of oxygen but is felt elsewhere.
- Shortness of breath, which can occur with or without chest discomfort and is symptomatic when it is unusual or unexpected.
- Other symptoms, such as sudden sweating, nausea and vomiting, lightheadedness, and undue, unexplained fatigue.

## Peripheral Artery Disease

Another form of cardiovascular disease, *peripheral artery disease* (PAD), is a common circulatory problem that limits blood flow to your legs and arms. Plaque can form in any artery, but when you get it in the arteries in your legs you may have end up with PAD. Having pain in your lower legs while standing or walking may be a symptom, but you would have to have the blood pressure in your leg or ankle measured and compared with your arm to have it diagnosed. If it is higher in your leg, you may have blockage there that is raising it. If you have symptoms like pain, find out for certain if you have PAD because it may be indicative of more widespread plaque formation in other arteries around your body.

PAD is treatable with certain prescribed medications that lower your blood pressure and dilate your leg arteries and relieve symptoms. Surgery can also improve blood flow to your legs by bypassing blockages. Exercising regularly is also highly recommended. Walking or other daily exercise helps you maintain optimal circulation in your legs. It may improve the blood flow to your feet, especially when combined with eating a more healthful diet and not smoking. Use pain as your guide and engage in easy or moderate walking and take rest periods as needed. If walking hurts too much, try doing seated exercises, water workouts, upper body resistance training, or stationary cycling.

# Hypertension

Regular exercise can lower your body fat and reduce insulin resistance, both resulting in modest decreases in your blood pressure, both your *systolic* (the higher blood pressure reading, such as 110 mm Hg) and your *diastolic* (the lower number, one like 70) readings. If you have high blood pressure (*hypertension*), avoid doing certain high-intensity or resistance exercises that may cause your blood pressure to rise dangerously high. These activities may include heavy weight training; near-maximal exercise of any type (this includes high-intensity intervals); activities that require intense, sustained muscular contractions in the upper body, such as waterskiing and windsurfing or kitesurfing; and exercises that make you involuntarily hold your breath (*Valsalva maneuver*) like power lifting.

If you have significant elevations in your blood pressure, you may have to stick with easier or moderate-intensity aerobic exercise. If you want to do resistance workouts, focus on lower-weight, high-repetition training, which usually causes less dramatic increases in blood pressure than heavy lifting. Avoid doing near-maximal efforts, isometric exercises, and breath holding because all these activities can cause an excessive rise in your blood pressure and increase your risk for a stroke or other cardiovascular event.

To lower your risk of stroke, if your systolic blood pressure (the higher number) is above 200 mm Hg or your diastolic blood pressure (the lower one) is above 110 mm Hg, avoid exercising until they are lower. During exercise, always watch out for stroke warning signs. Go to the emergency room right away for life- and brain-saving treatment within a couple of hours for the best possible outcomes if you do have any of the symptoms of a stroke. These include the following, all with a *sudden onset:*

- Numbness or weakness, especially on one side of your body (legs, arms, or face)
- Confusion
- Trouble with normal speaking or understanding
- Partial or total loss of vision in one or both eyes

- Trouble with walking, loss of balance, or lack of physical coordination
- Severe headache and dizziness
- Symptoms like sweating, nausea and vomiting, lightheadedness, or undue, unexplained fatigue

In closing, regardless of your personal health circumstances, think of your diabetes as a reminder to take better care of yourself, eat right, and exercise daily as much as possible. Find a way to be as active as you can because doing so can only help improve your diabetes management and prevent long-term health problems. Usually, exercise benefits you far more than it can hurt, but take precautions where necessary, especially if you have any complications, and use some common sense. You can safely participate in less strenuous forms of exercise even with almost any complication. Learn to manage your blood glucose effectively during any type of physical activity by following basic guidelines and safety precautions and by monitoring your body's response using whatever technology you have available to you.

## Athlete Profile: **Sean Busby**

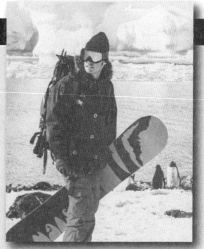

Courtesy of Sean Busby.
Photographer: Stan Pitcher.

**Hometown:** Mission Viejo, California (Residence: Northwest Montana, and Fritz Creek, Alaska)

**Diabetes history:** Type 1 diabetes diagnosed in 2003 (at age 19)—first misdiagnosed with type 2 before losing 30 pounds (14 kilograms) in 2 weeks and finally being put on insulin

**Sport or activity:** Professional snowboarder

**Greatest athletic achievement:** Within months of my correct diagnosis, I was able to get back on the pro tour to compete and regain my West Coast snowboarding championship title. Since then, I have backcountry snowboarded on all seven continents with first descents in some of the most remote mountain ranges in the world.

**Current insulin and medication regimen:** Insulin pump and CGM.

**Training tips:** Test, test, and test! Testing my blood glucose has been the key to my success in understanding how my body is acting in certain environments, including different climates, various humidity levels, competition stress and excitement, time zone changes, complex training schedules, and different altitudes. I now use a CGM to follow trends in new environments or climates and base my basal adjustments in how my CGM is reporting if I believe it to be accurate.

*Typical daily and weekly training and diabetes regimen:*

▶ *Monday:* Up early. I usually eat a healthy complex carbohydrate and reduce my basal. After breakfast I attend frontside training at the local ski resort. I warm up on easy terrain and build into complex technical terrain.

▶ *Tuesday:* Off day or coaching day of local snowboard athletes on technical skills. I typically have no reduction of my basal rates or a slight reduction pending training plans.

▶ *Wednesday:* Uphill day. I climb the ski area on a split board after hours. I eat simple and complex carbs along the way to stay balanced, with a moderate basal insulin reduction.

▶ *Thursday:* I spend the afternoon on the ski hill focused on technical skills in complex terrain. I implement a slight reduction of basal insulin.

▶ *Friday:* Free ride or backcountry day, using a slight to moderate reduction of basal.

▶ *Saturday:* Backcountry day climbing mountains outside the ski area, which usually lasts 6 to 12 hours. For that, I use a moderate reduction of basal and eat a complex carb breakfast and lunch sustained with protein. Dinner is focused on rebuilding and replenishing glycogen stores.

▶ *Sunday:* Same schedule as Saturday.

*Other hobbies and interests:* I love skijoring (a winter sport where a person on skis is pulled by a horse, a dog, or a motor vehicle—in my case, dogs) and dog sledding with our dogs. My wife and I live off the grid and are also into sustainable building/living and off-grid systems.

*Good diabetes and exercise story:* While I was trying to win back my West Coast championship title, my insulin ran out. I had brought an extra insulin cartridge with me that day but had accidentally left it down in the lodge. In first place and with one run left in the event, I began to develop the early stages of DKA, and the stress was making my glucose shoot even higher. Also, the high altitude was making me severely dehydrated. In the starting gate of my final run, I felt as though I was going to pass out, so I asked the start judge to hold the race so I could do an emergency rehydration. The event coordinators and judges put a 10-minute hold on the event to allow me to rehydrate and evaluate my situation. I was questioning whether I should disqualify myself from the event and my potential first-place medal or finish the final run and possibly hold on to first place. I knew that I had to get down the mountain either way, so I decided to get back in the gate and go for it. If I were to pull out of the course because of my glucose, I would know that I had at least tried to finish it. Also, I asked that a ski patrol crew be placed at the bottom. My final run quickly became one of my most challenging snowboard runs and races. I knew that my body could tolerate a little more stress but wasn't sure exactly how much more. As I raced, I reminded myself on every turn to turn quickly across the multiple fall lines throughout the course—usually effortless for me—but I could tell that my cognitive thinking was becoming slower. As I crossed the finish line, I nearly collapsed. Ski patrol then quickly rushed me down to my insulin by snowmobile. I later found out that I had gotten first place and went to stand on the podium. It was a rad feeling. That day I not only won and regained my West Coast title but also beat the hardest competitor I had ever faced—diabetes!

Before reliable CGM, I used to sing annoying kids songs on backcountry expeditions in places like Antarctica and regions of the Arctic. I would do this if it was too cold to get reliable blood

continued ➡

*Sean Busby continued*

glucose results or in areas where avalanche risks were very high and stopping to check was a poor option. By singing basic kids songs my expedition team members would recognize if I was low, such as if I was stuttering on a basic verse or forgetting what part of the song comes next. If that was the case, the assumption was that I was getting low (as it can be hard for me to spot my lows in extreme environments, especially with exercise), and we would instantly treat while continuing to keep moving. Looking back, it was absolutely ridiculous, but it worked in my situation and kept me safe as well as my teammates. Thankfully, there are now great CGMs on the market that have prevented me from continuing these annoying songs on many past and future expeditions.

# 6

## Thinking and Acting Like an Athlete

**A**thletes come in all shapes and sizes. In my opinion, an athlete is anyone who exercises regularly. You do not have to be continually competing in the Olympics or even in competitive or athletic events to qualify. If you only exercise recreationally, you are likely dealing with some of the same issues that elite athletes do when it comes to being emotionally and mentally fit for activity.

This chapter addresses how to know whether you are really an athlete (likely, you are), keep your mental stress under control (particularly when you are competing in events), relax more effectively, and use your mind to enhance your physical performance, keep your motivation for exercise strong, and deal emotionally with getting an athletic injury. You will also read an inspiring story about an athlete with type 1 diabetes who finished his first full-length triathlon dead last but still came out a winner. Finally, this chapter ends with some helpful troubleshooting tips to springboard your performance to the next level.

## ARE YOU REALLY AN ATHLETE?

A marathoner from Pennsylvania, Bill King says that being active and seeing yourself as an athlete is more about your spirit than your athletic capability. "I'm an athlete," he says, "because when I look in a mirror, I see myself as one. If you have an active lifestyle, you will immediately gain self-esteem." After more than 35 years with diabetes and a lifelong exerciser, he still runs marathons and trains doing a variety of activities 6 days a week, so he qualifies as a true athlete. But even if you train less, you can still benefit from seeing yourself that way. Use your vision of yourself as an athlete to stay motivated to be active every day of your long and healthy life.

Kerry White agrees with Bill King's approach and takes it a step further. In her 30s she won the solo female division of the Race Across America (RAAM), a grueling cycling road race that goes from the West Coast to the East Coast of the United States. She says, "I can attest to the fact that the most important quality of being a great athlete is not really athleticism. My various experiences as a road cycling team member and individual mountain bike and Nordic athlete in ultraendurance events have brought me to the realization that athleticism without integrity, honesty, and the ability to share the euphoria of exercise with others is nothing. The importance of being not just an athlete but also always maintaining a positive outlook for what you are doing and treating those who support you with the ultimate respect and integrity is paramount. Without those who support, the athlete is nothing."

Even if you have done nothing noteworthy or remarkable athletically—except for exercising with diabetes, of course—you can consider yourself an athlete. Joyce Meyers, an exerciser with type 2 diabetes from Chicago, Illinois, says that being regularly active is her greatest accomplishment. "After a period of time of exercising, you begin feeling better, which is self-fulfilling. When you feel better, you go exercise even when you don't really want to." She also advises people to treat exercise like you would diet: take it one step at a time and keep working at increasing it. "Add a walk and a healthy shared meal with a friend after exercise as reinforcement to good behavior. Work these aspects into your life so that you miss them when they are not there. Don't expect miracles overnight, though, and don't expect to necessarily become the perfect hourglass figure. Just exercise for the sake of exercising, feeling good, and having lower blood glucose."

# BEING COMPETITIVE WITH YOURSELF, OTHERS, AND DIABETES

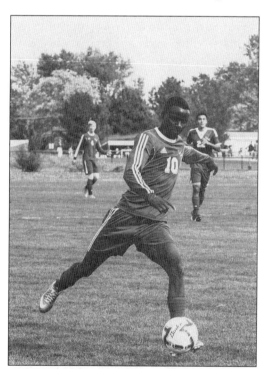

Dealing daily with diabetes can instill in you a determination and willpower to fight the odds and survive—the exact qualities that many elite athletes have.

Simply having diabetes can instill in you a determination and willpower to fight the odds and survive—the exact qualities that many elite athletes have and what it takes for them to reach the top of their sport. Thus, your desire and drive for some level of control over your diabetes parallels the desire to be a world-class athlete, and the two go hand in hand. Why can't you accomplish what others may tell you is impossible because of having diabetes? Remember, more than one successful Olympic athlete with diabetes was told he or she would never be able to compete at that level with diabetes but did! (For example, see Kris Freeman's athlete profile later in this chapter.)

Perhaps in some perverse way, diabetes makes all of us better and stronger. We say to ourselves, "I'm not normal because I have diabetes, so why should I strive to be only an average person?" Many athletes with diabetes are driven by the desire to prove that they can do it (whatever their unique "it" is) and that diabetes is not going to stop them. Take Canadian Al Lewis, a resident of Vancouver, British Columbia. He was a competitive master's swimmer and all-around athlete until an accident affecting his back forced him out of the pool a few years back, but he is still active today despite having had diabetes for over 80 years (since the age of 4). He still believes that being competitive is important. "I'm even more competitive with diabetes than I am with other swimmers," he says. "It's all about being successful with diabetes." For him, exercise has been a big part of his success, the element to which he attributes most of his longevity with diabetes.

Al Lewis contends that there are many considerations for getting ready for a competition, or even for a workout, if you have diabetes. You must consider the effects of any recent insulin doses, changes in pump usage (e.g., new infusion insertion, if you use a pump), recent meals, your mental outlook, the time of day, and concerns about other things. The athlete with diabetes who has done these things over and over tends to integrate the entire mix and guesstimate based on past experience and present circumstances. When you make a mistake, though, you may feel like you have screwed up. He reiterates, "Time and repetition are the keys to success, and they come only with experience. For the young athlete, the competitive attitude plays well not only for training and competition, but also for anticipating the effects of diabetes. Treat diabetes as another competitor, but also consider when it's more like a teammate. Saying that 'diabetes is on my team' is meaningful because then you have to consider its needs as well as your own during exercise and competition."

Sometimes, diabetes is more of a "team" sport. You may need outside help to perform your best, and you will find many people who will be supportive of your efforts to compete to reach your athletic goals with diabetes. Hailing from Mount Airy, Maryland, John Boyer says that one of his biggest challenges dealing with diabetes has been his awareness of his dependence on others. He says, "As much as endurance sports are very individual, educating my friends, training partners, and my wife has been critical to my ability to complete multiple Ironman triathlons, cross-country bike rides, and marathons, and to be as active as I am. I don't want to be a burden on anyone. It has taken a constant conscious awareness that people are most often not burdened by helping but get fulfillment from succeeding together. Immersing myself in a community of type 1 athletes by running Diabetes DESTINY, a camp for young athletes with type 1, has been a huge help. I love learning from the other volunteers and the kids. I also thrive on the accountability that I have to be a good example for the kids."

Likewise, Andy Duckworth of Stockport, England, says, "One of my biggest challenges with diabetes has been simply knowing I can deal with it. When I did my marathon, I also relied on the support of my diabetes specialist and my friends." Isn't that what teamwork is all about anyway? Don Muchow, an ultraendurance athlete from Texas, agrees that there are times when you really need an exercise buddy to help keep you safe. He advises, "On open water swimming, *always* train with a buddy who can help tell if you are having a low in the water. Sometimes it's hard to tell because you cannot feel sweat or chills when swimming. I've found that my form gets bad, I start feeling self-critical and fatalistic, and I clench my jaw. When that happens, you have no choice but to self-rescue while you are still capable. I also train with a bright orange visibility buoy, which serves as a flotation device as long as you are in conscious control of your activity. The last thing you want is to have seizures in the water."

Teenage athlete Patrick Peele, a resident of Cameron, North Carolina, recognizes the importance of thinking like a team, not just as an individual, during the sports he plays like basketball and American football. He advises, "Never ignore a low blood glucose because you want to continue playing. Get it back to normal as quick as possible and let your coach know you are all right to play again. Also, you and your parents should sit down with your coach and give a brief explanation of type 1 diabetes." Spreading your knowledge about managing diabetes with exercise is an important part of thinking and acting like an athlete.

Andy Bell from Missouri has overcome his perceived challenges to being active with diabetes as well. "There is nothing that I don't do," he says. "I exercise daily, play sports, and compete in submission wrestling tournaments." He also realizes the effect that having diabetes has had on his life, though, and on his desire to compete with himself and with others. "I love that I have competed in Brazilian jiujitsu tournaments. I feel like these are some of my greatest accomplishments as a diabetic athlete."

A half-century veteran of type 1 diabetes, Dwain Chapman from Illinois has a lot of good advice stemming from his life experiences. He says, "First of all, just do it! Exercise in some manner and at some level that works for you. Use the tools available whether it be a pump, multiple injections, CGM devices, blood glucose meters, CDEs (certified diabetes educators), fellow people with diabetes, fitness facilities, like-minded groups of bikers, walkers, golfers, etc. Learn what works for you—that's especially true if you are into endurance or very vigorous exercise. Everyone is different, and having diabetes in itself makes you different. That said, there's very little you cannot do versus a person without diabetes. You just have to do more planning, take better care of yourself, and stay safe."

John Boyer shares his unique viewpoint as well, stating, "My overall belief is that type 1 is a perspective. With it you have challenges and opportunities. It shows truly how your choice determines which is a challenge and which is an opportunity. One of the best questions I have ever heard was on a panel of type 1 athletes. A member of the audience asked the panel if they had the chance to go back to the moment they were diagnosed and chose if they had type 1 or didn't, what would they choose? It seems obvious on the surface, but each panelist paused. They reflected on the experience managing type 1 had provided and the people they had met through type 1, and the question was harder to answer than anyone could imagine. If the answer were always easy, you could say you haven't leveraged the opportunity."

At times, the physical changes associated with long-term diabetes and aging can alter your challenges and perspectives on being and staying active. Connie Hanham-Cain, a registered nurse from Albany, New York, has begun to feel the effects of living with diabetes for over 56 years. She has developed some neuropathy-related changes in her hands, feet, and lower extremities that make it harder. "Although I have danced since childhood," she admits, "I am still learning how to practice moving in different ways as the diabetes disease process takes a slow toll on my body. I can no longer do anything automatically without thinking about it, without figuring out how it is going to affect my blood glucose, and what to do about it so that I don't go too high or too low. I also have to focus on how to avoid harming or damaging my neuropathic joints and the bones in my feet, hands, wrists, and shoulders. This all has the potential to make the joy of engaging in physical activity a drag."

## Resources for Active People With Diabetes

# HypoActive (Australia)

HypoActive, a group based in Melbourne, Victoria, Australia, promotes an active lifestyle for people with type 1 diabetes. The group formed to provide information, ongoing support, and inspiration to people participating in exercise challenges, who can learn from other people with diabetes in the process. HypoActive has a strong commitment to assist in empowering all exercisers with type 1 diabetes, and each year they provide opportunities to participate in a number of select endurance challenges, lobby for more research into the effects of exercise on type 1 diabetes, and encourage others to exercise more often. The group meets monthly in Melbourne, but has key links throughout Australia and New Zealand.

Founded by Monique Hanley, a former Race Across America and Team Type 1 cyclist, this group features online articles about their athletes' latest endeavors, along with educational articles and links to research about diabetes and exercise. For more information, visit their website at www.hypoactive.org.

## EFFECT OF MENTAL STRESS ON DIABETES AND HEALTH

We often underestimate how significantly our minds can affect our bodies. You can undergo the hormone elevations that occur during intense training simply by experiencing mental stress or anxiety stemming from any source, which also releases adrenaline, cortisol, and other hormones that raise your blood glucose. As Ancuta Rosser of Arad, Romania, admits, "I always try to do and be better—more active, more dynamic, faster, more powerful—and at times that's stressful." Feeling upset or anxious additionally stresses your immune system, resulting in elevated levels of cortisol and blood glucose and a reduction in your ability to fight off colds and other illnesses. In fact, sometimes being too competitive can be bad for your mental health.

Stress can also stem from frustration and feeling a lack of control over situations. For example, Jeanette Styles, a resident of Eugene, Oregon, says she sometimes feels like she has everything figured out with her diabetes and being active, but on other days nothing seems to go right. She admits that she gets stressed out when her physical activities involve other individuals, and she ends up changing or stopping the activity all together. "My husband is extremely supportive and is happy and willing to help me carry supplies and glucose, never complains about stopping or resting to check my blood glucose, and has never made me feel bad," she says. "For that reason, I love to exercise with him, but I'm intimidated a little by larger group activities."

Joan Runke from Sun Prairie, Wisconsin, agrees that being active with diabetes can potentially cause a lot of stress. "Having been recently diagnosed at age 51, I could find almost no help (to figure out how to avoid exercise highs) even among medical staff as they mostly know about exercise lows. I bought tons of books, but could find almost nothing to help me. So I just started to experiment, even though my medical staff warned me not to take insulin before exercise. I work out late in the afternoon; I would be ready to eat dinner afterwards, and my blood glucose would be 170 to 180 mg/dL (9.4 to 10 mmol/L). No joy in exercising if you have anxiety about doing it the whole time! I still do not have it all down even remotely perfect."

If you can work past the mental stress often caused by managing exercise with diabetes, being physically active itself can have a positive effect on your mood, stress levels, and self-image, all of which positively influence your diabetes management when they are enhanced. The good news is that you can train and control your nervous system's response to mental stress by doing physical and other types of training. Moreover, you achieve optimal athletic performance only when you train both your body and your mind.

## "The One About the Gym"
### by Six Until Me Blogger, Kerri Sparling

UUUUUUUGGGGGGHHHHH, the one about the gym.

Dude, I wanted to start this post with a story about how hard it's been to regain traction with losing the baby weight and then end with a BAM I NO LONGER WANT TO BURN MY SHAPEWEAR IN A BONFIRE. But no. That is sadly not the case.

The road to my last pregnancy was paved with fertility drugs, miscarriage, depression, and other terrible crap. Ends eventually justified the means, and I was beyond grateful to find out I was pregnant after such a journey. (The Little Guy is my favorite guy.) My son was born 8 months ago, and he is exactly who we had been waiting for.

Table all the parental happies for a minute, though, because this post is not about infertility. Or The Little Guy. It's about the tarnish that's settled onto the word "just" in the sentence, "I've just had a baby."

No. I did not just have a baby. I had a baby 8 months ago. And I still feel like I'm trapped in the postpartum schlubby chub club.

So, I joined a gym.

I used to go to the gym a lot. It was kind of a family thing, and while I never sculpted a physique that would stop traffic (unless a vehicle actually hit me), I was stronger and healthier and slimmer than I am now. I didn't feel ashamed of my shape, and I wasn't avoiding my closet in favor of athleisure wear.

Oh, yeah. "Doing absolutely nothing in my active wear" has been a theme these last 8 months.

Postpartum anxiety didn't help (better now, though) and neither did the C-section recovery. I didn't feel great after my first C-section, and, despite rumors I'd heard that the second one is easier, I did not find that to be true. Add in some wrist and hand issues (I ended up with breastfeeding injuries, which feels silly as eff to type but is actually a thing), and my body felt like something I was renting out instead of taking ownership of.

That did not feel good. I want change. Can't wait around for change, though. Have to chase change. Change is exhausting. So is this paragraph.

So, about a month ago, I joined a gym. It wasn't a cheap decision, but the gym feels low pressure, has great hours, and also provides childcare for small baby people, so I have no excuse NOT to go. Also, something about paying for it makes me less likely to NOT go because I hate throwing money away. So I've been going. Despite feeling shy (is exercise timidity a thing?) and despite feeling frumpy, I've been going. I use the treadmill and the free weights, and I'm debating a class or two if I can find some glasses and a fake mustache to wear while participating. I'm trying not to weigh myself but instead using a particular pair of pants as my barometer for progress.

I hope to see some progress soon, but I'm trying to find small victories in the steadier blood sugars and increase of energy. And also in the "hey, I left my house and didn't spend the entire day juggling kid requirements only."

Hopefully, in time, I'll schedule my shapewear bonfire, but in the meantime, I'll try to find some pride in taking small steps now. Especially wearing these mad cool glasses and this fake mustache.

Reprinted from http://sixuntilme.com/wp/2017/04/26/the-one-about-the-gym/ with permission of Kerri Sparling.

# Exercise-Released Brain Hormones Lower Mental and Physical Stress

One of the most publicized mental benefits of exercise resulting from a bodily change is the release of brain hormones. The primary hormones released are called *endorphins*, of which there are 40 types. Basically, they are stress hormones with receptors throughout your brain and body that calm you and relieve muscle pain during intense exercise. In the brain, they contribute to your feeling of well-being or "runner's high" that usually arises during exercise, giving you a second wind. Exercise positively influences the same brain hormones (that is, endorphins, serotonin, dopamine, and norepinephrine) as antidepressant medications, but exercise is likely even more effective than drugs for treating depression. Each workout actually boosts your mood, at least for a little while. Some people are positively addicted to this release of endorphins and need to get their daily dose. Endorphins also likely improve your body's insulin action, thereby reversing or decreasing insulin resistance, which is why moderate aerobic training works so well for lowering it.

> *Exercise to get a maximal release of endorphins and other feel-good brain hormones on a daily basis. As a side benefit, you will feel less depressed and anxious and enjoy a greatly improved mood and better physical health.*

You also release *dopamine* in your brain during exercise, a key player in getting you to adopt an active lifestyle. When you release dopamine during exercise, it activates the pleasure centers in your brain, and you end up associating activity with an elevated sense of delight. That makes your brain recall pleasant feelings associated with training, and then you will be more likely to continue doing that activity to get your boost of feel-good hormones. *Serotonin* release, which physical activity causes, is associated with short-term improvements in your mood as well. As a bonus, you get the release of two brain *endocannabinoids*, which are brain neurotransmitters that dull pain. So aim to release endorphins, dopamine, serotonin, and other mood-enhancing brain hormones and neurotransmitters daily through activity to simultaneously manage your blood glucose and improve your outlook.

## Training the Mind and the Body

Although each workout you do causes some physical damage to your muscles, you ultimately end up stronger, faster, and better, and your body responds by releasing fewer stress hormones during subsequent workouts. Similarly, when you practice using relaxation techniques to control your mental stress levels, your mind learns to reduce your body's sympathetic stimulation as well. The more consistently you practice relaxation, the easier it is to avoid eliciting a strong stress response when "life happens" the next time. During recovery, your *parasympathetic nervous system* keeps your heart rate low and digestion high, so it is no wonder that a warm shower, a big meal, and a long nap after a workout make you feel more relaxed. You are in an *anabolic* (building and repairing) state then, and your glycogen is being restored while your muscles are being repaired and strengthened.

Philadelphia, Pennsylvania, exerciser Daniele Hargenrader, a personal trainer and diabetes coach, agrees that many of the benefits of being active for her are mental. She says, "The biggest challenge is being flexible and accepting that things won't always go the way you want them to. Being willing to experiment and not being hard on yourself when your blood glucose levels are not where you want them to be is crucial to your willingness to keep trying. Another thing that I overcame that made a big difference in my mindset was not telling myself that my workout was pointless if I had to eat or drink the calories back because of low blood glucose. The cardiovascular work, mental release, and so much more are still incredibly beneficial even if you have to replace the calories burned with glucose. Don't negate your efforts!"

## Relaxation Techniques to Help Control Your Stress

Sport psychologists recommend relaxation to enhance performance in athletic events and even speed up healing from injuries. Relaxation techniques can help you control the stress of competition as well as the stress coming from other avenues of your life. One method to relax is to sit quietly and focus your mind. But you can even use relaxation techniques while exercising. For example, punch the air with your fists to release your anger or anxiety and consciously relax the tense muscles in your body. Use your imagination to visualize more blood flowing to all the parts of your body that need it (like your heart, muscles, hands, and feet). You may be able to enhance the blood flow to your feet simply by visualizing it, verifying that a strong mind–body connection really exists. Also, take deep and steady breaths and release them slowly, particularly during your warm-up and cool-down periods when you are not working out as hard. Whenever you start to feel winded during a workout, take deeper breaths to bring more oxygen into your lungs and body.

# Yoga for Peak Performance

Other techniques for alleviating stress include stretching activities and yoga, which calm your mind and enhance parasympathetic activity, the branch of your nervous system that lowers your heart rate, breathing, and stress responses. If practiced regularly, yoga can balance your body and mind, enhancing both athletic performance and mental well-being by counterbalancing the effects of your sympathetic nervous system. Vigorous styles of yoga that are a workout in themselves are not as good for relaxing and maximizing the benefits of your parasympathetic activity; go for the kinder, gentler type for maximal relaxation. If you are mentally stressed, practicing such techniques can help train your mind and body to reduce its sympathetic drive, thus enhancing the quality of the often-limited time that you have for recovery. You may want to try some of the slower forms of martial arts, such as tai chi and qigong, to work on eliciting the same levels of relaxation as yoga and stretching.

Additionally, working your joints and muscles with yoga or stretching to maintain and increase your range of motion around joints helps prevent injuries and may enhance recovery from other workouts. Maggie Crawford from San Diego, California, is a firm believer: in addition to resting and hydrating well after her ultraendurance events, she does yoga. Thus, whether your goal is injury prevention or simply to be a better athlete, staying flexible can enhance your performance.

# ENHANCING YOUR PERFORMANCE WITH YOUR MIND

Visualization techniques get many athletes to the pinnacle of their respective sports. Moreover, they may improve your mental awareness and sense of well-being. Whether you call it guided imagery, mental rehearsal, meditation, or visualization, you can practice the technique by creating a mental image of what you want to happen or feel during an athletic event. Imagine a scene, complete with images of either your previous best performance or how you want to do the next time, and then become one, so to speak, with that desire. Try to imagine all the details, both physical and mental. Include visual images, physical sensations, and auditory cues (such as the cheering of onlookers). Call up these images repeatedly, just as you repeatedly do physical training.

> *With mental rehearsal you can train your mind and body to respond in the way that you are visualizing and better perform the physical skill or athletic event.*

Visualization can improve both physical and emotional responses. Imagining a positive outcome can build experience and confidence in your ability to perform when the time comes and the stress is greater. By reducing your response to the emotional stress of the event, visualization may help you keep your blood glucose better managed. Competition is tough, and athletes with diabetes have one extra (often overwhelming) variable to deal with, compared with the participants who do not have diabetes. In this case, effective visualization might be one way to gain back the advantage.

## A Diabetic Athlete's First Ironman (Finishing Dead Last, but Alive)

The true spirit of all athletes is exemplified by the story of Jay Handy of Madison, Wisconsin, doing his first full-length triathlon in 2003 (Ironman Wisconsin). He trained for months and did everything right, but it was only his mental visualization and sheer determination that ultimately got him through the race. The weather was unseasonably hot, which always means trouble for any athlete, with or without diabetes. His 2.4-mile (3.9-kilometer) swim went better than expected, given that he is more of a runner and cyclist. As he recalls, "A quick glance at my watch indicated I was out of the water 20 minutes faster than I had planned. It was the fastest I had ever swum in my life! This was going to be a great day, I remember thinking. Already ahead of schedule by 20 minutes and feeling great!"

His story continues with the 112-mile (180-kilometer) bike course that followed the swim: "I had rigged up a homemade contraption to hold my blood glucose meter on the bike itself to be able to check without slowing down. My blood glucose numbers were all perfect. All the hours of planning were paying off. I was so happy. Only then did it occur to me that the temperature was rising. I methodically counted my electrolyte pills and salt tablets inside their plastic bag. Every 30 minutes, I would take one salt tablet and two electrolyte pills. 'Perfect,' I thought. 'I have just enough for the remaining 5 and a half hours I need to finish the bike race.'" Friends and family kept his emotions high. "All sorts of people I knew had come out to cheer me on," he recalls. "They would yell as I passed, and I would raise my arm in a fist or give thumbs up. It was a mutual exchange of excitement. I felt like the luckiest person in the world."

Here's where his race began to go downhill (figuratively speaking, not literally). "By mile 80 (kilometer 130) the temperature was 90 degrees Fahrenheit (32 degrees Celsius), it was extremely humid, and I started to feel slight cramps in my legs. It was time to take another salt tablet and my self-prescribed electrolyte pills. I reached back toward my right jersey pocket where I kept them. It was empty, so I checked my center pocket. Not there. The left pocket? Only my emergency diabetes supplies. My heart sank, and my mind went completely blank for at least a mile. I also knew that, according to the rules of the event, there would be no tablets at the aid stations and that no one could give me any now that the race was in progress. I looked down at what I had taped to my handlebar. It was an e-mail a friend had sent me 2 days earlier saying, 'May God give you the strength and endurance to finish.' I thought to myself, 'I may need those two elements more than ever in my life today.'"

"Ten miles (16 kilometers) later, I started up the first of three tough climbs. I saw someone walking up the climb and thought that looked smart. I stopped, thinking I would simply jump off and begin walking. Instead, I fell over with locked legs due to severe cramping in both of my quads. It was excruciating, and I screamed into the treetops. I could see other bikers slowly ascending past me, none making eye contact for fear they might catch what I had." Finally, one cyclist stopped and asked what he could do for Jay. "I said, 'Kick. Kick me. Kick me behind my knees.' He did, and it broke the clenching spasms. As I lay on the ground in a fetal position,

I had an overwhelming desire to shut my eyes and go right to sleep, but instead I forced myself to get up. I lifted my bike and started to walk like a stick man, unable to bend my knees much. At the top of the hill, I slowly got onto the bike and began to spin my pedals with very little resistance." During the rest of the bike course, Jay's quads cramped up twice more, but he finished it with a minute to spare on the time cutoff to start the final 26.2-mile (42.2-kilometer) marathon-length run. "I was slightly delirious, but made it into the transition area. I saw several bodies on the ground moaning and in various stages of exhaustion."

After the final transition, Jay recalls, "I came out in my running gear—including my 'Running on Insulin' shirt—walking like a stick man. My legs kept locking at the knees. My wife Kim and my two daughters, Schuyler and Grace, were there. I could hear Grace begin to cry, and Kim said to me that I did not have to do this. I told her my legs would hopefully loosen up because different muscles are used for biking and running. I walked out of the chute onto the course. The crowds were cheering, not for me but for the finishers heading in the opposite direction, and I was just beginning a marathon. I had never felt so alone."

He recalls that the first mile of the marathon course seemed to take forever. "How am I ever going to do this?" he wondered. "My next thought was, 'Let's break it down; 1 mile done, only 25.2 to go.' But that was just too daunting. Instead, I focused on taking each step and pushing through the pain. My friend Mark called my cell phone when I passed mile 2. He was already at mile 13 (kilometer 21), and he suggested that I might want to consider doing just the half-marathon instead."

"By mile 6 (kilometer 10), my legs did loosen up some. I thought maybe I could run a little, just to speed things up. I tried a light jog for 100 feet (30 meters), but that was a major mistake. My legs stiffened right up. I knew the only way to propel myself forward was by speed walking, and I felt every step." At that point, he had about 20 miles (32 kilometers) to go. "With about 1.5 miles (2.4 kilometers) before the halfway mark, which is also at the finish line because there is a turnaround there, I called my wife. I told her I didn't think I could go on due to the pain. I told her I was sorry, after all she had done to support me, that I wasn't going to finish. I wanted to cry, but there were no tears. She said I had a lot to be proud of and that she'd meet me at my finish."

When Jay got there, all his supporters were there cheering the end of his race (albeit cut short). "When I hit State Street, I knew I had only seven blocks to finally decide to quit. I started to think again about having the strength and endurance to finish and of all the people who made an effort to see me through the race. Finally, I thought of the kids with diabetes. I couldn't DNF ("did not finish") this race. Yet I also couldn't fathom going back out there again and doing another 13.1-mile (21.1-kilometer) loop. When I was three blocks from my decision point, I saw Hans, a friend who is a former Olympic athlete. He had a different look in his eye. All he said was, 'Jay, you can do this.' I looked to my right, and there was my whole family and many others rooting for me. I heard the roar of the crowd; they all thought I was finishing, as did the official there. Right before the turnaround, I looked at my wife, raised my arm, and whirled my hand in a circle to indicate I was going back out. There was no way I could walk off. I had to keep going."

During the second loop, several people came along on bikes and met up with Jay to encourage him and keep him company, although he was still on his own, walking in the dark for most of it. He recalls the finish vividly: "I was finally approaching the last block to where the finishing arch was. I came around the corner and into the glow of spotlights, along with the roar of cheers. There were still hundreds of people there for me! The announcer said, 'And the final finisher is

continued ➡

*A Diabetic Athlete's First Ironman continued*

number 1076, Jay Handy, a type 1 diabetic!' The crowd's roar was unbelievable. I ran the last 50 yards (46 meters) to the finish. The pain had lifted, at least for a moment. I came across the line with my arms up and smiling. It was 12:07 a.m. Moments later, the medical team asked if I was okay. Other than the terrible pain in my cramped legs, I felt pretty good."

"Two volunteers came up, and one handed me a T-shirt," Jay recalls. "The other said, 'He needs his medal.' I protested, saying, 'No, no, I didn't earn one. It's after midnight, and I barely missed the time cutoff.' She looked to an official, who answered for her, saying, 'Yes, you do. You completed the distance. Therefore, you are a finisher and an Ironman.' The volunteer then draped the medal around my neck. I had finished—dead last, but still alive—and with a medal after all! Success." Jay, you did all athletes proud, not just those with diabetes!

The temperature that day reached 93 degrees Fahrenheit (34 degrees Celsius), and a quarter of the competitors sought medical attention. Also, 276 athletes dropped out of the race, the highest in the competition's long history. Jay's diabetes management was excellent throughout the race; his problems that day were the same as those of any other athlete. He has completed three more Ironman competitions since this first one with great success and many hours under the time cutoff.

# GETTING AND STAYING MOTIVATED TO EXERCISE

Even elite athletes have some days when they are not as motivated to exercise. You know those days—the ones when you have trouble putting on your exercise gear, let alone finishing your planned workout. For the sake of your blood glucose and your health, do not use one or two bad days as an excuse to discontinue an otherwise important and relevant exercise or training routine. Here is a list of motivating behaviors and ideas for regular exercisers and anyone else who may not always feel motivated to work out.

- Identify any barriers or obstacles keeping you from being active, such as the fear of getting low during exercise, and come up with ways to overcome them.
- Get yourself an exercise buddy (or a dog that needs to be walked).
- Use sticker charts or other motivational tools to track your progress.
- Schedule structured exercise into your day on your calendar or to-do list.
- Break your larger goals into smaller, realistic stepping stones (e.g., daily and weekly physical activity goals).
- Reward yourself for meeting your goals with noncaloric treats or outings.
- Plan to do physical activities that you really enjoy as often as possible.
- Wear a pedometer (at least occasionally) as a reminder to take more daily steps.
- Have a backup plan that includes alternative activities in case of inclement weather or other barriers to your planned exercise.

- Distract yourself while you exercise by reading a book or magazine, watching TV, listening to music or a book on tape, or talking with a friend.

- Simply move more all day long to maximize your unstructured activity time, and break up sitting with frequent activity breaks.

- Do not start out exercising too intensely or you may become discouraged or injured.

- If you get out of your normal routine and are having trouble getting restarted, simply take small steps in that direction.

As for other tricks that you can use, start with reminding yourself that regular exercise can lessen the potential effect of most of your cardiovascular risk factors, including elevated cholesterol levels, insulin resistance, obesity, and hypertension. Even just walking regularly can lengthen your life, and if you keep your blood glucose better managed with the help of physical activity, you may be able to prevent or delay almost all the potential long-term health complications associated with diabetes.

Natalie Koch, a competitive cyclist from Syracuse, New York, and a member of Team Type 1, explains how her motivation to be active has been shaped by diabetes: "Being physically active is really the best thing I can do to manage my diabetes. I usually feel pretty awful on days that I can't exercise (even though I know I need some rest days!). That said, because general training makes me feel so good, I feel less motivated to compete—race days make blood glucose management more complicated. So I've found that after getting diagnosed with type 1 diabetes 5 years ago (at age 27 when I was already doing bike racing), I am less inclined to race, but my motivation to get on the bike every day is so much stronger because I simply want to feel good physically and mentally. To deal with this, I have been very selective in choosing races and otherwise just not feeling bad about skipping others."

## Managing Depression, Anxiety, and More With Exercise

To motivate yourself to exercise, you also need to control your feelings of depression and anxiety. When you are depressed, the last thing you may want to do is exercise. The funny thing about physical activity, though, is that it reduces your feelings of depression and anxiety. If you can simply get yourself up and going, you may feel your depression lifting by itself. A resident of Glendale Heights, Illinois, Gin Carlin says, "I'm still struggling to figure out how to keep my glucose in range while I exercise; however, the energetic benefits of exercising help me avoid depression, so I'm going to continue working out and deal with the fluctuations in my readings." Studies have even shown that getting adolescents involved in organized youth sports may help reduce anxiety, improve and maintain a favorable sense of self-worth, and promote better coping strategies when dealing with everyday problems—and it may help even more when teens are dealing with having diabetes on top of the normal stressors of growing up.

It helps to keep everything in perspective if you can, and to not beat yourself up for not reaching perfection all the time. For instance, Rachel Zinman of Australia is not depressed or anxious, but she has found that exercising is about making choices and living with the outcomes. She says, "Too much exercise makes me high. I have learned which kinds of exercise work best for me, such as walking and yoga, and I mostly stick with them. If I do choose to do something like cardio or dance, I try to take it easy on myself about the high and ride it out. It's kind of like deciding to have chocolate: even though the after-effects are not as pleasant, the joy I feel during it (the exercise in this case) is worth it."

## Overcoming Barriers and Obstacles

Removing potential barriers to exercise can help as well—the excuses such as exercise being inconvenient or taking too much time, and being afraid of getting hypoglycemia. A resident of Boise, Idaho, Rhet Hulbert understands that having to consider diabetes in everything you choose to do can be inconvenient and an obstacle to being active. He says, "The biggest challenge is just planning your day and diet and medication around the exercise. It is difficult to just decide on a whim to go for a long run or whatever. You need to think ahead to make sure your blood glucose is in the right place." Whether you are a competitive athlete with diabetes or just a recreational one, we all face these same daily challenges when it comes to managing our sports and activities.

One of the most commonly cited barriers for everyone—with or without diabetes—is a perceived lack of time. However, if you stop thinking of exercise only as a planned activity and simply try to move your body more often, you will be more active all day long without feeling as though you have to come up with big blocks of time to fit it in. Most people expend the majority of their calories each day doing unstructured activities like standing and walking rather than during a formal exercise session. Doing something physically active during the day is always better than doing nothing, particularly when it comes to keeping your insulin action higher and your diabetes better managed. You may also benefit from just not sitting for long periods of time; instead, get up every half-hour or so and do 3 minutes of walking or easy resistance exercises at your desk at work or in your home.

As for diabetes-specific barriers, the most common reason why adults with type 1 diabetes choose not to exercise is being afraid of developing hypoglycemia. Camille Andre of Santa Barbara, California, still chooses to be active, but she finds getting low very frustrating because it usually forces her to stop her workout. To compensate, she has increased her exercise target blood glucose and is always very cautious about going low. She says, "This has resulted in more highs at the end of exercise, but for performance and my satisfaction with exercise I've decided that these highs are worth the decrease in lows." A resident of Redmond, Washington, Margaret Urfer says that one of her biggest challenges related to having diabetes has been her fear of getting low, which is less of a concern now that she uses the latest technologies to monitor her blood glucose. She recalls, "As a teen (who was out of shape), I never knew if I was low or just fatigued. That's why getting a CGM changed my life, allowing me to do more with less worry." Robin Leysen of Belgium admits that his only challenge related to being active with diabetes was his fear of getting low during sports, but he overcame that using technology as well (see more on this in the next section).

Tian Walker from Long Beach, California, had similar concerns about exercise-induced lows, but was able to come up with a solution that involved support from others. She recounts, "I was unable to do more than an hour of exercise 2 days in a row without lows that would completely stop me from walking around or getting anything done for hours at a time. I loved exercise, and I knew that it made my blood glucose levels better, but I was completely afraid of doing too much, and for good reason. I would notice my insulin needs decrease for up to 10 days after something intense like a 30-mile bike ride. I ended up lowering all my insulin and being in a situation of being forced to do exercise the perfect amount of time (somewhere between 30 and 40 minutes) every day in order to feel okay. I actually tried not exercising for a year because I was so frustrated, and I was surprised to discover that without exercise my blood glucose was less manageable." This all changed when she began running with a local group called Type One Run, which introduced her to my type 1 exercise coach who has it himself. She also learned how to better manage her basal rates to avoid lows after workouts of any sort.

## Taking Advantage of Available Technology

For some people, the availability of newer technologies like CGM (see the discussion in chapter 5) have made all the difference for them in overcoming some of their exercise barriers. For Robin Leysen, with his Libre (CGM) he feels that he does not have to worry about exercise-related lows anymore because he has immediate feedback on his blood glucose levels whenever he wants or needs it. Tian Walker of Long Beach, California, feels that with an insulin pump and a CGM, she has absolutely no reason to fear exercise anymore. For her, the ability to see her blood glucose in real time and make basal adjustments on her pump made it completely possible to figure out what adjustments she needs. Jeff Foot, a resident of Scotland, tells of other challenges that technology has helped him overcome. "It has given me the confidence to cycle alone in mountainous terrain with no phone signal or 3G, knowing I can manage my blood glucose okay using my CGM to monitor, pump to reduce insulin, and carbohydrates to cope with lows." Life with diabetes in this new millennium is definitely improving!

Zippora Karz from Los Angeles, California, had a long and successful career as a professional ballerina, but even she says, "When I was dancing professionally, the biggest challenge was being in the blood glucose range I needed to be to feel my best to perform, without going too low." Her performances would have undoubtedly been easier to manage with more immediate feedback on her blood glucose levels. Dwain Chapman, a long-time exerciser with type 1 diabetes from Highland, Illinois, is in full agreement. He recounts, "For the first 30 years, my biggest challenge with diabetes was simply not knowing—not knowing what my blood glucose was, and not knowing if that was even important. I really didn't know how to approach diabetes and exercise, and I didn't have any role models to follow. I was the first person with type 1 diabetes to run the Honolulu Marathon in 1978; when I ran it again in 1980, they'd included a special category for people with diabetes—but I was the only entrant for that!" He continues, "I only wish I'd have had the technology to better manage diabetes sooner in my exercising life. I completely believe that my determination to continue to participate in exercise and sports after my diagnosis at age 14 is the primary reason I'm alive and living an active life today"—over 50 years later.

## Building Your Self-Confidence to Boost Motivation

Keep in mind that having diabetes is the best reason to be physically active, maybe the only one that you need. Andy Bell of Columbia, Missouri, explains where diabetes played a role for him: "At 14 when I was diagnosed, I had already led a life of an athletic child, playing competitive soccer since I was 6, along with a lot of other sports. Getting diabetes struck me down. I lost the undeniable confidence (more like cockiness) that I had always had as a nondiabetic athlete. My self-esteem was shot, and I stopped competing in leagues and organized recreation because I didn't feel like I could do it anymore. It has been a very slow recovery process, one taken on by me and me alone. Now, I actually embrace having this disease. I have found that I am still the same athletic, competitive, little squirt that I was before my diagnosis. Not only do I have more confidence, but I'm now a better athlete than most people I know." For you diehard competitive athletes (and the wannabes), here are more tips about how to build your self-confidence and stay motivated to compete and improve your athletic performance even further:

- Manage mental stress and disappointment effectively.
- Stop all negative self-talk.
- Increase your ability to maintain and regain concentration.
- Mentally prepare well for competition.
- Improve communication with teammates and coaches.
- Set, reset, and manage your individual and team goals.
- Notice, avoid, and recover from competition burnout.
- Regain your mental fitness after an injury.

# RECOVERING FROM INJURY— EMOTIONALLY SPEAKING

Maybe an injury has left you unable to do your usual workouts. Taking some time to let your body repair itself (as discussed in the following chapter) is fine, but having a physical injury that keeps you from your normal routine can be emotionally devastating, especially for athletes with diabetes who have to deal with changes in their physical state when their exercise routines are altered. Physical activity may normally be your social outlet, your stress reducer, or a significant source of meaning and purpose in your life—even some of your identity. Athletes who lose their guiding light, so to speak, may have a negative reaction to injury that can lead to depression and lack of motivation.

An injury may not be life threatening or even permanent, but because your injury likely resulted in a loss of some kind, you may still find yourself going through the stages that people go through when a loved one dies. These stages—denial, anger, bargaining, depression, and finally acceptance—can be traveled in any order and sometimes repeated. Usually you have to reach the last stage, acceptance, to deal effectively with any physical injury (or diabetes complication, especially ones that interfere with being active). New research also shows that practicing mental skills during injury rehabilitation may help, including goal setting, positive self-talk and thoughts, relaxation techniques, and imagery. It may be worth trying one or more of these techniques to get yourself through it.

In times of injury, assemble people around you who can provide support, including physical therapists, health care practitioners, coaches, trainers, family and friends, counselors or therapists, and good doctors (especially if you need to have surgery to repair the damage). Next, set realistic goals for your recovery process, including the time that it will take and the necessary steps. (Giving myself the time to rest enough to recover fully from my injuries is not one of my stronger skills.) To minimize your fitness loss during your recovery, try to come up with alternative activities you can safely do. For instance, for many running injuries, athletes can spend time in the pool doing either aquatic running or swimming. Finally, think positively and set yourself on a road to faster recovery. As for the physical aspects of recovering from an athletic injury, those are discussed fully in the following chapter.

# TROUBLESHOOTING YOUR PERFORMANCE LIKE AN ATHLETE

As you have come to realize in this chapter, being an athlete is mostly a state of mind. However, sometimes your performance when you are an athlete with diabetes also depends on overcoming some regimen obstacles and other physical issues. In this final section, you will learn all you need to perform like a professional athlete.

As discussed back in chapter 2, many different factors can impact your blood glucose responses, and the more you know about them, the better equipped you are to figure out what works best for you in almost every situation. Regardless of how knowledgeable you are, this process always takes some trial and error. Consider using some of the following strategies if you are experiencing any of these issues with being active.

## Managing Exercise-Associated Hypoglycemia

Having to slow down or stop during an activity due to low blood glucose is annoying even to recreational athletes. It can also compromise your ability to complete your event, competition, or just your daily workout. It is worth keeping this from happening if you can. If you have been having any exercise-related lows, consider taking some of these actions or precautions to avoid them, especially if you use insulin.

### Lows During and After Exercise—Food Intake

- Treat lows with glucose or other rapidly absorbed carbohydrate first, and follow that up with other balanced foods and drinks if needed to keep from dropping later.

- Choose pre-exercise foods that require the smallest amount of (or no) insulin to cover them to keep your circulating insulin lower during activities.
- Take in extra carbohydrate before, during, and after activities (depending on your exercise intensity and duration, starting blood glucose, normal diet, and other factors).
- Consider using protein and/or fat intake during prolonged activities to help prevent lows, especially past the first hour of activity, because they take longer to digest.
- Consume some protein and/or fat shortly after exercise and possibly also at bedtime to counteract lows later on and overnight.

## Lows During and After Exercise—Insulin Adjustments

- Exercise when your insulin levels are lower, such as before meals or first thing in the morning before taking any bolus insulin.
- Before doing longer duration exercise, lower your insulin levels in anticipation by cutting back on your dose(s) of bolus and/or basal insulin.
- Lower the dose of any rapid-acting insulin you take within 2 to 3 hours before doing an activity (or set a lower basal rate on your insulin pump, if you use one).
- If using an insulin pump, consider lowering your basal rate for up to 2 hours before the start of exercise as well as during (and likely after) the activity.
- If you are prone to lows after exercise, reduce your dose of rapid-acting insulin given after any activity, or set a temporary lower basal rate on your pump for 4 to 12 hours.
- If you inject your basal insulin (Lantus, Basaglar, Levemir, or Toujeo), consider splitting the dose (although not necessarily evenly) to give it twice daily to allow for easier dose reductions before and after activity.
- If you use an even longer-acting basal insulin like Tresiba, watch out for possible insulin "stacking" on subsequent days, particularly when you are more active than normal.

## Training Effects and Other Considerations

- Check your blood glucose more often when doing a new activity or unaccustomed exercise because both are more likely to result in lows, both during and afterward.
- Check frequently if you have had a bad low or exercised hard in the 24 hours before your latest workout because both may blunt your release of glucose-raising hormones.
- Try doing an all-out sprint for 10 to 30 seconds to help counteract most lows during exercise, but only if your insulin levels are not too high.
- If you plan on doing both aerobic and resistance training during a workout, vary the order based on whether you want your glucose to stay more stable

(during resistance work) or possibly decrease (during moderate aerobic work, although intense training may raise it).

- Keep in mind that the rate of insulin absorption from skin depots depends on the size of the dose: smaller doses (1 to 3 units) are absorbed more rapidly than larger ones (5 or more units), which linger longer while you are active.

- Do not forget that your overall insulin needs are lower when you are regularly active; you may need permanently lower basal (and mealtime bolus) insulin doses.

- Avoid massaging the area where you just gave some insulin—massaging it can speed up its absorption.

- Remember that getting in a hot tub or having other prolonged heat exposure can speed up the absorption of any insulin taken (causing lows first, then highs later).

# Dealing With Exercise Hyperglycemia

If you have experienced high blood glucose related to being active, it can be hard to always pinpoint the source of the rise and take actions to prevent or manage it. Consider these possible scenarios and some solutions for troubleshooting.

## Highs Before Exercise

- If your blood glucose is over 250 mg/dL (13.9 mmol/L) and has been elevated for a few hours, consider giving yourself some insulin and waiting for the level to decrease before starting to exercise (especially with moderate or higher blood and urine ketones).

- If you take a dose of insulin to lower your glucose with a plan to start exercising shortly thereafter, take less than you normally would (50 percent or less) to prevent your blood glucose from dropping too rapidly during the activity.

- If your blood glucose is over 300 mg/dL (16.7 mmol/L) with no ketones, exercise only if you feel well and use caution because you can dehydrate more easily.

## Highs During or After Exercise

- Cut back on your carbohydrate intake during exercise, reduce your insulin less, or take extra insulin after exercise (albeit less than normal).

- Remember that eating a full meal within an hour of starting exercise can slow digestion and result in high blood glucose for 1 to 2 hours afterward, particularly when you have consumed lower glycemic index items (refer to chapter 4 for a discussion of the glycemic index).

- If you disconnect your pump during activities and your blood glucose starts to rise, reconnect at least once an hour and take at least a portion of your missed basal.

- Consider giving yourself some of your "missed" basal insulin in advance in some cases, such as when you have disconnected from your pump before a swim.

- Consider using an "untethered" pump regimen—that is, giving some of your insulin as an injection of long-acting insulin (e.g., Lantus, Levemir, Tresiba) and the rest via pump with a reduced basal rate; then if you disconnect, you still have some basal on board.

- For early morning exercise before eating, consider giving yourself a small dose of insulin (less than normal) and/or a small snack to break your fast to reduce cortisol levels that can lead to elevations at that time of day.

- If the stress or intensity of competitions affects you, keep your basal insulin higher and only give yourself 50 percent or less of your usual correction dose to lower glucose.

- Stay hydrated during activities because dehydration can make blood glucose seem higher (due to being more concentrated) and lead to excess correction dosing.

- Consider doing some easy aerobic exercise after more intense workouts to lower blood glucose naturally.

### Training Effects and Other Considerations

- After you have trained for a few weeks doing an activity, you may need fewer carbohydrates or smaller insulin reductions than before training due to a greater use of fat.

- Both endurance training and fat adaptation (from a low-carbohydrate diet) increase your body's efficiency at using fat as a fuel during aerobic activities that are submaximal.

- When you get very sore from exercise (peaking 2 or 3 days afterward), you may be more insulin resistant because you cannot restore muscle glycogen until your muscle damage from the activity is repaired.

- If you load up on carbohydrates before events, you should take enough insulin to cover them; otherwise, loading can raise your blood glucose and limit glycogen storage (check out the discussion on carbohydrate loading in chapter 3).

- You should keep your insulin from getting too hot or too cold; otherwise, its action may diminish and cause your usual doses to inadequately cover your insulin needs.

- Injected or pumped bolus insulin is absorbed faster in smaller doses; after a larger dose, you may end up too high first and then too low later on.

- Smaller doses of injected basal insulin are also absorbed more rapidly than larger ones (think 5 units versus 20), and they often do not last as long as expected.

# Avoiding Early-Onset or Excessive Fatigue

Did you ever DNF ("did not finish") a race or a competition? Certainly, that can happen if you twist your ankle, cramp up, or otherwise get injured. But sometimes your performance is affected when you get tired too soon during an event or if the fatigue is so bad you simply cannot go on. Here are actions you can take to prevent fatigue that comes on early or is bad enough to make you stop before you reach your athletic goals.

- Prevent both hypoglycemia and hyperglycemia (see the preceding sections) to delay or prevent fatigue when you are physically active.
- Keep your blood glucose as close to normal as possible for a day or two beforehand so your body can store optimal amounts of glycogen in muscle and liver.
- Consume carbohydrates during exercise to provide an alternate source of blood glucose (other than the limited amount your liver can release) and fuel for muscles.
- Avoid hyperglycemia by having adequate insulin in your blood to counterbalance the release of glucose-raising hormones during exercise.
- Try out new food or insulin strategies in advance during practices, not during the events or competitions themselves.
- Keep yourself adequately hydrated before and during all activities, especially if your blood glucose levels have been elevated (you may be dehydrated).
- If muscle cramps are causing you to stop early, consider supplementing with magnesium, electrolytes, and possibly a B vitamin complex.
- Have your blood iron levels checked because anemia can cause fatigue, particularly during exercise.

# Consider Other Factors Impacting Performance

Has your exercise performance been less than you had hoped for recently? Many different things can cause poor performance, but here are some potential causes (and solutions) to consider when you have diabetes and are athletically inclined.

## Inadequate Rest and Recovery Time

If you are doing well with your workouts but not with your performance during races and events, you may not be resting long enough to restore glycogen, repair muscle damage (caused by every workout), and fully recover beforehand. Cutting back on your workouts (tapering) for at least 1 to 2 days before a big event is critical. During that time, keep your blood glucose as close to normal as you can so your glycogen levels will be as full as possible for your race or event day.

## Compromised Blood Glucose Levels or Glycogen

Restoring your muscle glycogen between workouts takes eating enough calories or carbohydrates—and possibly extra time if you are eating a low-carbohydrate diet—and having enough insulin in your body that it works adequately. Doing longer and harder workouts can deplete your glycogen stores, and you may not be fully replenishing them fast enough because you are either not eating enough or not keeping your blood glucose in check. You must have an adequate amount of insulin on board to restore the glycogen in your liver and muscles.

## Low Body Iron Stores or Anemia

Having low body iron stores that result in *anemia* can cause you to feel tired all the time, colder than normal, and just generally lackluster. You can be iron deficient without having full-blown anemia. A simple blood test can check your *hemoglobin* (iron in red blood cells) and your overall iron status (*serum ferritins*). If your body's iron levels are low for any reason (such as having dialysis), taking iron supplements can help. So can eating more red meat, which has the most absorbable form of dietary iron.

## Low or Deficient Magnesium

Most adults with diabetes are magnesium deficient, especially when their blood glucose levels are higher than optimal, which causes more loss of magnesium through your urine. About 50 percent of the body's magnesium supply is found in the bone. Nearly another 50 percent is inside body tissue cells and organs, and less than 1 percent is in the blood. It is a critical mineral because it impacts over 300 enzyme-controlled steps in metabolism, including protein synthesis, muscle and nerve function, immune function, blood pressure regulation, and blood glucose management.

The symptoms of low body magnesium levels include agitation and anxiety, restless leg syndrome, sleep disorders, irritability, nausea and vomiting, abnormal heart rhythms, low blood pressure, confusion, muscle spasms and weakness, hyperventilation, insomnia, poor nail growth, and even seizures. Having a magnesium deficiency likely compromises your blood glucose and ability to exercise, and you may even experience some muscle cramping (unrelated to dehydration). Low magnesium can also lead to potassium imbalances.

Refining and overprocessing foods causes a loss of almost all the magnesium originally found in those foods, and the abundance of these magnesium-lacking foods has led to a widespread magnesium deficiency even among people without diabetes. You can eat more foods with magnesium in them naturally—such as nuts and seeds (especially almonds, walnuts, and Brazil nuts), dark leafy greens, legumes and beans, soymilk, yogurt, oats, avocados, fish, and even dark chocolate. However, taking a supplement may also help correct deficiencies in your diet. Magnesium in the aspartate, citrate, lactate, and chloride forms is absorbed better than magnesium oxide and sulfate. Slow-release magnesium supplements may also make it easier for you to keep your blood levels higher.

## B Vitamin Deficiency

With diabetes, thiamin (vitamin $B_1$) deficiency is also a likely culprit affecting your athletic performance, particularly if you are not eating a healthful diet. The eight vitamins in the B family are integrally involved in metabolism and even red blood cell formation. People who take metformin to control diabetes may end up deficient in vitamins $B_6$ and $B_{12}$, both of which are essential for proper nerve function and muscle contractions. Thiamin ($B_1$) is depleted by alcohol intake, birth control pill use, and more. Taking a generic B complex vitamin daily can help you avoid these issues, and excesses of most B vitamins are harmless (and simply urinated away).

## *Insulin Delivery Method and IGF*

Insulin pumps can help manage blood glucose and deliver rapid-acting insulin analogs like Humalog, Admelog, Novolog, Apidra, and Fiasp. The body metabolizes these altered insulins differently than it does long-acting Lantus, Toujeo, and Basaglar.

The rapid-acting insulin analogs that pumps use exclusively have little to no *insulin-like growth factor* (IGF) affinity, and most adults are reliant on IGF rather than human growth hormone (which is only higher in youth) to stimulate muscle growth and repair. Basically, IGF is critical to optimal recovery from workouts. Lantus and Basaglar apparently stimulate IGF activity more like human insulin, as does NPH. Levemir does not appear to have the same stimulation on IGF release, however.

If you are staying sore longer, feel like you are just not recovering well muscularly from your workouts, and are not using Lantus, Toujeo (Lantus at three times the concentration), or Basaglar, you may want to talk with your doctor about combining insulin pump use (for meal boluses or partial basal needs) with Lantus, Toujeo, or Basaglar (or possibly NPH) basal insulin injections to get more IGF activity to promote muscle repair between workouts.

> *Consider choosing Lantus, Basaglar, or Toujeo (all biosimilar) for your basal insulin needs because Levemir (another basal insulin) is less effective at raising your levels of IGF, which stimulates muscle growth and repair.*

## *Thyroid Hormone Issues*

Many people with diabetes also have thyroid hormone imbalances, some of which can be caused by another autoimmune condition. Having lower levels of functioning T3 and T4 (*thyroxine*) hormones can cause early fatigue and poor exercise performance, among other things. However, just checking the levels of thyroid hormones (T3 and T4) and the hormone that releases both (*thyroid-stimulating hormone*, or TSH) may not be enough. You may also want to consider getting your thyroid antibodies checked if your thyroid hormones are at normal levels and nothing else is helping your exercise training. Specifically, check for antibodies to *thyroid peroxidase*, especially if you have diagnosed celiac disease.

# What to Do If You Are Still Stumped

With diabetes as an added variable, the solution for improving your performance is not always simple and clear cut. If you have been through all the possibilities in the preceding sections and have had everything check out, consider other potential issues. The fix may be as simple as monitoring your hydration status and staying better hydrated, especially when your blood glucose runs higher. Or you may need to bump up your daily carbohydrate intake; adding even just 50 grams of carbohydrates per day to your diet may help get rid of fatigue. Also check for other possible vitamin and mineral deficiencies (vitamin D, potassium, and so on). If you use statins to lower your cholesterol, be aware that some statins cause unexplained muscle fatigue (see chapter 3), so you may need to talk with your doctor about trying a different one.

Your performance can also be affected by frequent hypoglycemia or hypoglycemia-associated autonomic failure (see chapter 2 for how to address that issue).

If you have made it this far in the book and learned even a little that helps you be a better athlete, then I have done my job well! The next chapter covers how to avoid injuries and best manage them (physically) when you do need to take some time to heal. Although all people serious about working out get injured at some point, there is nothing more annoying (to me at least) than getting yourself into the game only to be sidelined with an injury, or even with a low. Part II of this book (found in chapters 8 through 12) will give you real insight into how real-life individuals with diabetes manage their diabetes to perform at the top of their game during a variety of different fitness and recreational activities and sports.

## Athlete Profile: **Kris Freeman**

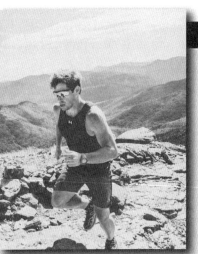

Courtesy of Kris Freeman.

**Hometown:** Campton, New Hampshire

**Diabetes history:** Type 1 diabetes diagnosed in 2000 (at age 19)

**Sport or activity:** Olympic cross-country skier, triathlete, adventure racer

**Greatest athletic achievement:** I was a 17-time U.S. national champion in cross-country skiing; in 2003, I won first place in the Under-23 division of the Classic Skiing World Championship; in 2003 and 2009, I was the fourth place finisher in the 15-kilometer Classic Event World Championship; and I finished fifth in the 2002 Olympic Winter Games as part of a U.S. 4-by-10-kilometer relay cross-country ski race (as the second leg of the race team). I raced on the U.S. Ski Team from 2002 to 2013 and at four consecutive Olympics, stretching from Salt Lake City in 2002 to Sochi in 2014. I had 10 individual top-10 World Cup results over the years and skied in eight consecutive World Championships.

**Current insulin and medication regimen:** I use an Omnipod insulin pump with a fairly simple basal regimen: overnight (8:00 p.m. to 7:00 a.m.) at 1.0 unit/hour, daytime hours at 0.7 units; these are my settings for when I'm training 1 to 2 hours per day.

**Training tips:** For me, having to train with type 1 diabetes means that every part of my day is planned toward my training. It makes it hard to be spontaneous. I try to eat my last meal 3 hours before I start training, and I eat a consistent, predictable amount. I reduce my basal rate some before going out, reduce it even more during the workout, but then raise it up again 30 minutes before ending. Waiting 3 hours after eating to train is not always feasible, so if I'm unable to wait that long for my insulin bolus to work its way out of my body, I will eat a lower carb meal that requires little insulin to absorb. Then while training I will plan to take on carbs since the small bolus in my system will demand extra carbohydrate as the insulin tail has a 3-hour duration. (The amount of carbs is modest, though, due to the small bolus needed for a high-protein/low-carb meal, and these extra carbs are really more like finishing my "meal" and not extra calories.)

I've got a constant math problem going on in my head on how to balance the insulin with the energy I need, along with my life stresses, what I did the day before, and whether I'm going hard or easy. It's a floating scale based on so many factors—a real balancing act. When I go into a race, I try to go into a controlled environment by controlling my food and my stress levels. It's still based somewhat on feel, on what's going on in my life, not always on one single formula.

*Typical daily and weekly training and diabetes regimen:* This is a typical week for me when I'm doing cross-country ski training, although I just retired from Olympic-level skiing, so I'm now mainly doing triathlon and adventure racing training.

► *Monday:* Morning workout, 3-hour roller skiing (which is as close to skiing as you can get with no snow as it's done on 2-foot-long skis with wheels); p.m. workout, 1-hour run (which is why I increase my basal rate at the end of my first workout so I can fuel back up between workouts).

► *Tuesday:* Morning workout, 2 hours of roller skiing including some speed work (20- to 30-second sprints); p.m. workout, 1-hour run followed by 45 minutes of low back and abdominal resistance exercises.

► *Wednesday:* Morning workout, 2-hour run with 45 minutes done at threshold (at "anaerobic threshold" or at 4 mmol/L lactate levels); p.m. workout, 1.5 hours of easy roller skiing.

► *Thursday:* Morning workout, 1-hour easy run or easy kayak recovery day (I do an easier recovery day after every 3 or 4 days of harder workouts).

► *Friday:* Morning workout, overdistance training consisting of a 4-hour run or 4 hours of roller skiing.

► *Saturday:* Morning workout, 2-hour run; p.m. workout, 1-hour kayak and 45 minutes of core strength exercises.

► *Sunday:* Morning workout, level 4 training (out of 5 levels; level 4 is done at race pace with lactate levels of 8 mmol/L) consisting of roller skiing 5 × 6-minute sprints for 30 minutes total (with 6-minute recovery periods between each one); p.m. workout, 1-hour mountain bike ride.

*Other hobbies and interests:* I like being outdoors and being active, so outdoor sports are most of my hobbies and interests. That's what I spend most of my time doing.

*Good diabetes and exercise story:* After my first Olympics, 2 years after being diagnosed with diabetes, I finally talked to my doctor about trends I was seeing during races. My blood glucose was climbing throughout my races despite my using a fairly aggressive basal rate. My doctor told me that it was due to the effects of stress hormones like adrenaline, coming from the exercise intensity being so high; he said that always happens. I asked him, "Why the hell didn't you tell me that before?" His reply was, "We didn't want to stress you out." Then I told him, "Withholding the information from me stresses me out. I need to know these things. Not knowing stresses me out!" Then he admitted to me that I was right, but that he never thought I was going to be able to compete in the Olympics anyway. He said, "I won't withhold info from you anymore." My reply was, "Good, then I won't have to fire you!" (He was a U.S. ski team

continued ➡

*Kris Freeman continued*

physician, not an endocrinologist by training, but still!) I did have a bad experience with the first two endocrinologists I saw; this one was actually more supportive than they had been.

My brother is also an Olympic cross-country skier and a runner—he's 4 years older. He used to like to map out hard trails in the New Hampshire mountains for us to train on. One time, he wanted to do this 32-mile run called the "Pemi loop" (short for Pemigewasset and hailed as the best multiday hike in the White Mountains). I agreed to do it—even though it was 7 hours long—and I remember spending a lot of time calculating how many carbs I needed to carry in my backpack and even brought along 50 percent extra just in case. My brother showed up to do it with only a 32-ounce Gatorade in his hand and said, "Let's do it!" I remember being envious of how much less planning he had to do to get ready to do anything athletic. Of course, with only a single Gatorade to refuel with during that 7-hour run, I was doing better than he was by the end of it.

# 7

# Preventing and Treating Athletic Injuries

If you exercise regularly, eventually you are likely to experience some kind of an athletic injury. Having diabetes also increases the likelihood of developing certain joint problems like frozen shoulder and trigger finger. The more you know about how to handle and prevent joint and other injuries—both acute and overuse ones—before they develop, the better off you will be. You will also benefit from knowing some tricks for preventing and treating delayed-onset muscle soreness and overuse syndrome discussed in this chapter, as well as exercise-associated muscle cramps. For the older athlete, arthritis can be another issue to deal with, along with simply dealing with other changes in your body as you get older.

## IDENTIFYING ACUTE AND OVERUSE INJURIES

Acute injuries are sudden, sharp, traumatic injuries that occur immediately (or within hours) and cause pain, most often resulting from obvious causes like an impact, fall, sprain, or collision or even carelessness (e.g., dropping a weight on your foot). Some examples are spraining your ankle, dislocating your shoulder, or pulling your hamstring muscle. Diabetes is not usually a contributing cause to these sorts of injuries unless you fall and injure yourself due to getting low or having changes in how you walk when you have neuropathy in your feet. In any case, if you experience sudden-onset joint pain, swelling, reduced range of motion, weakness, numbness, or tingling, stop what you are doing and treat your injury sooner rather than later.

*Never ignore acute pain in your knee, ankle, elbow, or wrist joints, which is most likely related to ligament (connection between bones) or tendon (muscle to bone) damage.*

If a specific point on a bone, muscle, or joint is painful (which you can check by pressing your finger on it), you may have a significant injury, especially if pushing on the mirror image spot on the other side of your body does not hurt. As for swelling, it is usually obvious and present with almost all acute sports injuries, such as twisting an ankle. The injury causes the affected areas to swell, which results in pain, stiffness, or a clicking sound as *ligaments*, which connect bones to other bones across joints, snap over one another when they have been pushed into a new position by the swelling. You will lose mobility around swollen joints and not be able to move them as far. Weakness on one side of your body but not the other is also a sign, along with numbness or tingling, likely related to compression of a nerve.

On the other hand, longer-term (chronic) injuries often result from excessive or repetitive training that causes an *overuse injury* or *overtraining syndrome*. These injuries are nagging and persistently uncomfortable. For instance, shoulder rotator cuff tendinitis tends to feel worse at night after you lie down, at which point you often experience a dull ache in the affected shoulder. Other common examples include tennis elbow (*lateral epicondylitis*), swimmer's shoulder (*rotator cuff tendinitis* and *rotator cuff impingement*), Little League elbow, runner's knee, jumper's knee (*infrapatellar tendinitis*), Achilles tendinitis, shin splints, and *plantar fasciitis*. In most sports and activities, overuse injuries are the most common and challenging to diagnose and treat, and they often worsen over time if neglected.

# IMMEDIATE AND CHRONIC TREATMENT OF INJURIES

Treatment of acute injuries is best handled with RICE—rest, ice, compression, and elevation. You never want to heat an acute injury because heat increases circulation and causes it to swell, which is what you are trying to limit with the ice, compression, and elevation.

Follow these steps for treatment of an acute injury:

- Immediately stop whatever activity you are doing.
- Wrap the injured area in a compression (Ace) bandage.
- Apply ice (using a bag of crushed ice or even a bag of frozen peas) for 15 minutes, let the area warm back up, and reapply the ice two or three times total, as much you can tolerate it.
- Elevate your injured joint to reduce swelling; if it is your ankle, try to get it up higher than the level of your heart (or at least even with it).
- See a physician for proper diagnosis and treatment of any serious injury.

## Reducing Inflammation With Medications

Taking anti-inflammatory medications, otherwise known as *nonsteroidal, anti-inflammatory drugs* (NSAIDs), many of which are available in drugstores without a prescription, is often helpful. Aspirin, ibuprofen (sold as Advil or Nuprin in the United States), and naproxen (Aleve) all fight inflammation and reduce pain, but acetaminophen (commonly sold as Tylenol) limits only pain. Your doctor may also prescribe stronger anti-inflammatory medications to use initially. Some inflammation is probably helpful to and necessary for speedy healing, so sparingly use any anti-inflammatory medications and try to get by with as few as you can to avoid slowing down the natural healing process.

> *Follow RICE to treat both acute and overuse injuries (after workouts that aggravate the latter), and consider (sparingly) treating them with NSAIDs.*

If an affected area becomes inflamed enough that you cannot control it with rest and NSAIDs or prescription pain medications, or if it is painful for several weeks without any improvement, you may want to look into having a cortisone injection to relieve pain and joint tenderness. Keep in mind that although such injections are localized, they can affect your whole body, and most cortisone preparations increase insulin resistance (and, therefore, your blood glucose levels). For instance, Kenalog, a common steroid, may bump your blood glucose up into the range of 300 to 400 mg/dL (16.7 to 22.2 mmol/L); others, like Depomedrol, may cause fewer problems, raising them only into the 200s (11.0 to 16.0 mmol/L) until the steroid wears off after a few weeks. Whether you take insulin or other medications, you may need to increase your doses temporarily to cover these glycemic effects.

## Using Cold Therapies

Ice therapy is arguably the best immediate treatment for acute injuries because it reduces swelling and pain by causing blood vessels in the iced area to constrict, which also limits fluid influx into the area. When using this therapy, you should apply ice to the affected area for 10 to 15 minutes at a time, several times a day, and for up to 3 days. If you treat a chronic injury with ice, use it after (not before) activities to prevent or reduce inflammation and pain. The easiest method is to use an ice or cold pack that conforms to the shape of the area that you are icing down, but you can also use a bag of frozen veggies (like peas), ice frozen in a paper cup (you peel down the edge of the cup as the ice melts), or a bag of ice wrapped in a thin towel for comfort.

> *Ice or cold therapy works well on acute injuries and for reducing pain after workouts with chronic injuries. Only use heat therapy for chronic injuries and other conditions where you do not have any inflammation and swelling (like for sore joints or stiffness).*

## When Should You Heat Your Injuries?

Most athletes know to apply ice to an acute injury like a sprained ankle but are not so sure when to use heat instead. If anything is hurting (either an acute or chronic injury) after a workout, use ice. Heat is better for chronic injuries or injuries without inflammation and swelling, such as sore joints, stiffness, or nagging pain. Using heat therapy before exercise may even increase the elasticity of your joints' connective tissues, stimulate blood flow, or relax tight muscles and spasms. Apply heat for 15 to 20 minutes at a time, and put enough layers between your skin and the heating source to prevent burns, particularly if you are heating an area in which you have lost some of your sensation (e.g., neuropathic feet) and would be unlikely to realize if it is too hot. Moist heat is best, so you can use a hot wet towel. You can also use special athletic hot packs or heating pads, but never leave them on for more than 20 minutes at a time or while sleeping. Heated whirlpools and spas are also effective, but avoid using them if you have open sores or ulcers on your feet or lower legs.

# OVERUSE INJURIES AND OVERTRAINING: CAUSES AND TREATMENT

By definition, an *overuse injury* is caused by excessive use of a particular joint. Overuse injuries are, unfortunately, more common if you have diabetes because of structural changes in your joints caused by spikes or elevations in your blood glucose over time. But regardless of the cause, all overuse injuries are treated the same way. What's more, their onset can usually be linked to changes in athletic endeavors or training techniques. For example, if you have been running 3 miles (5 kilometers) several days a week at a moderate pace and then you suddenly start running 5 miles (8 kilometers) 6 days a week at a faster pace than before, you are setting yourself up for an overuse injury. Make only gradual increases in your training duration, frequency, or intensity so that your body will have time to adapt. Exercise is all about causing damage to your muscles to stimulate rebuilding them stronger, faster, or fitter—a result that can occur only if you allow adequate time for recovery and recuperation of both muscles and joints.

> *All athletes have a higher chance of getting an overuse injury at some point due to overstressing muscles, joints, and bones with repetitive or damaging movements, particularly by rapidly increasing their training. Having diabetes raises your risk of getting one as well.*

Some people are prone to developing overuse injuries, but their development is often related to anatomical, biomechanical, or even training considerations. For instance, imbalances between your strength and flexibility around certain joints (e.g., quads versus hamstring strength) can predispose you to hamstring pulls. Uneven body alignment, such as knock-knees, bowed legs, unequal leg lengths, and flat or high-arched feet, can also contribute to a greater risk. Even having old injuries leads to a greater likelihood of overuse injuries. Other factors matter as well, such as the type of running shoes you use, the terrain you work out on (hilly, flat, or uneven), and whether you exercise on hard surfaces like concrete roads or hard floors or softer ones like grass, dirt or gravel trails, asphalt, or cushioned floors.

Many overuse injuries involve inflammation of an area, or redness, soreness, and swelling, which you can identify by the use of "itis" at the end of its name. In general, *tendinitis* is inflammation of any *tendons*, which attach muscles to bones—it is a very common overuse injury that results from a tendon rubbing repeatedly against a bony structure, ligament, or another tendon or from being impinged. *Tennis elbow* is a type of tendinitis located on the outside of the elbow common in tennis players, along with rowers, carpenters, gardeners, golfers, and other exercisers who repeatedly bend their elbows forcefully. Swimmers often develop tendinitis and other impingement syndromes in the *rotator cuff* (shoulder) because of the overhead movement required by the sport. In sports that involve running and jumping, tendinitis often occurs in the knee, foot, and Achilles (heel) tendons. The more common athletic overuse injuries, symptoms, and treatments are listed in table 7.1.

**Table 7.1   Common Athletic Overuse Injuries, Symptoms, and Treatments**

| Injury | Area Affected | Symptoms | Treatment and Prevention |
|---|---|---|---|
| Carpal tunnel syndrome | Wrist (inside) | Pain, weakness, or numbness in hand and wrist, loss of grip strength | Rest, ice, NSAIDs, surgery if lasts longer than 6 months |
| Tennis elbow | Outside of the elbow | Painful to touch or bump, pain when shaking hands or turning a doorknob | Rest, ice, NSAIDs, use of a strap around the upper forearm, using a two-handed tennis backhand, exercises |
| Rotator cuff tendinitis | Shoulder | Pain when lifting arms, or brushing or combing hair | Rest, ice, NSAIDs, stretching and strengthening exercises |
| Chondromalacia patella | Knee | Knee pain made worse by bending the knees, doing full squats, or sitting for long periods with bent knees | Rest, ice, NSAIDs, strengthening the inner quads with weight training |
| Iliotibial band syndrome (ITBS) | Knee | Pain along the outside part of the knee or lower thigh | Rest, ice, gentle stretching (iliotibial band and gluteal muscles), running on both sides of the road, wearing proper shoes |
| Shin splints | Front of lower legs, along the tibia bone | Generalized pain along the bones of lower leg | Rest, ice, NSAIDs, slow progression of training program, avoidance of running on hard surfaces |
| Stress fractures | Metatarsal bones of the foot, lower leg bones (tibia, fibula), calcaneus (heel bone), talus (ankle bone) | Localized pain at the point of fracture (tender to the touch), swelling | Rest, ice, use of supportive shoe or boot, limited or modified activity for 6 to 8 weeks |
| Plantar fasciitis | Heel, bottom of foot (arch) | Heel pain during first steps each morning and after periods of inactivity | Rest, ice, NSAIDs, stretching and massaging the plantar fascia, exercises |
| Achilles tendinitis | Heel and calves | Pain in the heels and tight calf muscles | Rest, ice, NSAIDs, frequent stretching of the calves and thighs, limited wearing of high-heeled shoes |

Having diabetes makes you more prone to developing overuse injuries with a slower onset that can limit movement around joints, ones that may not be specifically related to any exercise training that you are doing. Common injuries are shoulder *adhesive capsulitis* (frozen shoulder), *carpal tunnel syndrome* (wrist pain), *metatarsal fractures* (broken foot bones), and neuropathy-related joint disorders (e.g., Charcot foot) in people with peripheral neuropathy. *Trigger finger*, which results in a curled finger due to shortening of ligaments, usually requires cortisone injections or surgery to release the contracture. People who have had diabetes for a long time are additionally prone to nerve compression syndromes at the elbow and wrist that may be aggravated by repetitive activities, prolonged gripping, or direct nerve compression during weight training, cycling, and other activities. In most cases, good management of your blood glucose can reduce your risk for developing these injuries.

> Remember these words of wisdom from former ultradistance runner with type 1 diabetes Missy Foy: "Try everything in practice that might come up in a race. My coach always said that they call it practice for a reason. Also, do not always assume that diabetes is the problem. We still have to train our way to achievement, and we end up with the same problems and injuries that athletes without diabetes encounter."

## Preventing Overuse Injuries

If your nagging aches and pains are only minor, simply cutting back on how hard, how often, and how long you do the activities that irritate your joints may bring relief from your symptoms. In other words, give your joints a rest! One way to prevent problems in the first place is to adopt a hard–easy workout schedule in which you alternate and vary your workouts by the day to avoid stressing your joints in the same way with every workout. If your problems are being caused by anatomical concerns, fix what you can (such as getting orthotics to correct leg-length discrepancies) and then consider doing other activities that do not cause as much risk of injury, such as working out on an elliptical trainer a few days a week instead of always running outdoors on concrete or asphalt. In addition, working with a coach or taking lessons may help you improve your training and techniques to lower your injury risk. Make sure to do a proper warm-up and cool-down, ice down inflamed joints after workouts, and use NSAIDs when absolutely necessary to control inflammation and pain.

You may also benefit from cross-training while you are recovering from an injury. Do other activities to maintain your fitness as long as they do not overly stress any injured areas. For example, if you have lower-leg pain, work out your upper body by doing activities that allow your legs to recuperate and heal. Even before you ever get an overuse injury, try alternating weight-bearing activities like walking or running with non-weight-bearing ones, such as swimming, upper-body work, and stationary cycling so that you can avoid overworking and injuring any areas of your body. Doing cross-training (i.e., not doing the same type or intensity of activity every day, but rather alternating workouts on different days) allowed me personally to go over 25 years at one point without an overuse injury of any type, even though I had gotten them frequently earlier in my athletic career.

*After you resume your normal activities, work to strengthen the muscles around the previously injured joint to prevent recurrence of overuse, especially after tendinitis.*

Strengthening the muscles around an affected joint, after the pain is gone, is critical to preventing the return of the problem. For example, after a shoulder joint injury like rotator cuff tendinitis or impingement, focus on doing resistance work using all sections of the deltoid muscle in the shoulder in particular, along with strengthening exercises for your biceps, triceps, pectoral muscles, upper-back muscles, and neck muscles. Here are some other helpful suggestions for preventing injuries.

- Never bounce during stretches because doing so can cause injuries, although dynamic stretching (stretching during gentle movement) is fine.
- If you have not exercised in a while, start slowly and progress cautiously to avoid delayed-onset muscle soreness (DOMS) or an acute injury.
- Warm up with easier work before you begin to exercise more vigorously to get your joints more mobile and blood flowing to active muscles.
- Choose an exercise that suits your condition; for example, swimming might be suitable if you are recovering from an ankle or knee injury.
- Vary your exercise program or try out new activities; doing so emphasizes different muscle groups and joints and increases your overall fitness.
- Cross-train to reduce the risk of injury by varying muscle and joint usage.
- Alternate hard and easy workout days to allow adequate recovery and repair to occur between harder workouts.
- Wear appropriate shoes and socks, and check your feet daily after you exercise for areas of redness or irritation.
- Avoid going back to your normal activities until your injury symptoms have almost completely gone away.
- For best results do not forget to always cool down after workouts; stretching afterward (or anytime muscles are warmer) may also be easier to do.

# Choosing the Proper Footwear

Wearing proper shoes is critical to preventing many lower-extremity and foot problems. The best type of shoes to wear varies by the activity. Walkers and runners generally need some cushioning, whereas tennis players require footwear with greater stability during their side-to-side movements. For most fitness activities, you will also benefit by picking your shoes based on whether you rotate on your feet toward the arch of your foot or toward the outside edge.

To determine how you step, look at the wear pattern on your shoes. For example, exercisers who are *pronators* (meaning that they rotate their feet too far toward the inside arch) or who have flat feet or carry a lot of extra body weight will wear out the insides of their soles first. If you have this problem, motion control shoes may help. Generally heavy but durable, they are rigid, control-oriented running shoes that have firm midsoles designed to limit overpronation; they also come in varieties with more cushioning. If your shoes do not compensate for overpronation, you may place extra stress on your knees, hips, and ankles that can result in injuries.

Conversely, *supinators* usually have high arches and more rigid feet and thus wear out the soles of their shoes along the outside edge. If you are a supinator, you will generally do better wearing highly cushioned shoes with plenty of flexibility to encourage foot motion. If you have normal arches, you will want to aim for shoes with moderate control, such as those with a two-density midsole. If you are unsure which type of arches your feet have, wet your feet and make a footprint to see how much of the arch region of your foot shows (the less that shows, the higher your arch).

## Recognizing and Treating Overtraining Syndrome

*Overtraining syndrome* frequently occurs in athletes who are training for competition or a specific event without allowing adequate time for rest and recuperation. Becoming more fit and improving your performance is a balancing act between training and recovering from it. You are never stronger or faster right after your workout, but rather after your body has repaired the damage that you did with the exercise. Overloading your body excessively without enough recovery time can result in both physical and psychological symptoms.

The symptoms of overtraining are not hard to recognize when you know what to look for. They include chronic tiredness, lethargy, soreness and aches, chronic pain in your muscles and joints, an unexpected drop in your performance, insomnia, an increased number of colds and upper-respiratory tract infections, mild depression, and general malaise (not feeling well).

> *To determine whether you have overtraining syndrome, measure your resting heart rate first thing in the morning. If it is increasing over time, you are likely overtraining.*

Getting sick more frequently means that excessive training is compromising your immune function, and because overtraining results in elevated levels of cortisol, you may have more problems managing your blood glucose as well. If you start feeling chronically tired, drained, and lacking in energy, cut back on your training schedule a bit and see whether that helps—if you are overtraining, it will. Cross-training (or just doing different activities) can also help if you are overworking certain muscles or joints, and it may help you maintain or improve your psychological outlook. Total recovery from overtraining can take several weeks. Make sure you get proper nutrition and reduce your stress to aid your recovery.

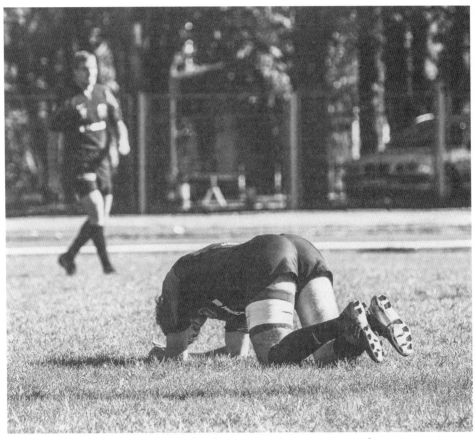

Ignoring minor overuse injuries can lead to more serious ones, so make sure to rest appropriately or cut back on the intensity of your exercise to give your body a chance to heal between workouts and events.

# Common Arm and Shoulder Issues

The most common problems affecting the arms and shoulders are carpal tunnel syndrome (wrist), tennis elbow (lateral epicondylitis), rotator cuff tendinitis in the shoulder, and frozen shoulder (i.e., adhesive capsulitis). Most, but not all, involve tendinitis, which occurs more commonly in diabetes because the glycation of collagen structures in your joints can limit their mobility and result in minor swelling and inflammation of tendons. Other problems stem from impingement syndromes or inflammation of other joint-related structures and tissues such as ligaments, fascia, and bursas.

## *Carpal Tunnel Syndrome*

*Carpal tunnel syndrome* results from a squeezing of the *median nerve*, which runs from your forearm down into the palm of your hand. That nerve controls sensations to your thumb and most fingers, as well as impulses to some small muscles in the hand that allow your fingers and thumb to move. The carpal tunnel is a narrow passageway that contains ligaments, tendons, and the median nerve. When the area becomes inflamed from overuse, your nerve is compressed, resulting in pain, weakness, or numbness in your hand and wrist that can radiate up your arm.

Symptoms often first appear in one or both hands during the night because sleeping with flexed wrists aggravates the condition. Your grip strength will suffer, and you may have trouble forming a fist, grasping small objects, or doing other things with your hands. Carpal tunnel syndrome is more common in the dominant hand and in women because their carpal tunnel area is smaller. Contributing factors include trauma or injury to your wrist that causes swelling, mechanical problems in your wrist joint, repeated use of vibrating hand tools, and fluid retention during pregnancy or menopause, among others. Carpal tunnel problems can be treated by wearing a wrist brace (to prevent wrist flexion, which I had to wear during some of my first pregnancy), by icing the area, by taking NSAIDs, and sometimes by having surgery when your pain lasts longer than 6 months. Doing stretching and strengthening exercises for your wrist can help prevent its recurrence.

### Tennis Elbow

Technically known as *lateral epicondylitis*, this overuse injury is literally a pain in your elbow, mainly where your forearm muscles attach to the bony prominence on the outside (*epicondyle*). The symptoms include pain that radiates from the outside of your elbow into your forearm and wrist (especially if you touch or bump that area) or that occurs when you extend your wrist, a weak grip (not good for your tennis game!), and discomfort in that area when you shake hands or turn a door-knob. Repeatedly contracting your forearm muscles can cause it, as can playing tennis and using poor technique with your backhand stroke; if you use a two-handed backstroke, you are much less likely to develop tennis elbow. But it is not just tennis that you have to worry about. You can get tennis elbow from repeatedly twisting a screwdriver, hammering, painting, raking, weaving, playing string instruments, and more. The typical treatments apply, such as rest, ice, and use of NSAIDs to reduce pain and inflammation. Many athletes find that wearing an adjustable strap or brace around the top of the forearm helps keep the pain from coming back again. You will also want to do elbow stretches and strengthening exercises after the pain is gone as a preventive measure.

### Athletic Shoulder Issues

Your shoulders can experience a variety of problems resulting from athletic pursuits, such as rotator cuff tendinitis, bursitis, and impingement syndrome. These conditions have similar symptoms and often occur together. For instance, if the rotator cuff and bursas are irritated, inflamed, and swollen, they may become impinged, or squeezed, between the head of the *humerus* (the long upper-arm bone) and the *acromion process* (a bony structure in the shoulder). Repeated motion involving your arms over many years may also irritate the tendons, muscles, ligaments, and surrounding tissue.

In tendinitis of the shoulder, the rotator cuff and biceps tendons can become inflamed, usually due to being pinched by surrounding structures. When the rotator cuff tendon becomes inflamed and thickens, it may become trapped under the acromion process. If squeezing occurs, you get impingement syndrome. Tendinitis and impingement syndrome are often accompanied by inflammation of the bursa sacs that protect the shoulder, or *bursitis*. Sports that involve overuse of the shoulder (like swimming and volleyball) and occupations that require frequent overhead movements are other potential causes of irritation to these structures and may lead to inflammation and impingement.

Slow onset of pain in the upper shoulder or upper arm and difficulty sleeping on that shoulder are symptoms, as is pain when you try to lift your arm away from your body in certain directions or overhead. Treatment normally includes rest, ice, and NSAIDs, but it can also involve physical therapy, gentle stretching, and exercises to strengthen the muscles surrounding your shoulder joint. If you do not experience improvement in 6 to 12 months, you may be a candidate for arthroscopic surgery to repair damage and relieve pressure on the tendons and bursas.

### Frozen Shoulder, or Adhesive Capsulitis

Frozen shoulder is a condition that usually results from inflammation, scarring, thickening, and shrinkage of the capsule that surrounds your shoulder joint. Any injury to your shoulder can lead to frozen shoulder, including tendinitis, bursitis, or rotator cuff problems. Unlike those overuse injuries, however, frozen shoulder (*adhesive capsulitis*, which is also possible in the hip joints) usually limits the ability to move your shoulder in all directions, not just specific ones.

Frozen shoulder usually involves three stages. Initially, the pain increases with movement and is usually worse at night, much like you get with rotator cuff tendinitis. But you will likely experience a progressive loss of motion around your shoulder joint in all directions, with increasing pain for 2 to 9 months. Stage 2 involves diminishing pain and more comfortable movement of your arm, but the trade-off is a more limited range of motion for 4 to 12 months. Finally, in the last stage, most people experience gradual restoration of motion over the next 12 to 42 months, although some may need surgery to restore more normal movement.

Treating a frozen shoulder often involves a combination of anti-inflammatory medications, cortisone injection, and physical therapy. If you do not treat it aggressively, a frozen shoulder can become permanent. Physical therapy is often the key and includes treatments like ultrasound, electrical stimulation, icing, and range-of-motion and strengthening exercises. Months of physical therapy may be required for full recovery, depending on the severity of the scarring of the tissues around your shoulder. You should also try not to reinjure your shoulder during its rehabilitation—avoid sudden, jerking motions or heavy lifting.

## Knee and Shin Issues

Knees are critical joints for movement. They are made up of a conglomeration of tendons, ligaments, cartilage (meniscal padding), a joint capsule, a sliding kneecap (*patella*), synovial fluid, and more. Your athletic knees can get all sorts of aches and pains, including chondromalacia patella, iliotibial band syndrome (ITBS), ligament and meniscal tears, and shin pain, to name a few. The origin of each is different, although most of the treatments for these injuries are similar.

## An Athlete's Account of Frozen Shoulders

Delaine Wright of Hopkinton, Rhode Island, recalls her experience with getting frozen shoulders: "In truth, with my first frozen shoulder, I had no idea what was going on. It came on gradually, and by the time I realized what was happening, I couldn't put my hands in my back pockets, struggled with bra clasps, and eventually couldn't put a coat on without cringing (and even at times bursting into tears) from the pain. I couldn't lie down flat at night because of it, and for more than a year, I slept sitting straight up in bed propped up on five or more pillows because it felt better when I was nearly upright. I felt 80 years old! My husband and I had a few laughs over it, but sometimes even the shaking of a laugh hurt.

My shoulder range of motion was so bad that with my arms out straight, I couldn't raise my hand any higher than just below my shoulder. But the worst part was the pain. I tried everything: physical therapy (the most painful thing), chiropractic manipulation (which I do not suggest), and more. The only thing that got me past the most painful point was a cortisone injection that included novocaine, and I had two of those months apart. During that time I kept up with the physical therapy—doing active and passive stretches, especially the gravity-assisted ones, light-weight one-arm hangs, and others. I found valerian root and heating helpful at night to sleep, and I regularly got a massage. I also used flaxseed (oil and ground up) and still do to assist in decreasing inflammation (I think it helps). I experienced about a 4-month painful freezing stage, followed by eventual regression and slow return of my shoulder movement, but the whole process took about a year.

"Just as I was getting over the one shoulder, the other started. The second time wasn't as bad, although whether that was because I knew what to expect and immediately did what worked for me the first time (the analgesic and cortisone injections, stretching, but no formal physical therapy) or because the second shoulder was a milder case, I'm not sure. Although I have never fully returned to my pre–frozen shoulder motion and am definitely stiff, at least the pain is gone. Regular yoga practice helps, along with my trapeze and aerial exercise. I've just accepted that there are some things that I will never be able to do anymore even though I'm not that old. I can't externally rotate my shoulders like most people can—I can barely accomplish a backbend because I can't get my arms in that rotated, over-the-head position, and I can't exactly manage some of the Ashtanga yoga arm wraps and such—but I suppose that's okay. I accept my body and its limitations.

"I was always looking for the answer as to why my frozen shoulders happened, but I never found it. I had never had a prior shoulder injury, and my blood glucose has always been well managed. The whole experience certainly allowed me to appreciate the complexity of the shoulder. The good news is that it does go away eventually (with some intervention), but I'll never take my shoulders for granted again."

### *Chondromalacia Patella*

Also known as *patellofemoral syndrome*, this overuse injury is the most common cause of chronic knee pain. It results from poor alignment of the kneecap as it slides back and forth over the lower end of the *femur*, or thigh bone, whenever you bend your knee. If you have this, your patella tracks abnormally during bending, sliding toward the *lateral* (outside) edge of the femur instead of straight. You may feel some discomfort in your inner knee area related to the resulting inflammation that is made worse by activities like running, jumping, climbing or descending stairs, and prolonged sitting with bent knees (like in airplane seats). If you are experiencing pain, you will want to avoid activities that irritate it and use ice and NSAID therapy. One thing that can help is selectively strengthening the inner part of your quadriceps (front of thigh) muscles with resistance training. In addition, you should avoid doing full squats (bending your knees to a 90-degree angle), particularly when you are using weights; do quarter squats instead.

If you have "runner's knee" and are unsure of the cause of the pain, you can start by assuming that it is an overuse injury and treat it as such. Treatments include rest, icing your knee, doing quarter squats to strengthen the quadriceps muscles, stretching your iliotibial band, replacing your running shoes every 350 to 500 miles (550 to 800 kilometers), and possibly getting orthotics for your shoes.

## Iliotibial Band Syndrome

*Iliotibial band syndrome*, also known as ITBS, is an overuse injury that causes an ache or burning sensation on the outside of your knee, most often during physical activity but also later or if you turn your knee. The iliotibial (IT) band consists of tough fibers that run the length of the outside of your thigh, attaching to your buttock (*gluteal*) and hip abductor (*tensor fasciae latae*) muscles at the top, crossing the knee, and attaching to the *tibia*, or shin bone, at the lower end. Its primary function is to act as a stabilizer during movement.

This syndrome is common among runners and cyclists, but is also associated with weightlifting (especially doing squats), practicing the lotus yoga posture (sitting with your legs crossed, your feet on top of your thighs), hiking, excessive hill or stair running, rowing, breaststroke, and treading water (eggbeater kick). Running on a sloped surface (on the side of the road or the beach) can aggravate the IT band because it tilts your pelvis, but so can excessive pronation of your foot, leg-length discrepancy, lateral pelvic tilt, bowed legs, and tight gluteal or quadriceps muscles. Apparently, friction occurs as or just after your foot hits the ground when you are running. Downhill running in particular reduces the knee flexion angle and can aggravate it, whereas sprinting increases the angle and is less harmful.

Treatment includes rest, ice, correcting your training errors, wearing good shoes and orthotics, massage, and gentle stretching, particularly of the IT band itself and gluteal muscles. To stretch your IT band, cross your right leg over your left while standing and extend your left arm against a wall or another stable object. Push your right hip in the opposite direction while leaning your weight to your left toward the wall. Your right foot should remain stable, but allow your left knee to flex. If you are doing it correctly, you will feel the stretch in your right hip and down the outside of that leg (along the IT band).

## Knee Ligament and Meniscal Tears

Although usually more of an acute injury, tears in either the ligaments supporting your knee or the cartilage cushion there require prolonged treatment and often surgery. Ligaments are more easily injured in sports with rapid starts and stops and quick directional changes, such as basketball. The *anterior cruciate ligament* (ACL) and the *medial collateral ligament* (MCL) are the most often injured, but the *posterior cruciate* (PCL) and *lateral collateral* (LCL) ligaments can also be affected. During an acute injury, you will often hear a loud popping noise that may or may not be accompanied by pain. A magnetic resonance imaging (MRI) scan is usually required to confirm these tears, and nowadays arthroscopic surgery, which is minimally invasive, is used to treat partial tears.

If you tear the cartilage in your knee, you have usually torn a *meniscus*, which is a small, *C*-shaped piece of cartilage that serves as a cushion between the thigh (femur) and tibia (shin) bones on both sides of your knee; the *lateral meniscus* is the outside one, the *medial meniscus* is on the inside. You can tear these alone or along with one of the ligaments (most often the ACL) as a result of twisting or pivoting with your foot planted, by decelerating, or by a sudden impact. Manual tests can determine whether it is torn, but often your tear must be confirmed (and treated) arthroscopically.

### Shin Splints

Although not a specific diagnosis, *shin splints* result from generalized pain that occurs in the front of the lower leg along the shin bone (tibia). This injury has a number of different potential causes, but it is most likely a cumulative stress injury that occurs from overtraining or excessive running on hard surfaces, resulting in inflammation in those areas or stress fractures in the tibia or fibula (lower leg bones). Your bones can heal themselves over time, but if you do not rest them after a crack starts to appear, they can fracture fully. If you are a beginning runner, you have a higher risk of developing shin splints and stress fractures because you are less accustomed to the high impact of running.

How can you tell whether you have shin splints? Watch out for pain on the medial (inside) part of your lower leg that gets worse with running or other weight-bearing exercise (especially on hard surfaces). Other symptoms are an aching pain that lingers after exercise, as well as increased pain with activity such as running, jumping, hill climbing, or downhill running. Taking all your runs along the edge of the ocean on the packed sand while barefoot is a sure way to get this type of overuse injury!

Generally, icing your shins after workouts, taking NSAIDs, and resting are effective ways to treat it. Return to your activities gradually, using pain as your guide. Get new, well-cushioned shoes with adequate support to lower your risk. Also, make sure you stretch properly, warm up effectively, train moderately, progress your workout schedule conservatively, and avoid running or jumping on hard surfaces or running for long distances on tilted or slanted surfaces. If the pain does not subside using these treatments or if you have a single point of intense pain, consider seeing a podiatrist with expertise in lower extremities and diabetes to pinpoint the exact cause.

## Foot and Ankle Injuries

Given the large amount of stress placed on your feet and ankles, they are also a common site of overuse injuries, including plantar fasciitis, chronic sprains, Achilles tendon problems, blisters, calluses, and ulcers. For people with diabetes, particularly if they lose some of the feeling in their feet, blisters, calluses, and ulcers can lead to larger problems, possibly even gangrene and the need for amputation. In some cases, foot deformities (e.g., *Charcot foot*) are more likely to develop after a sprain and continued walking when you have neuropathy; at such times, you may need a foot cast to heal properly. In addition, people with diabetes have a greater risk of fractures of the long bones of the feet (*metatarsals*), likely because of the potential for loss of calcium and other minerals from long-term diabetes. In athletes without neuropathy, though, plantar fasciitis is the biggest concern, followed by problems with your Achilles tendons and stress fractures.

## Plantar Fasciitis

An inflammatory overuse injury, *plantar fasciitis* is the most common cause of heel pain. It is usually recognizable by your first steps in the morning being painful. Your feet are extended when you sleep (in a position called *plantar flexion*), which allows the fascia that makes up the underside of your foot to shorten. You may feel pain when you start an activity, which generally goes away and then returns after a long rest when you restart being active. Plantar fasciitis is common in runners and in those who gain weight quickly, because the plantar fascia runs the length of the inside of your arch; it is stretched to flatten your arch slightly each time your heel hits the ground. The plantar fascia is not very flexible, so repetitive stretching from impact can result in small tears in the fascia that become inflamed.

You are more likely to get this injury if you have very flat feet or high arches, excessive pronation (tipping your ankle inward), a tight Achilles tendon, obesity, or a sudden weight gain. You can also get it from a rapid increase in your workout intensity or duration, wearing shoes with poor cushioning, changing your usual running or walking surface, or standing for excessively long periods. An athlete from Mesa, Arizona, with type 2 diabetes found out the hard way that you can also develop this problem from not wearing shoes at all. Her fitness routine includes doing an active video game on Wii Fit, which she did in her socks until she developed plantar fasciitis. After taking 2 months off, she now only does the game wearing proper athletic shoes.

If you find yourself with plantar fasciitis, taking NSAIDs can help control the inflammation and pain. In addition, take some time off from the activities that are most irritating, including walking barefoot on hard surfaces. It may also help to stretch the plantar fascia and massage that area by rolling your foot over a 3- to 4-inch (8- to 10-centimeter) diameter tube like a rolling pin or a soup can or tennis ball. You can also try taping your heel and arch and using inside arch supports and supportive athletic shoes.

A new stretching technique may reduce heel pain when performed several times a day. To do it, you need to cross one leg over the other, pull your toes toward your shin for a count of 10, and repeat 10 times. To prevent recurrence, try doing strengthening exercises, such as scrunching up a hand towel with your toes or pulling a towel weighted with a soup can across the floor. After exercise, ice your heel for 15 to 20 minutes to relieve pain.

## Achilles Tendinitis

This type of tendinitis is caused by inflammation, irritation, and swelling of the Achilles tendon, which connects your two calf muscles (*gastrocnemius* and *soleus*) to your heel bone (calcaneus). You use these muscles for pushing off your foot or going up on your toes and for walking and running. As an overuse injury, this type occurs most commonly in walkers, runners, and basketball and volleyball players because of the large amount of stress that jumping puts on this tendon. As you age, you can also experience Achilles tendon problems from arthritis, which can cause extra bony growths on the heel (spurs) that inflame the tendon. Having an inflammation in this area also increases your risk for experiencing rupturing of your Achilles tendon, correctable only with surgery.

The usual treatments include rest, ice, NSAIDs, exercises, and occasionally a cast, boot, or brace worn to keep this tendon from moving and becoming more inflamed before the swelling goes down. To prevent Achilles tendinitis, progress slowly when starting an exercise program after being inactive for a while and make sure to stretch your calves and thigh muscles properly. Also keep in mind that long-term statin use may weaken this tendon in some people and make it more prone to rupture.

Another point of caution is relevant if you have been wearing high-heeled shoes and switch to flats. Your Achilles tendon and lower leg muscles adapt to a shortened position because the high-heeled shoes prevent your heel from stretching down to ground level; putting on flat shoes to exercise causes your tendon to stretch farther than it is accustomed to, which can cause it to become inflamed. If you wear high heels regularly, stretch your calves every morning and night to keep this tendon a more normal length to prevent problems.

## Stress Fractures

A stress fracture is a small, incomplete crack in a bone or severe bruising within it. Most are caused by overuse and repetitive activity and are most common in runners and athletes who participate in sports like soccer and basketball. You are most likely to get a stress fracture when you change your activities—such as doing a new exercise, ramping up your workout intensity, or using a different workout surface—but also if you train with improper form or worn out shoes with less cushioning. Sometimes thinning bones (from osteoporosis) can contribute to your risk of getting these, along with use of certain medications (like insulin sensitizers) that can weaken bones. But even just doing everyday activities can lead you to get a stress fracture.

Bones are in a constant state of turnover (*remodeling*), where new bone is constantly being formed after being stressed during physical activity. If your training is more than your bones can handle—meaning that the breakdown of bone occurs more rapidly than its replacement—then your bones may thin and weaken. Overuse stress fractures typically occur when you repeat an athletic movement so often that your weight-bearing bones and supporting muscles do not have enough time to heal between training sessions. The most susceptible bones are the ones in your feet, ankles, and lower legs (see the prior discussion on shin splints for the latter). Stress fractures in the second and third metatarsals (long bones) in the feet are common because that is where you get the greatest impact from pushing off when you walk or run. When you are active, you can also frequently get them in your heel (*calcaneus*), outer lower leg (fibula), ankle (*talus*), and midfoot (*navicular*) bones.

How should you treat a stress fracture? It typically takes from 6 to 8 weeks to fully heal. In addition to initially following the RICE protocol and taking NSAIDs, you may benefit from using crutches to keep weight off your foot or lower leg until most of the pain subsides. Depending on the site of the fracture, you may also need to wear protective footwear, such as a stiff-soled shoe or sandal or a removable short-leg fracture brace shoe or boot. Stress fractures in the fifth metatarsal foot bone (on the outer side) or in the navicular or talus bones may require a foot cast to keep your bones in a fixed position for a time.

You can remain active during the healing process by doing modified activities. Refrain from doing any high-impact exercise until it heals because going back too soon to your activities that caused it to fracture may delay the healing and increase your risk for a complete fracture (which can take even longer to recover from). Switch to activities that place less stress on your foot and leg, such as swimming, walking in a pool, cycling, or seated exercises. Personally, I have usually been able to come up with reasonable activity alternatives that let what needs to heal get better without overstressing another part of my body—but clearly not always because I just got a stress fracture in an outside metatarsal bone from walking funny (and too far) on it for weeks when the plantar fascia in the arch of my same foot was having problems. Use common sense to avoid this sort of scenario from happening to you!

## Muscle Cramps: Are They Preventable?

If you experience a painful, involuntary contraction of your muscle, you are having a muscle cramp. Cramps can occur in any muscle, but they are most common in the legs, feet, and muscles that cross two joints, such as your calf muscle (gastrocnemius, which crosses your knee and your ankle joints), quadriceps and hamstrings (front and back of your thighs), and your feet. Not all of them are that painful; they range in intensity from a slight twitch to severe cramping that makes the muscle feel rock hard and that can last from a few seconds to several minutes. They can also ease up and then cramp again several times before disappearing.

Although the exact cause of muscle cramps remains unknown, they are likely related to poor flexibility, muscle fatigue, or doing new activities. Athletes are more likely to get cramps in the preseason when they are less conditioned and more subject to fatigue. Cramps often develop near the end of intense or prolonged exercise or during the night afterward. Of course, if you are exercising in the heat, cramping can also be related to dehydration and depletion of electrolytes (sodium, potassium, magnesium, and calcium) lost through sweating. When these nutrients fall to certain levels in your blood, you are more likely to experience muscle cramps.

Cramps usually go away on their own without treatment, but there are effective ways to deal with them. For starters, stop the activity that is causing your muscles to cramp (if you can). Then, gently stretch and massage the cramping muscle, holding your joint in a stretched position until the cramp stops. To prevent them, increase your fitness level and avoid becoming excessively fatigued during an activity. Warm up before you start intense workouts and stretch regularly when you are done exercising, focusing on your calves, hamstrings, and quadriceps muscles.

## Treating and Preventing Muscle Soreness

Feeling stiff or tight after training is neither uncommon nor cause for alarm. Stretch out all your muscles and joints after workouts. If you find yourself slightly sore the day after exercise, low-level exercise, light stretching, and gentle massage can help. But if you are still sore a day or two later and you feel stiff and weak, you are likely experiencing delayed-onset muscle soreness (DOMS), which peaks in intensity 24 to 72 hours after an activity. You may even be so stiff and sore that you find it difficult to walk down stairs or fully straighten out your joints.

Although unpleasant, DOMS is different from an acute injury and requires no special treatment. It is a common occurrence, particularly if you are just beginning an exercise program or doing a new or unusual activity. The cause is likely minute tears in your muscles and connective tissues. As these damaged areas become inflamed and swollen, your nerves are sensitized, and you feel the pain. Two or 3 days may pass before you reach the maximum point of pain, and it may take a week or more to resolve completely. Mild activity, stretching, gentle massage, hydrotherapy (such as getting into a hot tub), and NSAIDs can all help relieve discomfort, but they do not speed up the healing process—the best healer is simply time. The good news is that your body responds with *stress proteins* that it builds into the repaired muscles, almost eliminating the possibility that you will reach that level of soreness in the same muscles for 6 to 8 weeks afterward, even if you overdo it again.

The amount of tearing (and resulting soreness) you may experience depends on the activity, intensity of your workout, and its duration. Any unaccustomed movement can lead to DOMS, but *eccentric* muscle contractions (when your muscles are contracting while lengthening) cause the most soreness. Examples of eccentric contractions include going downstairs, running downhill, lowering weights, and doing the downward (gravity-assisted) part of squats and push-ups. As far as diabetes goes, the bad part about DOMS is that you will not be able to restore glycogen in affected muscles until they are fully repaired, which can lead you to be insulin resistant and cause your blood glucose to be harder to manage. In addition, certain muscle pain or soreness can be a sign of a serious injury, so if the soreness does not get better within a week, consult your physician.

> *You can gain strength similarly from resistance exercise and other training programs done correctly without getting undue muscle soreness. Getting excessively sore is not necessary to reach your fitness goals and can be harmful to your health in the short run.*

## Avoiding Extreme Muscle Soreness

You might have heard about a serious condition called *rhabdomyolysis* ("rhabdo" for short), which can result from extreme soreness after unaccustomed exercise training. Rhabdo is the actual death of muscle fibers, which leads them to release the contents of damaged muscle cells (like myoglobin) into the bloodstream. Severe symptoms like muscle pain, vomiting, and confusion are indicative of greater muscle damage and possible kidney failure. If you have severe muscle pain and dark colored urine, seek immediate medical treatment because you can end up in kidney (*renal*) failure. In rare cases, this can even cause death.

By way of example, a young woman who was a physical therapist and a regular CrossFit participant woke the morning after a particularly grueling session consisting of hundreds of repetitions of arm exercises and found she could not bend her elbows. She was shortly thereafter diagnosed in the emergency room with rhabdo and treated in time to prevent more severe complications. Many other reports of rhabdo from similar types of strenuous exercise have surfaced, albeit it is still rare. CrossFit and similar intense training is not inherently bad or ineffective, especially if it is done appropriately, but if you are just starting out with it, do not do too much too soon and follow the proper form to prevent injuries. Just be aware of this possibility and its symptoms.

## Resources for Active People With Diabetes

## Team Novo Nordisk

Team Novo Nordisk is a global, all-diabetes sports team of cyclists, triathletes, and runners, spearheaded by the world's first all-diabetes professional cycling team. It is composed of nearly 100 athletes from over 20 countries who compete for the team in more than 500 international events each year. Their mission is to inspire, educate, and empower people affected by diabetes and to show them all that is possible, even when you have this chronic condition.

Phil Southerland, cofounder and CEO of the team, and Novo Nordisk came together to create Team Novo Nordisk to empower people with diabetes. In 2006, Phil Southerland and Joe Eldridge started out as Team Type 1, a group of eight cyclists with diabetes who took on the grueling 3,000-mile Race Across America. They won the whole event in 2007, 2009, and 2010 and quickly attracted more endurance athletes with diabetes. Nowadays, Team Novo Nordisk competes on a global scale, and its athletes are vehicles of empowerment for people with diabetes worldwide. You can find more information about the organization on their website at www.teamnovonordisk.com.

---

# ARTHRITIS

Although exercise is good for you, too much exercise may increase your risk of joint injuries and *osteoarthritis*, the most common form of arthritis. Trauma to, or overuse of, the joints can cause this condition. If you have ever had an injury to one of your joints, you are more prone to developing arthritis there. But it is unclear whether long-distance running causes knee and hip joints to deteriorate. Some endurance athletes have been tested and found to have an increase in arthritis-related changes, but they do not necessarily have more symptoms. Long-distance running apparently does not increase your risk of osteoarthritis of the knees and hips if you are healthy, and it might even have a protective effect against joint degeneration. Diabetes does not increase your risk for arthritis either, although hip fractures may be more common among those with diabetes, particularly if you do not regularly participate in weight-bearing exercise that helps stimulate and strengthen your hips and leg bones.

If you have already developed some arthritis in your joints, do not despair—you can still exercise safely doing something. Being regularly active likely reduces the pain in your affected joint or joints, although stopping activities may cause you to revert to your pretraining pain level. But your activities should not cause pain in your joints while you are exercising. Obviously, activities of higher intensity or longer duration have greater potential to cause pain, so use pain as your guide to know how much to do. Also, avoid sports with a high risk of joint trauma, such as contact sports and others with frequent directional changes like racquetball. Sometimes it is all about finding alternative activities, as Cathy DeVreeze of Ontario, Canada, knows well. "I have severe arthritis in my right knee," she says. "Walking is difficult, and I am unable to use the treadmill and elliptical. This makes it harder to exercise to help manage diabetes. But I have dealt with this by reaching out for help from trainers at my gym. They have been great to help me plan an exercise routine using strength training and other cardio machines as well as swimming."

# INJURIES AND THE OLDER ATHLETE

No one likes to think or talk about it, but everyone has to face the fact that getting older in itself is likely to cause changes in your physical performance. For instance, the world record in the clean-and-jerk power lift is 20 percent lower in men and 40 percent lower in women in athletes over 50 years of age. Even if you continue to compete in athletic events past your mid-20s, after that you will be past your peak for most sports and at greater risk for getting acute and overuse injuries—but that does not mean you should give up on working out and competing, just that you need to be realistic about it.

From your mid-20s on, you will experience a slow decline in your maximal heart rate, aerobic capacity, lung function, and nerve function (unrelated to diabetes). Although being active lowers your risk for colds, certain cancers, heart disease, and other illnesses, these other physiological changes cannot be entirely prevented. The result is that you will have lower overall strength and endurance as you get older. You are likely to experience selective loss of the fast-twitch muscle fibers used for power and speed, although using those fibers regularly through exercise training will prevent you from losing them as quickly. We used to assume that people became more insulin resistant due to loss of muscle mass with aging, but research has shown that master athletes maintain their insulin sensitivity as high as younger athletes and that the declines in insulin action seen are more likely due to physical inactivity and obesity, not aging per se.

Unfortunately, the loss of calcium and other minerals from bones accelerates with age, particularly in postmenopausal women, but weight-bearing and resistance

*The decline in insulin sensitivity experienced by many older individuals is more strongly associated with physical inactivity than aging alone. Stay active to keep your insulin action higher and to retain more of your muscle mass as you get older.*

exercise can slow and reverse those losses to some extent. Especially with diabetes, you will want to use weight-bearing and resistance exercise as a tool to help you retain your bone mineral density and prevent fractures. Although your body's maximal ability to use oxygen during exercise also declines—typically by 1.5 percent per year—highly trained older athletes show a slower, though steady, rate of decline of only 0.5 percent annually. Moreover, training will keep your breathing muscles stronger and fitter.

Although runners of any age who exercise moderately tend to be physically better off than less active people their age, extensive training for marathons, ultramarathons, and triathlons can increase the risk of injury. Doing that level of training may cause your joints to wear out more quickly than they will if you do more moderate amounts of activity. Many older athletes spend up to a month each year unable to exercise because of injuries. As Bill King, a long-time marathon runner from Philadelphia, Pennsylvania, recounts, "Injury has been more frequent for me than for others in my family. My connective tissues (ligaments and tendons) seem to now be less flexible and heal more slowly. Getting old and staying active with type 1 diabetes is not easy." Actually, it is not easy for anyone, whether or not diabetes is an added variable that may add to injury risk.

Older athletes face some general physical problems that make specific injuries more common. For instance, your joints become less flexible with age, and changes in your body's connective tissues combined with arthritis mean that your knees, hips, and other joints must bear greater stress during exercise than your muscles do. Such changes make running a particularly damaging activity for your joints over time, but so can other intense activities. A long-time resistance training athlete, Guy Hornsby from West Virginia laments, "Arthritis in my hip led to a replacement. It does limit flexibility, especially in achieving low positions to catch the snatch and clean lifts, but all of us old people are seeing declines in competitive performance."

Diabetes itself can cause you to lose flexibility faster over time, even if your blood glucose is well managed. With injury prevention in mind, include an adequate warm-up period with stretching exercises to stay as flexible as possible to lower your risk. Stretching regularly can help slow the loss of flexibility but cannot prevent it completely, so at some point most runners have to choose alternative activities like walking or working out on lower-impact conditioning machines.

For various sports, you may have to make other adjustments as you age to prevent injuries. For instance, master swimmers are more likely to experience rotator cuff tears and should avoid excessive use of hand paddles (which increase stress on the shoulders) and swim fins (which aggravate knee problems), and they should increase swimming distances gradually. Older cyclists are more likely to suffer from compressive or inflammatory syndromes involving nerves in the upper body, but these problems are largely preventable by reducing training. Aging cyclists should use the correct seat height, wear padded gloves, use a padded seat (like a gel pad), wear padded cycling shorts, and avoid resting on their hands on the handlebars. Golfers can develop shoulder problems; neck, lower-back, and wrist pain; and golf or tennis elbow over time. If you golf, warm up properly, stretch, and do strengthening exercises, especially for your back muscles.

You should now realize that despite the risk of injuries, both acute and overuse, that comes with being physically active, your joints, muscles, bones, and body as a whole will be better off if you stay fit and active. You can prevent overuse injuries by varying your training and treat any injuries that you do get by following the advice given in this chapter.

## Athlete Profile: **Sébastien Sasseville**

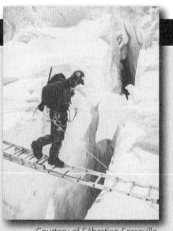
Courtesy of Sébastien Sasseville.

**Hometown:** Québec City, Québec, Canada

**Diabetes history:** Type 1 diabetes diagnosed in 2002 (at age 22)

**Sport or activity:** Mountain climber, long-distance runner, triathlete

**Greatest athletic achievement:** The two athletic endeavors that I am most proud of are my Run Across Canada and climbing Mount Everest. In 2014, I did a solo cross country run from St. John's (the capital of Newfoundland in the far northeastern corner) to Vancouver, British Colombia. The distance I covered was 7,500 kilometers (roughly 4,660 miles), which was the equivalent of running 180 marathons in 9 months. I also summited Mount Everest in 2008 on my first attempt.

**Current insulin and medication regimen:** I use an insulin pump and a CGM device.

**Training tips:** My main tips are (1) collect data, (2) prepare for exercise, and (3) trust the data. Collecting data is very important, which I do with my CGM. Preparing is equally important. As a person with type 1 diabetes, if I'm going to go for a 90-minute run, I have to start planning it out 60 to 120 minutes ahead of time. What basal rate do I need? What insulin do I want to have on board or not? What should I eat? I may have to plan as far as the day before and decide things like what is the best time of day for my run and plan accordingly. Finally, it's important to trust your data. We make so many decisions based on fear (of lows), but you should base your decisions on data instead. If you're about to start working out and you take that extra gel or juice just in case, that's based on fear, not data. Athletes need to fuel—you need insulin and carbs, and you need to manage those carbs with enough insulin. It's counterintuitive to take insulin before working out, but sometimes you have to.

**Typical daily and weekly training and diabetes regimen:** It's always different. What works may only work once with diabetes. I try to understand the formula with all the changing variables. I generally have a higher volume of exercise when I'm training for a triathlon. I try to build endurance throughout the year and then focus more on event-specific training leading up to an event. Here's a general idea of how I may train, though.

▶ *Monday:* Rest day (do some sort of movement and stretching for about an hour).

▶ *Tuesday:* Speed work (if rested) and work out for an hour, once or twice.

▶ *Wednesday:* Some longer workouts of some sort (such as swim in morning and cycle later).

▶ *Thursday:* Power workout of some sort (maybe cycling).

▶ *Friday:* Swim for an hour or so (but not too hard).

▶ *Saturday:* Bike for 3 to 6 hours followed by a run afterward.

▶ *Sunday:* Long run of 1 to 3 hours.

*Other hobbies and interests:* I like writing a lot. I spent close to a year working on my book (*One Step at a Time*), which chronicled my run across Canada and my climb of Mount Everest. I also like watching movies.

*Good diabetes and exercise story:* I think it's important to talk about having diabetes. When you talk about it, people really want to understand it. We need to remember that we didn't know much about type 1 diabetes when we were diagnosed either. There are no dumb questions, and if people ask you about it, it's because they are concerned.

So my story is that I was racing an Ironman triathlon once and made a mistake by taking too much insulin. I was about midway through the marathon run (about 9 hours into my 11-hour race), and my blood glucose was just crashing. I thought the next fueling station was closer than it was, but I was wrong. It was nowhere in sight, and I was so low. When I finally found the courage to ask someone around me for help, I grabbed the first person I could find, a woman in the crowd of spectators. I said to her, "I have type 1 diabetes, and I'm low. I need help." She said, "I have type 1, too. Stay here, and I'll be right back." Of all the thousands of people to ask, I randomly picked someone else who totally understood my dilemma. She ran over to a friend somewhere nearby who must have been keeping a bunch of sweets for her, and she came chasing me on the course with a ton of carbs in her hands. She saved the day and my race. I was able to finish the last 2 hours of the race.

# Guidelines for Specific Activities

# 8

# Fitness Activities

**B**eing physically fit is the way to go—both for better health and to live long and well with diabetes. Whether you participate in aerobic dance classes, learn martial arts, pump up with weights, or push your limits on the conditioning machines, you are headed in the right direction for your fitness, health, and diabetes management goals. We all want an athletic, toned, fit look, and most of us acknowledge that we have to sweat some to get it. Besides, being physically fit has many health benefits, especially when you have diabetes (if you have forgotten what they are, go back and read up on them in chapter 1). As I always say, having diabetes should be your excuse to exercise regularly, not a misguided reason for staying a sedentary couch potato!

The activities included in this chapter run the gamut from low-intensity activities (e.g., yoga and balance training) to power ones like heavy weight training and kickboxing to endurance-based race walking and stationary cycling. Most of these with a fitness focus are endurance activities using the aerobic system (see chapter 2 for a review of the body's energy systems). You can participate in most fitness endeavors in a health club or fitness gym, although others like walking can be done inside on a treadmill or outdoors. Stretching and yoga can be done in a class or on your own. Many bodyweight resistance exercises and balance training can be done just about anywhere.

All the remaining chapters in this book, including this one, give some general recommendations for managing your blood glucose during and after the included activities (in this case, fitness ones), separated out by insulin changes for anyone using a pump or injections, dietary changes, or a combination of both. For each activity, you will also find real-life examples of diabetes management by athletes based on changes to their insulin, diet, or both. If exercise intensity, duration, timing, environment, or other things can have an effect, you will find examples of how athletes deal with those factors as well.

> *A few examples from athletes with type 2 diabetes who use no medications or only noninsulin ones are given throughout part II. They are listed under "diet changes alone" for a specific activity.*

# GENERAL RECOMMENDATIONS FOR FITNESS ACTIVITIES

Fitness activities vary widely with respect to the energy systems and fuels that your body uses while you are doing them. For example, aerobic dance is mainly an endurance activity, but it may also contain elements of muscle toning, strengthening, and stretching. Some martial arts may involve only short, intense movements. Conditioning machines like stationary cycles or rowers can provide aerobic and anaerobic conditioning, depending on how hard and how long you use them. For a review of the various energy systems and fuels, refer back to chapter 2.

Regular participation in fitness activities can cause you to lose fat weight, gain muscle mass, and improve your overall blood glucose. Your insulin sensitivity is likely to improve, resulting in a need for lower doses of insulin or other diabetes medications. The actions of different types of insulin and oral medications are covered in chapter 3, as well as what you need to know about them regarding exercise.

*Although you may be proficient in regulating your insulin doses on your own or with some input from your diabetes care providers, you should adjust the prescribed doses of other medications only on the recommendation of your health care team.*

# GENERAL ADJUSTMENTS BY DIABETES REGIMEN

How you adjust your medications and food intake for any activity will vary with which diabetes regimen you use, the type of exercise you do, and how long and intensely you exercise. In general, the guidelines in this section simply let you know whether you will likely have to change your medications, possibly eat more, or both.

If you use an insulin pump, the first section that follows is for you. Others taking insulin via pens, syringes, or inhalation will find the second section on basal–bolus regimens more relevant. If you still use NPH insulin instead of a longer-lasting basal type, just think of that insulin as being a basal one except around the time that it peaks, when it acts more like a bolus dose that may need adjusting in advance (e.g., the breakfast dose for after-lunch exercise). If you do not use insulin, go right to the third section, "Noninsulin and Oral Medication Users," for advice that applies to you.

## *Insulin Pump Users*

If you reduce your basal insulin doses by 0 to 100 percent during most of these activities, you will likely prevent your blood glucose from going too low. Remember, when people without diabetes exercise, their bodies reduce the amount of insulin circulating during the activity, thus keeping their muscles from taking up too much glucose. With an insulin pump, you have the option to more easily lower your basal insulin by reducing the rate before and during exercise or by disconnecting it altogether.

Depending on your activity, you may also need to keep your basal insulin rates lower for a while after exercise. But for most weight training or stretching activities you may need to make only minimal changes, or you may have to take additional insulin to prevent or correct exercise-induced elevations in your blood glucose.

Depending on what the activity is, how much you lower your basal insulin, and the time of day, you may still need to eat some extra carbohydrates. If you exercise right after you eat, you have the option of lowering your meal bolus as well as eating more. Of course, what works best varies with the activity and its duration, intensity, and timing. You may need more carbohydrates or other food if you do not lower your insulin on board (see table 2.3 for bolus insulin reductions), but you could possibly need up to 75 grams of carbohydrates per hour to enhance your performance and/or prevent lows.

## Basal–Bolus Regimens

For most fitness activities (except prolonged ones), you can simply lower your doses of bolus insulin if you eat within 2 hours of when you start an hour of moderate exercise (see table 2.3). You may also need to increase your carbohydrate and other food intake, depending on your bolus insulin dosing and your starting blood glucose level (refer back to table 2.2 for carbohydrate recommendations). If you are working out more than 2 or 3 hours after your last dose of rapid-acting bolus insulin, it is easier to have less insulin on board, which means you just have to focus on your carbohydrate and other food intake. You may need less food if you have only basal insulin in your system (depending on the time of day), or you may get by with eating nothing at all for shorter activities. You may need to lower the dose of your next injection of basal insulin after prolonged workouts as well to prevent later-onset lows.

## Noninsulin and Oral Medication Users

If you do not use insulin, doing most of these fitness activities is unlikely to make your blood glucose go too low. To get a better idea of how your body responds, check your blood glucose before and after your activities at least for the first few weeks or whenever your medications change. During prolonged activities, you may benefit from consuming some carbohydrates—even athletes without diabetes often eat up to 75 grams of carbohydrates during prolonged, more intense workouts to help provide muscles with alternate fuels to enhance performance. If you start to experience lows more often after you have been exercising regularly, talk with your physician about lowering the doses of your noninsulin diabetes medications. If any of these interfere with your ability to exercise, check to find out whether it is possible to reduce your dose or adjust the time of day you take them.

## Other Effects to Consider

Other factors impact your glucose responses as well, including how long and hard you work out, the time of day you are exercising, how much insulin you have in your body, your starting blood glucose level, whether you are practicing or competing, your hydration status, and many more (also refer back to figure 2.1). Sometimes you may have to deal with effects coming from doing combinations of training or environmental factors or even the effect of using various technologies to manage your glucose when you are active. Look for specific athlete examples addressing some of these, and learn to manage them all for yourself.

The duration and intensity of your workout, the time of day that you exercise, and your starting blood glucose levels have the biggest effect on your responses to fitness workouts. In general, longer bouts of exercise have the potential to lower your blood glucose more than shorter ones, and to compensate you may have to make more adjustments in your diabetes regimen before, during, and afterward. As discussed in chapter 2, intense activities may initially maintain your blood glucose levels more effectively (or even cause them to go up due to glucose-raising hormones), but you will have a much higher risk of getting low later because you will have used up more muscle glycogen.

As for the time of day, any activity that you do early in the morning when your insulin resistance is higher and your insulin levels are lower is less likely to cause your blood glucose to drop compared with exercising later in the day or at any time that your insulin levels are higher. Exercising right after a meal, even breakfast, results in your muscles using more blood glucose. If you exercise after your bolus insulin is mostly gone (2 to 3 hours after your last meal or correction dose), you will need fewer adjustments to keep your blood glucose stable and in a more normal range.

*Exercising with minimal insulin on board (other than basal) is one of the most popular trends for working out among the athletes surveyed for this book (except when it comes to doing heavy or intense weight training, which may require taking more insulin).*

Your blood glucose level when you start a workout will significantly affect whether you need to eat or reduce your insulin and how much. To avoid getting low, some athletes still try to bump their glucose up to 180 mg/dL (10 mmol/L) or higher before they start, but more exercisers nowadays are simply choosing to exercise at times when their insulin levels are lower to avoid having to eat extra or deal with getting low. Avoid being too high (e.g., above 250 to 300 mg/dL [13.9 to 16.7 mmol/L]) at the start, or else you may have to wait to exercise or take an insulin bolus to reduce your level.

## AEROBIC CONDITIONING (FITNESS) MACHINES

Workouts done on a treadmill, elliptical strider, cross-trainer, stepper, stationary cycle, ski machine, rower, or rebounder predominantly use your aerobic energy system. These activities can be easy, moderate, or vigorous intensity and generally involve either large-muscle groups in your legs or your full-body musculature. Some, like ski and rowing machines, also involve significant upper-body work. Your regimen changes will depend primarily on the intensity and duration of your workout, as well as the time of day.

**Treadmills.**  As far as your blood glucose is concerned, treadmill walking or running is similar to walking, race walking, or running outdoors. The main differences arise from the environment and foot-strike stress, which is less on a treadmill than outdoors on concrete, asphalt, or cement. Compared with using a treadmill indoors, exercising outdoors will lead you to expend more energy, particularly in hot, cold, or windy conditions. For examples, refer to walking and race walking later in this chapter, running in chapter 9, and exercising with environmental extremes in chapter 12.

**Elliptical Striders and Cross-Trainers.**   An elliptical strider is a cross between a treadmill and a stair-climber, whereas cross-trainers often emphasize more of a leg-lifting action than striders do. Although it is typically more intense than treadmill walking, exercising on striders and cross-trainers is less taxing on your lower-leg joints because your feet are constantly in contact with the footpads, thereby lowering the stress on your lower limb joints. It is possible to pick programs on such machines that allow you to do faster intervals or hill work to increase the intensity of portions of your workout.

**Stair-Steppers or Stair-Climbers.**   Working out on a stair-stepper or stair-climber is much more aerobic than, say, sprinting up stadium steps. Although the intensity of stair-climbing varies with the program that you choose (hills, manual, random, and so on), your blood glucose will respond mainly to how long you work out because climbing stairs is typically harder than treadmill walking and other activities. If you climb for a relatively short time (10 to 15 minutes), you may not need any regimen changes. Doing this activity for longer will use more muscle glycogen and may have a greater immediate and longer-lasting impact on your blood glucose.

**Stationary Cycles.**   The intensity of stationary cycling can vary widely. It can involve sprinting and intermittent increases in intensity with hill climbing, both of which provide significant stress to your anaerobic metabolism, especially the lactic acid system. Doing "spinning" on a cycle (a fast pace with lower or variable resistance—see more on this activity in the next section) is less taxing than pedaling as hard as possible against a heavier resistance. How hard you work out on a stationary cycle will affect your blood glucose. A longer duration at a higher intensity generally lowers your glucose levels more, but the time of day also plays a role; intense stationary cycling in the morning may cause your level to rise compared with the same workout later in the day. Recumbent stationary cycles are a good alternative to regular ones because the angle formed at your hip while riding in a recumbent position is more natural and is less likely to cause hip joint pain.

**Rowers.**   The biggest effects of rowing come from how hard and how long you work out. Short, intense rowing will maintain your blood glucose more effectively because of a greater release of glucose-raising hormones. If you row for longer at a more moderate or an easy pace, you may have to make more adjustments to prevent hypoglycemia. Rowing outdoors, however, may increase your body's blood glucose use because of a greater intensity elicited by temperature and wind effects (as discussed in chapter 10).

**Ski Machines.**   "Skiing" indoors on a ski machine has almost the same fitness and blood glucose benefits as cross-country skiing if you use good technique. Most people, though, do not work out on a ski machine for as long as they would cross-country ski outdoors (see the next chapter), and they do not have to deal with the effects of a cold and sometimes windy environment. As a result, this fitness activity will generally lower your blood glucose less than skiing outdoors will for a similar length of time.

**Rebounders.**    Walking, jumping, or just moving on a mini-trampoline (rebounder) may work well for some people who prefer to exercise at home. Rebounders may also have a bar attached to hold on to for anyone who has balance issues. This fitness activity can vary in intensity based on how you do it, but it may lower your blood glucose if you work out on it for long enough.

## Athlete Examples

Although the fitness activities vary, these examples show that comparable adjustments can be made for all of them, depending on your exercise intensity, starting blood glucose, time of day, and circulating insulin levels. For some, insulin or dietary changes are enough, while others may require changes in both or neither.

### Insulin Changes Alone

Combinations of changes in basal and bolus insulin delivery are used by exercisers, especially those with insulin pumps. For instance, for fitness machines, Hannah M. from Winona, Minnesota, turns down the hourly rate of insulin on her pump by 50 percent starting an hour before working out and avoids taking an insulin bolus within 2 hours of her workouts. If she needs a correction bolus, she reduces it by 50 percent before exercise. Rebekah Lindsay of Sevierville, Tennessee, handles her workouts similarly, lowering her basal rate by 50 percent 1 hour before starting aerobic conditioning and suspending basal insulin delivery while working out.

A resident of Philadelphia, Pennsylvania, Gary Scheiner reduces his preworkout meal bolus by 33 percent before engaging in vigorous cardio workouts lasting 45 to 60 minutes. Before doing 30 to 60 minutes on fitness machines, Todd Daugherty from Carthage, Missouri, typically suspends his basal insulin delivery up to an hour beforehand and during exercise, depending on how hard he works out. Likewise, Kris Maynard of Mead, Washington, usually sets his basal rate at 30 percent of normal 2 hours before starting a 90-minute, intense cardio workout.

For 45 minutes of moderate exercise with fitness machines, resistance training, agility, or aerobics, Corianne Blotevogel from Oklahoma City, Oklahoma, works out on basal insulin only until about halfway through each session. By then, her blood glucose is usually on the rise and will spike well over 200 mg/dL (11.1 mmol/L) without more insulin, so she boluses with about 2 units and finishes her workout. For 45 minutes of moderate stationary cycling, Melodie Savoca of Margate, Florida, makes sure her blood glucose is over 140 mg/dL (7.8 mmol/L) when she starts and suspends her pump's insulin delivery until she is done exercising, which some days includes doing weight lifting for 30 minutes after cycling.

### Diet Changes Alone

An exerciser from Laramie, Wyoming, Brown finds that her blood glucose levels need to be between 95 and 115 mg/dL (5.3 and 6.4 mmol/L) for her to start aerobic conditioning workouts and have good results. She tries to work out 1 to 2 hours after she eats, and she will typically have 2 teaspoons of peanut butter or two peanut butter crackers to compensate.

Conversely, Sarah Richard of Fort Walton Beach, Florida, exercises for 60 to 90 minutes vigorously 4 days per week, but does not do anything different on the days that she exercises. If her blood glucose is lower than 70 mg/dL (3.9 mmol/L), she treats it with glucose tablets or a glucose gel. If it is higher than 140 mg/dL (7.8 mmol/L), she corrects with insulin—in the gym and out of the gym alike.

A resident of Levittown, Pennsylvania, Bobbie Silber eats lunch at noon, boluses normally, and goes straight to the gym after work. Based on her afternoon blood glucose, she decides how much to supplement before a 30- to 40-minute intense workout on an elliptical strider. For a starting glucose of 120 to 130 mg/dL (6.7 to 7.2 mmol/L), she eats four glucose tablets. If she is in the range of 130 to 170 mg/dL (7.2 to 9.4 mmol/L), she needs two to three tablets. For 180 mg/dL (10 mmol/L), she just eats one, and for 200 mg/dL (11.1 mmol/L) she takes none. Her blood glucose starts to drop after 10 minutes, and she usually finishes in the range of 80 to 90 mg/dL (4.4 to 5.0 mmol/L). In addition, she often uses a temporary basal reduction of 20 percent on her pump for the 3 hours before bedtime on her workout days.

For 1 hour of vigorous conditioning, Mark Rosenbaum of New Bern, North Carolina, eats glucose tablets and granola bars right before he starts to raise his blood glucose to 125 mg/dL (6.9 mmol/L) or higher. During his workouts, he will treat himself with glucose tablets if he reaches 80 mg/dL (4.4 mmol/L) on his CGM or even 90 mg/dL (5.0 mmol/L) if it is trending down rapidly, but he says it also depends on how much additional exercise he will be getting.

Barry Toothman from Lake Charles, Louisiana, an exerciser with type 2 diabetes, takes only metformin and Jardiance to manage his diabetes. However, for intense, 1-hour aerobic and interval workouts on a treadmill, elliptical, and other machines, he checks his blood glucose and then typically consumes four Smarties candies (24 grams of glucose) before starting. He is also careful to drink enough water (usually 40 ounces) to avoid dehydration.

### Combined Regimen Changes

Aaron Kowalski, a runner from Somerville, New Jersey, often works out on fitness machines—treadmills, rowers, or stair-climbers—early in the morning while he is still fasting (before breakfast). He bases his carbohydrate intake on his CGM starting glucose and its trend or direction. During these 45-minute vigorous workouts, he often removes his pump.

For 45-minute vigorous workouts on conditioning machines, Michelle from Wayne, Pennsylvania, takes a 50 percent bolus correction if her starting blood glucose is greater than 150 mg/dL (8.3 mmol/L), but none if it is less than that. She eats her breakfast or snack without taking a bolus and then takes 75 percent of her normal meal bolus 10 to 15 minutes after her workout.

Similarly, Jeff Foot of Scotland works out moderately on a cross-trainer machine for at least 30 minutes, usually after breakfast. For this activity, he reduces his basal rate by 30 percent starting about 1 hour before breakfast (but only for 15 minutes) and docs not bolus for his breakfast (containing ~20 grams of carbohydrates).

For Jason D. of Colorado Springs, Colorado, doing any conditioning machine workouts requires him to decrease his basal rate to 25 to 50 percent of normal starting 1 to 2 hours before exercise. If his blood glucose goes below 120 mg/dL (6.7 mmol/L), he eats a packet of fruit snacks and finishes his workout.

For 1- to 1.5-hour moderate workouts, Hanna Kinder from Germany makes sure she is starting out a bit higher if her last bolus injection for a meal is within 2 hours of starting her workout. If it is longer than 2 hours, a starting blood glucose of 120 mg/dL (6.7 mmol/L) is usually fine to maintain. If she is starting sooner than that after eating, she lets her glucose rise to 250 mg/dL (13.9 mmol/L) when doing cardio (or 200 mg/dL [11.1 mmol/L] before weight workouts). She always carries glucose and a banana, but she does not need to make adjustments to her basal (Lantus) insulin.

Javad Ramezani from Iran works out for an hour or so about 3 to 4 hours after lunch, for which he takes regular insulin. He has very little insulin left from lunch on board by then, so he does not have to worry much about going too low. Depending on the intensity and type of exercise, he may decrease the amount of insulin he takes later or eat more for dinner to prevent overnight lows.

## Other Effects to Consider

**Effect of Workout Intensity.**   Hailing from the United Kingdom, Jennie B. finds that light cardio training invariably drops her blood glucose after 30 to 40 minutes, so she reduces her basal rate on her pump half an hour or so before she starts, and she carries jelly babies in case of need. For harder workouts, she finds that her blood glucose may go up temporarily but then drop later in the activity or afterward (she uses her CGM to judge how to react). Most of all, she aims to have as little insulin on board as possible when starting any activity, unless she is actively trying to lower her blood glucose with activity.

**Effect of Starting Blood Glucose.**   For pumper Courtney Duckworth from Washington, D.C. (profiled in chapter 10), what she needs to do depends on the type, intensity, and duration of the activity, as well as her starting blood glucose and insulin on board. If her blood glucose is above 120 mg/dL (6.7 mmol/L) and below 180 mg/dL (10 mmol/L), sometimes suspending her pump suffices. If it is below 120 mg/dL (6.7 mmol/L), she typically supplements with 15 to 30 grams of a GU energy gel, a banana, or some cereal.

Canadian Lynn Witmer of Toronto, Ontario, usually reduces her insulin basal rate by 50 percent during running, cycling, or elliptical trainer workouts, starting 15 minutes before and continuing until about 30 minutes after she finishes. But if her starting blood glucose level is below 126 mg/dL (7 mmol/L), she eats some dried fruit; for 198 mg/dL (11 mmol/L), she does not eat or reduce her basal rate; and when it is above 252 mg/dL (14 mmol/L), she takes a small insulin bolus.

**Effect of Time of Day and Circulating Insulin Levels.**   Bec Johnson of Perth, Australia, always aims to train with her system clear of food and rapid-acting insulin to minimize the variables in play and keep things simple. Before breakfast is ideal for her, but if she works out in the evening, she eats lunch early so there is no food or meal-related insulin in her system before training. Daniele Hargenrader, an exercise enthusiast from Philadelphia, Pennsylvania, always tries to do her 1-hour sessions of harder conditioning exercise while fasted (before breakfast) with minimal insulin on board so her blood glucose stays more stable.

Christel Oerum, a fitness enthusiast from Santa Monica, California (profiled at the end of this chapter), knows that for moderate cardio fitness training for an hour or more while fasting, she does not need any insulin corrections because her morning hormones keep her steady. When she is doing a similar workout later in the day, she makes sure not to have more than a half-unit of insulin on board from her last bolus to avoid lows.

Similarly, K. Mathias from Toronto does not need adjustments for working out for 30 minutes on varying fitness machines (stair-stepper, treadmill, elliptical strider, or stationary cycle) if she works out first thing in the morning. For the same exercise in the evening, she takes only half of her usual dinner bolus beforehand.

To use an elliptical trainer for a half hour three or four times a week, Kateri Routh of Chicago, Illinois, takes off her insulin pump when she works out in the afternoon and drinks a small juice box before starting. For similar exercise in the morning, she has to leave her pump on, but she lowers her basal rate by 50 percent and does not drink any juice.

**Effect of Combined Cardio and Resistance Work.**   Dwain Chapman from Highland, Illinois, finds that doing a combination of treadmill walking and weight training has lingering effects that lower his blood glucose later when compared with only working out on the treadmill or stationary cycle. Treadmill walking by itself has less of a residual effect, although he finds it can still cause lows during the activity if he has not prepared properly by lowering his basal and/or eating more carbohydrates for the activity. Before most cardio work, he consumes some carbohydrates if his starting blood glucose is 150 mg/dL (8.3 mmol/L) or less.

## AEROBIC FITNESS CLASSES (DANCE, SPINNING, HIP HOP, PILATES, AND STEP AEROBICS)

These activities are mainly aerobic in nature, with interspersed periods of greater intensity work and easier stretching and toning exercises. Even if you use light weights or do repetitions like abdominal crunches during the classes, the workouts are still mainly aerobic because most classes last at least 45 minutes and emphasize muscular endurance over strength. Classes also vary in intensity based on how hard you push yourself and the nature of the class (e.g., high impact, low impact, cycling, step, and others).

Aerobic fitness crazes come and go, with spinning being one of the more popular ones at present. Spinning classes take place on specially designed stationary cycles. You pedal to motivating music (like in other fitness classes), while the class instructor often talks you through a visualization of an outdoor cycling workout. You vary your pace during the class—sometimes pedaling as fast as you can against lower resistance and other times cranking up the tension and pedaling slowly from a standing position—but you should always be able to finish simply by turning the resistance down to a workload that you can handle. Using a Peloton bike with online video connection to a class instructor and other participants is a novel way to do these types of classes without ever leaving home or having to do them alone.

For most of these aerobic classes, how hard, how long, and when you work out have a big effect on your blood glucose responses. For example, higher-intensity workouts that last an hour or more will generally reduce your blood glucose more than doing easier ones for the same amount of time. If you take classes in the early morning, such as before breakfast when your insulin resistance is higher and insulin levels lower, you will be less likely to experience hypoglycemia than after a meal when you have more insulin on board. Working out more than 2 or 3 hours after your last bolus insulin helps maintain your blood glucose. But you may still need to eat something, depending on where your glucose starts and on the intensity and duration of the workout.

## Athlete Examples

Aerobic fitness classes come in all types and intensities, but you can manage your diabetes so that you can do all of them. Consider class intensity and duration, as well as timing of exercise, when making regimen changes.

### Insulin Changes Alone

Iulia Latiffa from Romania finds what works best for her is to check her blood glucose level before and after aerobic classes and complete them disconnected from her pump. Emily Marrama, an exerciser from Lynn, Massachusetts, judges what she needs to do at the start of each activity. If her blood glucose is around 150 mg/dL (8.3 mmol/L) at the start of a high-intensity workout, she needs to lower her basal by at least 30 percent for 2 hours.

Before participating in an hour-long aerobics class (with 20 minutes each of step aerobics, kickboxing, and weightlifting), Cynthia Fritschi of Chicago, Illinois, cuts back her preactivity meal bolus by about 1 unit and sets her pump at 25 percent of her normal basal rate. Rachel Lanclos of Lubbock, Texas, teaches fitness classes, including step aerobics, kickboxing, yoga, and Pilates. She finds it easiest to simply remove her pump during the hour-long classes. For aerobics classes, Adelaide Lindahl from Bloomington, Minnesota, prefers to reduce her basal rates during the activity rather than cut back on her premeal boluses, but for her doing that tends to lead to postprandial spikes. However, if she reduces her basal rates to 0.5 unit per hour starting an hour before and during the class, she does not need to eat extra.

Fatima Shahzad, a Cambridge, Massachusetts, resident, finds that she needs to watch her blood glucose more closely when doing aerobics or other fitness classes because they tend to make her blood glucose go low. She also checks afterward and overnight, cutting back her basal insulin in the evening and setting her CGM alert thresholds higher to pick up nighttime lows sooner. Aline Verbeke from Bruges, Belgium, reduces her basal insulin by 50 percent 30 minutes before starting a fitness class, and she keeps it lower until she finishes working out.

On the other hand, Catalina Perieteanu from Bucharest, Romania, does 1-hour indoor cycling classes for which her main adjustment is to give a small insulin bolus if her starting blood glucose is over 150 mg/dL (8.3 mmol/L). If she is lower than that, she does not need to make any adjustments because the high intensity of the class raises her blood glucose.

## Diet Changes Alone

A resident of Charleston, West Virginia, Kelly Rowan Wymer teaches spinning classes and does other daily workouts. She works hard to stay on target but sometimes has blood glucose highs after teaching a very vigorous spin class. Since type 1 diabetes was diagnosed for Kelly at age 55, she has taken minimal insulin daily and limits her carbohydrates to no more than 25 grams per meal.

For an hour of Pilates, Michelle McCotter from Los Angeles, California, usually eats 10 to 15 grams of carbohydrates if she starts with a normal blood glucose level. If her glucose is around 120 mg/dL (6.7 mmol/L), she will not eat anything.

## Combined Regimen Changes

Hailing from Stockport, England, Andy Duckwork reduces his meal before an hour-long exercise class, and he takes half of his usual bolus afterward, along with reducing his basal dose by 50 percent during the activity. He aims to start with a blood glucose of about 180 mg/dL (10 mmol/L), and he drinks a bottle of Lucozade (an English sports and energy drink containing glucose and caffeine) every hour for activities lasting longer.

Jennifer Burt from Calgary in Canada simply eats a meal before classes and cuts her bolus insulin dose in half to compensate. Occasionally she may need a glucose gel or GU energy gel packet every 30 minutes during long, intense workouts to prevent lows.

A resident of Cleveland, Ohio, Jorden Rieke has a set protocol for dealing with aerobic conditioning classes, fitness machines, and more. She has some coffee before her workout while stretching for 30 to 45 minutes. She admits that her MiniMed 670G (hybrid closed-loop system) takes care of a lot of her glucose management during exercise; however, if her blood glucose is below around 120 mg/dL (6.7 mmol/L) before starting or she will be doing cardio training, she does not take insulin to cover the usual bump in her glucose caused by the caffeine in her coffee. If she is above 160 mg/dL (8.9 mmol/L) before a workout, she takes a small bolus for correction. During exercise, if she drops below 70 mg/dL (3.9 mmol/L), she treats it with 20 to 40 grams of carbohydrates from juice, depending on how fast she is dropping. Otherwise, she does not change her food intake for this activity.

A resident of West Roxbury, Massachusetts, Lulu Morrison does step aerobics 4 to 5 days per week. For this activity, she suspends her pump during the class and takes four glucose tablets before it starts if her blood glucose is less than 150 mg/dL (8.3 mmol/L). If it drops during class, she eats another two to four tablets to compensate. Likewise, fitness instructor Catherine Cunningham of Lexington, Kentucky, suspends her pump during aerobics classes. She additionally eats some protein and carbohydrate before starting classes.

For spinning classes, Karen Tank of Princeton, New Jersey, lowers her basal rate by 50 percent before starting and keeps it there until the end. She also checks her blood glucose about halfway through the hour-long class and eats carbohydrates if she starts going too low. For morning workouts, she tries to eat a breakfast higher in protein, fat, and fiber (but low in carbohydrate) so that she does not have to bolus much, if at all, beforehand.

Vic Kinnunen from Lawrenceville, Georgia, reduces his basal dose by 65 to 75 percent for twice the length of class time (which usually lasts 45 minutes to 1 hour). He also eats a banana or peanut butter crackers on the way to the gym (30 minutes before the spinning workout), and he drinks chocolate milk afterward with a full bolus to cover the carbohydrates.

## Other Effects to Consider

**Effect of Exercise Intensity.**   An exerciser from Melbourne, Australia, Andrew Baker takes a weekly Pilates class but does not find it too hard or stressful for him. He does not need to make any major modifications to his insulin or diet to participate. (Normally he eats something before most workouts, though.)

When she does high-intensity spinning or F45 (high-intensity interval) workout classes during which her heart rate goes up significantly (at least 170 beats per minute), Bec Johnson, a Humalog and Levemir user from Perth, Australia, knows she needs to have more insulin in her system to manage her blood glucose. She takes 0.5 to 1.0 units of Humalog, depending on her starting blood glucose, between 30 and 40 minutes before the workout to stay stable.

Naomi, a Spokane, Washington resident, attends a 1-hour barre method exercise class and does not need to adjust anything or eat during for it. She speculates that the combination of cardio and resistance training likely helps stabilize her blood glucose.

**Effect of Time of Day.**   Jeanne LeBow from Tempe, Arizona, does all her exercise classes in the morning because her morning glucose levels are less volatile than at other times of day. Nina Horvath, a resident of Vancouver, British Columbia, Canada, also does her exercise classes first thing in the morning, so she does not eat anything before, but she boluses 2 units afterward to avoid blood glucose spikes, followed immediately by breakfast.

Likewise, Kathleen Johnson of Lake St. Louis, Missouri, finds that she has to make fewer adjustments for the early morning step aerobics classes that she instructs. She does not eat before the class and takes no insulin boluses. An exerciser with type 2 diabetes, Arlene Pearson from Springfield, Oregon, works out while fasted every day as well. Because she takes no diabetes medications, she does not need to do much to keep her blood glucose in check.

## BALANCE, FUNCTIONAL, AND AGILITY TRAINING

*Balance training* can be as easy as practicing standing on one foot at a time or doing simple exercises (like a three-way leg swing or picking up a towel with your toes) that work on lower leg and core body strength and basic stability. All resistance training exercises that work these areas also double as balance training. Most *functional training*, such as practice walking on uneven surfaces, also works on balance as well as the ability to perform activities of daily living and self-care.

Physical movements that are part of activities like tai chi and yoga involve varying combinations of resistance and flexibility training that can help build functional fitness and balance. Older athletes may undertake balance, functional, and agility exercises to help them remain more stable and be less likely to fall.

*Agility training* is more about improving power and managing quick directional changes, which leads you to be more powerful for sports participation along with being steadier on your feet. Younger athletes may be involved in agility training as part of training for speed and rapid directional movements (as occur in many team sports). Some agility practice may be more intense, but most exercises are shorter in duration. Depending on the kind of balance, functional, or agility training, you may not need any immediate regimen changes to manage your blood glucose, but intense, prolonged agility training has the greater potential to impact blood glucose later.

## Athlete Examples

The impact of any of these types of training is more related to successful sports performance or aging well with diabetes and less related to diabetes management, except possibly when it comes to agility training. Sean Busby (see his profile in chapter 5) views balance exercises as part of his training to maintain his body from past injuries and keep his performance high for snowboarding.

To participate in agility training, Dan Stone from Middletown, Pennsylvania, approaches it like any other anaerobic activity (including weight training, rock climbing/bouldering, and agility training). For the activity itself, he does not make any changes; after the activity is finished, he reduces his pump basal rate by 30 percent for a while based how long his activity lasted or he increases his fat and/or protein intake during his postworkout meal.

## BOWLING

This activity involves extremely short bursts of activity (e.g., swinging and releasing the ball) and relies on your short-term energy (phosphagen) system. Most of the time, you do little activity between your turns. Consequently, the total energy that you use in bowling is minimal, its effect on your blood glucose is usually insignificant, and you probably will not need to adjust your regimen. But if you bowl competitively for 2 or 3 hours or more, you might need to make some changes, especially if you are bowling after a meal.

## Athlete Examples

The intensity of this sport can vary depending on whether you are doing it recreationally or professionally. Most of us fall into the former category. Kory Seder of Madison, Wisconsin, concedes that he hardly considers bowling to be a physical activity. When he bowls, it is low enough in intensity that he does not make any adjustments. Mason Klahn from Colorado just treats bowling like any other activity; he checks his blood glucose during games and treats lows immediately.

## BOXING

This activity involves short, powerful jabs and quick (anaerobic) movements, as well as constant motion of your legs during a given round. Training for boxing usually involves a combination of power and endurance moves. For most people, this is a fitness training activity rather than a competitive sport. For recommended changes, refer to the section on kickboxing later in this chapter.

## CLIMBING, INDOOR

Climbing and bouldering indoors at a gym on a specially designed wall involves muscular endurance and strength as you have to hang onto the handholds with your fingertips for extended periods without rest and push off the wall and find footholds with your legs. Artificial climbing walls allow boulderers to train indoors in areas without natural boulders. Higher climbs usually require equipment to allow you to belay up the side of a wall. Your muscles are working while staying the same length (doing isometric contractions), which involves both muscular strength and endurance. For short climbing attempts, the intensity of this activity will likely keep your blood glucose stable, but if you climb for long periods, you may need some regimen changes to compensate, both during climbs and later to prevent lows. For other athlete examples, read the sections on bouldering and rock and ice climbing (all done outdoors) in chapter 12.

## Athlete Examples

Due to the anaerobic nature of this activity, you may need no immediate changes in your regimen, or you may need to make adjustments later to prevent lows after climbing. How you respond depends on how long you climb and how much glycogen your body uses.

### No Changes Necessary

When Patrick Bowyer in the United Kingdom does indoor climbing for about 2 hours, he checks his blood glucose before, during, and after the activity. He mainly expects his blood glucose to drop lower about 2 hours after he finishes, not during the activity. He often just lets his glucose come down on its own afterward if it is on the high side when he finishes.

### Insulin Changes Alone

Dean McColl of Bremerton, Washington, finds that rock climbing indoors requires her to reduce her basal insulin by 25 percent while she is climbing. Afterward, she keeps it 25 percent lower for the same number of hours that she spent climbing to prevent lows. Conversely, for outdoor climbing, she may not need to reduce her insulin at all.

## DANCE: MODERN, SOCIAL, BALLROOM, SWING, AND OTHERS

Dance activities often combine aerobic and anaerobic components, depending on how hard and long you dance. An extreme example is ballet (covered in chapter 10), which requires power moves such as jumping, and sustained muscular contractions when holding dance positions, along with hours of training and practice. Other types of dance are generally more aerobic in nature, but they are usually lower-level activities that necessitate fewer adjustments. Social or recreational dancing (e.g., line or swing) may not lower your blood glucose much.

## Athlete Examples

These exercisers often make changes in their diet and insulin dosing, but the actual adjustment depends largely on the type of dancing that they do. How long they dance and what they typically eat can also impact their blood glucose during dancing.

### Insulin Changes Alone

For Irish set dancing, Andrea Limbourg of Paris, France, lowers her basal rate when she is dancing all day, but for helping with beginner or intermediate classes she does not need many changes in her regimen. She takes more of a situational approach to dancing: she looks at her glucose trends a few hours beforehand then makes the decision of whether to reduce her basal rate, eat something, or take a bolus (if she is on the high side). If she cannot anticipate her trends, she checks at the start and adjusts from there, treating with food rather than reducing her basal rate if her blood glucose is on the low side because she finds that carbohydrates kick in faster to raise her glucose.

### Diet Changes Alone

New Yorker Judith Jones-Ambrosini tries to keep her blood glucose in the 100 mg/dL (5.6 mmol/L) range during a Movement Speaks dance class that lasts an hour and a half. If her blood glucose (monitored with her CGM) drops down to 80 mg/dL (4.4 mmol/L) during the class, she drinks a juice box.

Connie Hanham-Cain from Albany, New York, has a Greek yogurt (mixed with spring water to equal ~12 to 18 grams of carbohydrates) before a dance or movement class and/or as a recovery drink after an intense class. Sometimes she has a protein/carbohydrate bar (Transend Protein Snack Bar containing 15 grams of carbohydrates) instead. For belly dancing, she aims to keep her blood glucose in the range of 80 to 140 mg/dL (4.4 to 7.8 mmol/L); if her starting blood glucose is on the low side, she may have a tablespoon of honey with her yogurt drink.

### Combined Regimen Changes

A Richmond, Washington, resident, Margaret S. Urfer decreases her basal rate before dancing for a couple of hours. For that activity, she eats slowly absorbed carbohydrates beforehand and has snacks on hand (such as granola bars or chocolate).

For Courtney Duckworth of Washington, D.C., her regimen changes depend on the type, intensity, and duration of dancing as well as her starting blood glucose and insulin on board. If her blood glucose is above 120 mg/dL (6.7 mmol/L) and below 180 mg/dL (10 mmol/L), sometimes all she needs to do is suspend her pump during dancing. If it is on the low side, she often eats 15 to 30 grams of a GU energy gel, a banana, or some cereal beforehand.

During swing dancing lessons, Sarah Soper of West Lafayette, Indiana, lowers her basal rate down to 65 percent of normal for an hour. For weekly jam sessions, she lowers it even more, to 45 percent for 2 hours. If her blood glucose is going lower before she starts, she often eats a granola bar, for which she sometimes gives herself a very small bolus.

For Tian Walker of Long Beach, California, her regimen changes depending on the type of dance she is doing. For House dancing (an intense form derived from hip hop that involves a lot of jumping), she completely suspends her pump, and if she has any residual bolus insulin on board, she often eats Honey Stingers to keep from going low. For hip hop or popping, she puts her pump at a 50 percent basal rate because her heart rate is still increased and her insulin needs are definitely reduced.

## HOUSEWORK

Housework is an activity that has elements of strength and endurance, depending on what specifically you are doing. Most aspects of housework minimally involve standing; others, such as sweeping or vacuuming, require you to hold out your arms away from your sides for potentially long periods while walking around. The best training for housecleaning and other domestic chores is to do fitness activities regularly. Doing housework for an extended period can require you to make some adjustments to prevent hypoglycemia.

## Athlete Examples

Although not a sport per se, housework does involve manual labor, and it can affect your blood glucose—particularly when it is intense or prolonged. Often regimen changes only involve making one adjustment at a time, however.

### Insulin Changes Alone

When Julie Heverly of Richmond, Virginia, cleans her house two Saturdays a month for 4 to 6 hours, she has to lower her basal rate down to 50 percent of normal. Her cleaning is physically active, including going up and down steps many times, moving furniture, vacuuming, and more. Likewise, Corianne Blotevogel of Oklahoma City, Oklahoma, finds that housework drops her blood glucose pretty quickly. She either turns her basal down to 50 percent of usual or suspends insulin delivery while cleaning.

A resident of Annapolis, Maryland, Shiela Bostelman finds that while she cleans house for 2 hours, she must lower her basal rate on her pump down to 30 percent of normal. Similarly, Gayle Land of Minnetonka, Minnesota, finds that vacuuming usually takes a toll on her blood glucose, forcing her to reduce her basal rate on her pump during the activity.

Leanne Full from Ocean Grove, Victoria, Australia, always needs to use a lower temporary basal rate during activities, except for during housework and gardening.

If she does happen to start getting low during these activities, she relies on her hybrid closed-loop pump (used on auto mode) to suspend her basal insulin delivery for her.

### Diet Changes Alone

Australian Warwick Sickling finds that vacuuming and mopping floors drops his blood glucose levels very quickly. He has to check his blood glucose while cleaning and often must take in additional carbohydrates. He also finds that looking after his young kids is another activity that quickly drops his blood glucose, especially when it involves some unplanned exercise. He never knows in advance how much exercise he will end up doing with the children because it very much depends how energetic they are feeling and how much involvement in their play they want from him on any given day.

For housework, Katherine Owen from Tallahassee, Florida, finds she needs to eat snacks containing 10 to 12 grams of carbohydrates if her sensor reaches 80 mg/dL (4.4 mmol/L). Likewise, for doing moderate housecleaning for an hour or more, Sheri Ochs of Santa Barbara, California, finds that she may have to eat an extra 10 to 15 grams of carbohydrate per hour to prevent lows if she is cleaning soon after a meal. If she cleans for more than 2 hours after her last bolus injection, she needs to supplement only during the second hour of cleaning, not the first.

## ICE SKATING AND INLINE SKATING

These activities are mainly aerobic in nature, much along the lines of walking. The gliding effect of the skates reduces some of the energy required to cover any given distance. Ice and inline skating, if you do them at a high skill level, may involve powerful, quick movements such as jumping or spinning, which are more anaerobic activities.

The intensity and duration of either type of skating will affect your blood glucose response. For instance, recreational ice or inline skating requires minimal aerobic effort and, like slow walking, uses little blood glucose or muscle glycogen. Competitive skating (speed or figure, usually done on ice) is much more intense than recreational skating and will certainly require you to make some adjustments (as discussed in chapter 10).

## Athlete Examples

The following example stresses how many people can make minimal adjustments for recreational skating. Because figure skating and speed skating are not typically done recreationally or for fitness reasons, they are not included in this section.

### Insulin Changes Alone

For inline skating, Sarah Soper from Indiana disconnects from her pump during the activity but not before, giving herself about 20 percent of the basal insulin that she is going to miss up front. When she reconnects, she gives herself the other 80 percent.

## Diet Changes Alone

Jay Handy, a distance athlete from Madison, Wisconsin, who follows a low-carbohydrate diet, finds that because his inline skating often lasts over an hour, he may need an occasional Clif Shot Blok. He just makes sure his CGM is working to monitor his blood glucose.

A resident of the Czech Republic, Klara Pickova usually does longer duration inline skating. For anything over an hour, she replenishes her carbohydrates in the form of a 5 percent glucose solution in the amount of 15 to 30 grams per hour.

## KICKBOXING

Kickboxing is mostly anaerobic, involving short, powerful movements. It may also involve repeated movement of your legs if you are doing quick kicks. Training for this activity involves power and endurance movements designed to increase the strength and endurance of your leg and trunk muscles. Higher-intensity, more anaerobic workouts often require you to make fewer changes than you would expect because of the release of glucose-raising hormones. Having low insulin levels during this kind of high-intensity activity will further lessen your need to adjust, except that if your blood glucose is higher when you finish you may need a small amount of insulin to bring it down.

# Athlete Examples

This activity is most similar to intense martial arts with regard to its effect on your blood glucose (that is, the intensity tends to keep glucose stable or make it rise). To compensate, you can make a variety of regimen adjustments, depending on the time of day you do it and your insulin on board.

## Insulin Changes Alone

For Dessi Zaharieva of Canada, boxing, kickboxing, martial arts, and jiujitsu all fall under the same category of blood glucose response. She exercises with as little insulin on board as possible to manage it, and she removes her insulin pump for 1 to 2 hours, depending on the training. She checks her blood glucose halfway through and may take 1 to 2 units, depending on her level; otherwise, she checks at the end of training and takes 1 to 2 units then if she did not need it halfway through exercise. For her, it is easier to train in the evenings and eat her dinner late or after training because she does not like training, grappling, or full-contact sparring on a full stomach.

## Combined Regimen Changes

Klara Pickova of the Czech Republic tries to start kickboxing or muay thai (Thai boxing) with blood glucose levels between 80 and 144 mg/dL (4.4 to 8.0 mmol/L), with a small amount of active insulin on board to prevent or decrease her adrenaline-based glucose spikes. She usually eats a light snack (fruit or a sports bar) 2 hours before and takes her regular bolus. Sometimes if she sees her glucose rising, she gives a small correction bolus during exercise. Afterward, she has her regular dinner and decreases her meal bolus by 20 percent. Overnight, she uses a temporary basal that is 20 percent lower all night.

Stephanie Malmstrom of Salt Lake City, Utah, goes into this and other intense activities knowing what her blood glucose is and having eaten protein with fat (without needing to bolus before exercise). She checks her blood glucose or CGM during exercise to ensure that her blood glucose is staying level. If it goes below 80 mg/dL (4.4 mmol/L), she eats 8 grams of a fast-acting carbohydrate to bump her blood glucose back up; if it rises too high, she does not correct it because she knows it will come down shortly after exercise.

When she is doing more vigorous activities like kickboxing or kettlebell training (causing her heart rate to go over 140 beats per minute for an extended period), Michele Storr of North Carolina typically eats before exercise. She takes a bolus that is 50 percent of what her insulin pump wizard recommends, extended over 90 minutes. She tends to need to bolus at the end of her workout with another 1 to 2 units, however.

### Other Effects to Consider

**Effect of Time of Day.**   Patti Murphy Cerami chooses not to do kickboxing in the morning because its intensity and her body's resistance to insulin at that time of day make her blood glucose go extremely high. Instead, she works out later in the day when her insulin resistance is lower.

Karen O'Mara from Wakerly, Queensland, Australia, does boxing, walking, and other fitness activities. Usually, she works out exercise early in the morning before eating or taking any boluses. If she uses a lower temporary basal rate on her pump during these activities, she rarely gets low. If she does get low, she treats it with jelly beans. If her glucose is below 108 mg/dL (6.0 mmol/L) before starting, she may eat a banana as well. If she is exercising after breakfast, she is much more likely to have her blood glucose drop, so she reduces her prebreakfast bolus, along with lowering her basal rate during the activity.

## MARTIAL ARTS

The martial arts category of activities is composed of karate, judo, taekwondo, jiujitsu, tai chi, aikido, qigong, and more and covers a wide range of exercise intensity. Most involve power moves like kicking, chopping, and punching, although disciplines like tai chi and qigong include slower, more controlled movements that are more prolonged and less intense. The intensity of the activity will have the greatest effect on your blood glucose levels. Extremely intense workouts will be more anaerobic in nature and may not cause much of a decrease in glucose during them; in some cases your blood glucose may increase instead because of the greater release of glucose-raising hormones. If you work out long and hard, however, your risk of experiencing delayed drops in blood glucose is heightened by your depletion of muscle glycogen. Activities like tai chi and qigong are lower in intensity and may require no adjustments.

## Athlete Examples

These examples demonstrate the need to modify regimens differently according to the type, intensity, duration, and timing of martial arts workouts. In most cases, the intensity of the workout results in a rise in blood glucose rather than a fall during the activity.

### *Insulin Changes Alone*

For his martial arts participation, Tom Seabourne of Mount Pleasant, Texas, no longer finds he has to make any regimen changes since he switched to a low-carbohydrate diet (no starchy carbohydrates). He has minimal insulin in his body during the activity.

Tom Shearer of Carlsbad, California, studies kung fu. During the 30- to 60-minute classes, he simply removes his insulin pump because it gets in the way. But that also serves to lower his basal insulin delivery to none while he keeps it off.

Canadian Dessi Zaharieva experiences some challenges associated with doing mixed martial arts for 2 hours in the evening, 6 days per week. These include having to disconnect her pump during training, taking a small bolus of insulin (1 to 2 units) halfway through training or sometimes at the end of training instead, and often setting a temporary (lower) basal rate overnight to help prevent exercise-associated hypoglycemia. She aims to work out with as little insulin on board as possible.

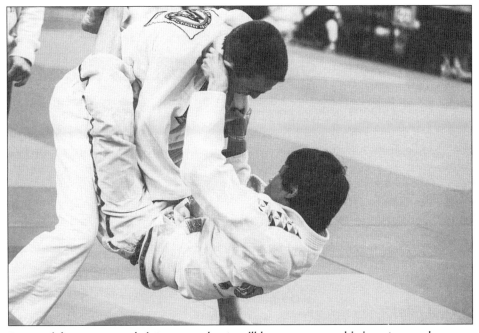

For martial arts, extremely intense workouts will be more anaerobic in nature and may even cause an increase in blood glucose. But if you work out long and hard, your risk of delayed drops in blood glucose will be heightened by your depletion of muscle glycogen.

A Lumberton, New Jersey, resident, Chris Creelman takes a mixed martial arts fitness class at a jiujitsu gym. The workout is different every day, but it amounts to high-intensity interval training that includes a variety of weightlifting exercises, body-weight exercises, and cardio training (jogging, burpees, ladder climbing, sprinting, tire flipping, battle ropes climbing, and punching or kicking a bag). For this activity, if her blood glucose is 100 mg/dL (5.6 mmol/L) or lower before starting, she adjusts her basal rate down to 50 percent for 2 hours. If higher than 200 mg/dL (11.1 mmol/L), she gives herself a small bolus to bring her glucose down but then lowers her basal rate after training by half for the first hour after her workout.

For tai chi chuan participation, American Christopher Gantz reduces his dinner bolus by half (he uses regular insulin because he is on a high-protein diet). He eats his normal dinner before working out because the class is in the evening. He would prefer, however, to exercise without any active insulin in his system whenever possible.

## PHYSICAL EDUCATION CLASSES AND GYM (SCHOOL BASED)

School physical education (PE) activities can vary widely, depending on which sport or activity (e.g., basketball, soccer, running, dance, or health instruction) the PE instructor is focusing on for the day or week. These activities may be done indoors or outdoors, depending on the weather, available facilities, the nature of the sport, and other factors. Not all schools offer PE classes daily anymore, making their effects even more unpredictable at times. Because these classes are so variable, compensating for the activities in advance can be difficult. Your best bet may be to make sure that you have carbohydrate snacks available to eat before and during more intense activities to prevent low blood glucose. Adjustments may need to be made on a daily basis to compensate for different activities done in PE and gym classes.

## WALKING AND RACE WALKING

Walking is an endurance activity that uses your aerobic energy system. Your body uses fat and carbohydrate when you walk at a moderate pace, but it uses carbohydrate (both blood glucose and muscle glycogen) almost exclusively for brisk and race speeds. How long you walk will also make a difference, and you may need to alter your insulin, diet, or both for longer walks at certain times. For additional ideas, refer to hiking in chapter 12.

## General Adjustments by Diabetes Regimen

Because walking is such a common activity for everyone, an outline of some general recommendations for walking and hypoglycemia prevention for specific groups is useful.

### Insulin Pump Users

If you use a pump, you have the most flexibility in lowering your insulin levels because you can suspend or reduce basal insulin when walking, giving you the most normal physiological response. If you walk at a slow or moderate pace (either walking comfortably or briskly), you may need no or minimal reductions in your basal rates, depending on the time of day. For more intense or extended walks, such as maintaining a race-walking pace or walking for an hour or more at a faster pace, you may need to lower your basal delivery more, along with taking smaller boluses for any snacks during or meals after walking.

## Basal–Bolus Regimens

If you walk more than 2 or 3 hours after a meal, you will have to make fewer regimen adjustments than if your exercise closely follows bolus insulin injections. You may not need any adjustments for slow or short walks at any time, but longer or faster ones may require you to eat to prevent lows because your muscles will be using more blood glucose as fuel. If you know that you will be taking a substantial walk soon after a meal, you may want to lower your meal injection of insulin to prevent lows.

## Noninsulin and Oral Medication Users

If you take no meds or only noninsulin ones, walking may have very little effect on your blood glucose levels. In fact, in a study I conducted, when exercisers with type 2 diabetes do 30 minutes of self-paced (slow to moderate) walking either before or after a meal, the after-meal activity keeps their blood glucose more stable with less of a postmeal spike. If you make your own insulin, your levels of this hormone will be higher after you eat than before, and by walking you get the double effect of exercise and insulin on lowering your blood glucose. Any exercise also slows your digestion of food, which can help prevent those postmeal spikes. If you walk briskly first thing in the morning, your blood glucose may go up. To combat this, have a small snack before you start your exercise to cause the release of enough insulin to break the higher insulin resistance present before breakfast.

# Athlete Examples

The following examples illustrate a variety of changes to compensate for everything from slow strolling to race walking and walking the dog (or cat, in one case).

## Insulin Changes Alone

For walking moderately, A.J. Krebs of Medford, Oregon, changes her regimen based on her starting blood glucose levels. If it is in the range of 100 to 125 mg/dL (5.6 to 6.9 mmol/L), she suspends her basal insulin delivery for the duration of her walk. If the range is 125 to 150 mg/dL (5.6 to 8.3 mmol/L), she sets her temporary basal rate at 15 percent of normal. If the range is 150 to 170 mg/dL (8.3 to 9.4 mmol/L), she puts her basal rate at 50 percent, but keeps a close eye on her CGM. At over 170 mg/dL (9.4 mmol/L) she leaves her basal rate alone but checks every 5 minutes and lowers it if her blood glucose starts to drop.

Emma Baird of Scotland does a lot of walking. If she times it right, she does not need to make many changes, especially when walking in the morning or right after a meal with no bolus insulin with the meal. She can start with her blood glucose in the range of 90 to 126 mg/dL (5.0 to 7.0 mmol/L), and it consistently lowers her blood glucose, whereas other exercises, especially those with intensity, push it up.

For power walking, Michael Krupar of Silver Spring, Maryland, walks when his insulin levels are already low, and he tries to stay in the range of 90 to 110 mg/dL (5.0 to 6.1 mmol/L). If his CGM alarm goes off, he stops his activity to double-check his blood glucose, correcting with carbohydrate intake as necessary.

A resident of Huntingdon Valley, Pennsylvania, Marc Blatstein does moderate walking for 20 minutes for exercise most of the time because he had both knees replaced in the past couple of years. Two hours before his walk, he lowers the basal rate on his pump by 20 percent, and he keeps it lower until 2 hours after his walking ends. Similarly, Martin Berkeley from Cardiff, Wales, puts his pump on a temporary basal rate that is 60 percent of normal while walking moderately for 45 minutes.

Sarah McManus, a resident of Pittsburgh, Pennsylvania, walks briskly for fitness, usually an hour at a time. For that activity, she reduces her basal rate by 50 percent about 45 minutes before she starts and leaves it lower until she has about 30 minutes of walking left.

Dessi Zaharieva from Canada finds that walking often helps her with weight-cutting before competitions with weight categories, such as boxing, kickboxing, and martial arts (in addition to managing her diet with low-carbohydrate eating). For walking, she reduces her basal insulin 60 to 90 minutes pre-exercise by 50 to 80 percent, but she makes sure to resume her normal basal rate right after she gets done walking. Overnight, she may set a temporary basal that is 20 percent lower for 6 hours.

## Diet Changes Alone

While on a 5- or 6-mile beach walk, Judith Jones-Ambrosini of New York tends to have her blood glucose drop because of the intensity of walking fast in the sand. She prefers to keep her blood glucose around 110 mg/dL (6.1 mmol/L) or even a little higher so she does not have to worry about dropping faster than she can handle. If she gets down to 80 mg/dL (4.4 mmol/L) while walking, she drinks a juice box.

Another long-timer with type 1 diabetes (over 72 years), Richard Vaughn of Kingston, New York, uses modern technology to exercise effectively. He watches his CGM and checks it frequently during all fitness activities, including walking. His glucose target is 110 to 130 mg/dL (6.1 to 7.2 mmol/L) during walking, gym workouts, and yard work. He eats as needed (usually Skittles or jelly beans) or stops exercising if his blood glucose drops below 80 mg/dL (4.4 mmol/L) then waits until it rises to start back up.

A Seattle, Washington, resident, Danielle Okuly finds that she needs a small snack like a nectarine before walking because even short walks tend to drop her blood glucose quickly. She carries Skittles with her during walks and eats two to three at a time, although she seldom needs more than 5 grams of carbohydrates to treat her lows.

United Kingdom resident Helen Cotton is more likely to have her blood glucose decrease during prolonged low-level exercise like walking around shops all day (for which she takes a 20-gram glucose gel). She forgets to think ahead and plan for this type of activity like she normally does for swimming.

For walking for 2 to 3 hours at a moderate pace, Sheri Ochs of Santa Barbara, California, often has to supplement with 6 to 15 grams of carbohydrate during the second and third hours only due to the effects of the activity and her basal insulin (Basaglar), even when she starts walking at least 3 hours after her last injection of Humalog. For walking an hour or less, she does not need to make any adjustments.

Stetson Siler from Oak Park, Illinois, has a volunteer job that involves a lot of walking—often 3 hours a day. To manage this, he usually has a midmorning muffin before starting, followed by a late lunch, which almost always keeps his blood glucose levels in a normal range. When doing low-intensity, long activities (e.g., walking and yard work), Naomi from Spokane, Washington, requires some carbohydrates as well. She can also do them when her blood glucose is higher and she wants to bring it down. During these activities, she watches her blood glucose on her CGM closely and eats when her level is trending down.

Bonny C. Damocles, a type 2 exerciser from Midland, Michigan, has been able to manage his diabetes with exercise and diet for over 25 years. He does physical activities like walking, power walking, or jogging in place immediately before each meal, before bed, and when he gets up in the morning for no fewer than 15 minutes each time to keep his blood glucose in a more normal range.

## Combined Regimen Changes

A resident of Excelsior, Minnesota, Bren Gauvin-Chadwick deals with walking by making sure that she is not trending down on her blood glucose. She then treats it with a Clif Shot Blok (8 carbohydrates per block) or snack. Occasionally she needs to decrease her basal rate.

For Kerri Sparling from Providence, Rhode Island, her main exercise is walking with her toddler son or doing free weights. To do either, she aims to have as little insulin on board as possible (preferably none) because exercise always has a tendency to cause sharp declines in her blood glucose. When working out, she is never without fast-acting glucose sources on hand. Her treadmill always has a jar of glucose tablets in the cup holder, or she keeps a juice box in her son's stroller, or she keeps fruit snacks crammed into her SPIbelt (small personal item belt) while walking. Lows have always hit her fast and hard, and she takes the risk of hypoglycemia very seriously (and remains vigilant about treating it).

Orangeville, California, resident Mark Conley always checks his blood glucose before he starts walking or doing a fitness class, as well as sometimes during and immediately after working out. He eats fruit leather or sports bars as needed during exercise and may have one before starting unless his glucose is 150 mg/dL (8.3 mmol/L) or higher. During most activities, he suspends his insulin pump as well.

## Other Effects to Consider

**Effect of Intensity (Pet Walking).**   A resident of Denver, Colorado, Daniel Schneider says that walking the dog for him rarely lasts more than 30 minutes, and he just makes sure to have snacks with him in case of emergency. On the other hand, Marialice Kern of Moraga, California, takes her dog hiking in the hills. For this activity, she makes sure that her blood glucose is above 150 mg/dL (8.3 mmol/L) when she starts, and by the end of the first hour she usually has to eat a Quest Protein Bar or a few glucose tablets, depending on how much longer she and her dog will be out.

A resident of Long Beach, California, Tian Walker, does not change her basal insulin for walking the dog—she walks her cat. They do a 10-minute walk and a 5-minute run, which is a short enough exercise span to not require any adjustment.

**Effect of Time of Day.**   For Ginger Vieira, a resident of Burlington, Vermont, doing 30 minutes to an hour of walking in the morning before breakfast (while still fasting) works like a charm. She starts with a blood glucose of 80 mg/dL (4.4 mmol/L) and finishes at 80 without needing to take in any extra carbohydrates. If she does start to get low, how much she takes in depends on the amount of insulin she has on board and the time left in her walking workout. She may take in 5 to 8 grams of carbohydrates for a mild low that is not dropping quickly, or closer to 15 to 30 grams if she is going down faster and wants to keep walking.

Riva Greenberg of Brooklyn, New York, also finds it is easier for her to walk in the morning, although she does her hour of moderate walking after breakfast because that time of day is when she is still most insulin resistant. She likes to start with a blood glucose of around 160 mg/dL (8.9 mmol/L), and if she is going low by the end of her walk, she may take in a glucose tablet or two (4 to 8 grams of carbohydrates). In general, she just takes a little less bolus insulin if she is going to walk and sticks to her low-carbohydrate diet. (To cover her basal insulin needs she takes Tresiba, which cannot be adjusted easily for exercise.)

**Effect of Spontaneity.**   For Canadian Sarah McGaugh of Brampton, Ontario, it makes a difference whether she has time to plan ahead. If she is doing planned walking, she reduces her basal or bolus insulin before walking. If the walking is unplanned, she reduces the basal rate on her pump when she starts and typically consumes fast-acting sugars throughout to keep her blood glucose stable.

## WATER AEROBICS AND AQUATIC EXERCISE

Water aerobics and aquatic exercise are similar to aerobic dance except for their intensity. Workouts in the pool are not weight-bearing like regular aerobic workouts are, making the water-based ones less intense for that reason alone. The good thing about water exercise is that it places less stress on your lower limb joints and feet, which can be particularly good if you have any neuropathy. It is still aerobic in nature, with periods of greater and lesser intensity depending on how hard you want to work. Like most other aerobic activities, doing them first thing in the morning allows you to maintain your blood glucose more easily. Otherwise, to prevent lows you can lower your basal doses or cut back on premeal boluses if you plan to do this activity within 2 hours of eating.

## Athlete Examples

These examples show that anyone can safely engage in various types of aquatic exercises and classes, although you should abstain from water activities if you have an unhealed ulcer on your foot or lower leg secondary to peripheral neuropathy.

### Diet Changes Alone

Cathy DeVreeze, a resident of Ontario, Canada, checks her blood glucose before she goes in the pool and when she gets out. Unless she is running higher than desired, she does not change her insulin. She finds it better to have a snack than to reduce her insulin (which is Fiasp for boluses and Tresiba for basal needs).

### Combined Regimen Changes

A Jensen Beach, Florida, resident, Judy Unger does laps in the pool using foam barbells and various techniques (e.g., body row, body bicycle, and kicking) for about 25 minutes at a time. After finding that completely removing her pump led to high blood glucose, she now keeps it on (it is waterproof) and simply lowers her basal or boluses to compensate. She will not exercise with a blood glucose over 180 mg/dL (10 mmol/L); if it is below 100 mg/dL (5.5 mmol/L) at the start, she eats 15 to 20 grams of carbohydrate.

Grace from Coral Gables, Florida, aims to have her blood glucose in the range of 80 to 120 mg/dL (4.4 to 6.7 mmol/L) before either water aerobics or other pool exercise. She takes in 15 grams of carbohydrates if she is at 80 mg/dL (4.4 mmol/L) or below (taken as juice or glucose tablets according to the severity of the low). If she is running high (250 mg/dL or higher [over 13.9 mmol/L]), she takes an insulin bolus to correct it. For anywhere in between, she finds her blood glucose is usually lowered naturally by the activity. But if not, she gives herself an appropriate correction between 30 minutes to 1 hour after finishing her workouts.

## WEIGHT AND CIRCUIT TRAINING

Weight, or resistance, training involves short, powerful repetitions and mainly uses your anaerobic energy sources (stored phosphagens and muscle glycogen). More often than not, such training causes a greater release of glucose-raising hormones than most aerobic activities. Doing any intense activity may require you to make minimal adjustments to prevent lows, at least during the activity, and your glucose may go up instead of down. Doing prolonged or heavy weight training can use up a lot of muscle glycogen, thus increasing your risk of later-onset lows, even if your blood glucose rises initially.

If you do your workout with lower levels of insulin on board, such as 2 or more hours after eating or in the early morning, you may need some insulin to prevent a rise in glucose or bring it back down. The majority of athletes surveyed who do resistance training found that it is more likely to raise their blood glucose than any other of their regular activities, especially when done fasted with minimal insulin on board. The solution that many have found to work is to give more insulin before or during this activity.

Others choose to do weight training in combination with an aerobic workout to help reverse this rise (or they give more insulin afterward to bring it down). An alternative is to do circuit weight training, which usually emphasizes a greater number of repetitions with lower resistance and is slightly more aerobic in nature (meaning that it usually causes less of a rise in your blood glucose levels). By way of example, Stephanie Winter from Fayetteville, North Carolina, finds that circuit training works best for maintaining a steady blood glucose when working out with minimal insulin on board.

## Athlete Examples

As you will see from these examples, how you choose to do your weight training affects the changes that you will need to make to maintain your blood glucose levels.

If you just have basal insulin on board when you go to train or you have access to a hybrid closed-loop system, you may not have to do anything. For instance, Katherine Owen of Tallahassee, Florida, does nothing to compensate for her weight training because the sensor and auto mode of her hybrid system will release enough basal insulin to keep up with any increases from the intensity of her training. Even though her pump does not have an auto mode, Canadian Sarah McGaugh has found that she does not need to make any regimen changes to do resistance training. Type 2 exerciser John Stover from Charleston, South Carolina, uses a combination of resistance training and rowing workouts to lower his blood glucose levels so that he does not have to take insulin to treat his diabetes.

### Insulin Changes Alone

American Christopher Gantz follows a very low-carbohydrate, high-protein (Dr. Bernstein) diet for which he finds his insulin needs are greatly reduced, although he covers his protein intake with regular insulin due to its slower peak and longer duration. On a typical morning, after his weight training he takes 1 unit of regular insulin for 6 grams of carbohydrates and lots of protein, and he stays stable all morning. He rarely boluses before weight training. If his glucose does spike from his workout, he chooses to finish up with some cardio work rather than an insulin injection to bring his blood glucose back to normal.

When Christel Oerum from Santa Monica, California (who is profiled at the end of this chapter), does resistance training in the morning after breakfast, she needs to reduce her pre-exercise meal bolus by 50 to 75 percent, depending on whether she does any cardio training afterward (which brings her glucose down more). Similarly, Philadelphia resident Gary Scheiner lowers his preworkout meal bolus by 20 percent before doing resistance training.

Guy Hornsby, a master weightlifter from Morgantown, West Virginia, rarely makes any adjustments for his morning or afternoon training routine, although both times tend to raise his blood glucose by 20 to 40 mg/dL (1.1 to 2.2 mmol/L) because of the intensity of his workouts. If intense training raises his glucose more than 40 mg/dL (2.2 mmol/L), he gives a correction bolus to bring it down. Otherwise, he needs insulin adjustments only if he is sick or injured and cannot train as he normally does. He never exercises within 2 hours of eating and injecting any insulin other than his basal one (Basaglar).

Kory Seder from Madison, Wisconsin, finds that each activity is different, but he does not really consider most fitness activities as exercise, other than kettlebell training and resistance workouts. Before doing any high-intensity strength training, he does a 10-minute aerobic warmup to prevent the rise in his blood glucose that happens when he does not do that first. He may also bolus 1 to 2 units before training that is heavy.

For Jennie B. in the United Kingdom, weight training tends to raise her blood glucose if it is intense, so she may bolus in advance or just keep an eye on her CGM as she works out. She also finds she often must bolus in the hour or so after training to bring her blood glucose down. Likewise, for intense weightlifting, Dalton Merryman from Fresno, California, has to increase his basal rate of insulin by 50 percent starting 15 minutes before his workout.

Unlike when she does aerobic workouts, Rebekah Lindsay needs to keep her basal rate the same as normal for weight training and then increase it by 25 percent for an hour or 2 afterward to combat postworkout glucose elevations. Conversely, Leslie K. from Raleigh, North Carolina, finds that she needs a 50 percent decrease in her basal rate during weight training when it is moderate in intensity.

Jack Borck of West Ellis, Wisconsin, finds he needs to reduce his basal rate starting 1 hour before heavy weightlifting, but how much depends on his blood glucose. Right before he starts lifting, he further reduces his rate (down to about 80 percent total). He may need to leave it lower by 25 to 50 percent for 2 hours after working out as well, depending on his glucose values. Similarly, D. Jones of LaGrange, Illinois, has to reduce his basal rate by 50 percent 1 hour before starting an hour's worth of heavy weight training.

Philippines resident Sally Clark does weight training 4 days a week while fasting. She has to take 1 to 2 units of Humalog first, though, to prevent the rise in blood glucose that her morning workout causes. Occasionally, she also needs extra insulin afterward for correction.

## *Combined Regimen Changes*

A resident of Apple Valley, Minnesota, Aaron Gretz does full-body weight training and stretching three afternoons a week, which starts around 3:00 p.m. and lasts about 2.5 hours. On those days, he eats lunch (a big salad loaded with meats and eggs) and takes a larger than usual Humalog injection due to his extra carbohydrate intake. After training, he drinks a low-carbohydrate protein shake (20 grams of protein and 5 grams of carbohydrates) without taking a bolus. Dinner follows an hour after the shake, and it is low carbohydrate (typically grilled chicken or steak and a veggie), for which he takes very little insulin. Before going to bed, he takes a lower dose of Basaglar (25 units) than normal or else his blood glucose goes low in the middle of the night.

American Shelby T. eats a preworkout meal 1 hour before doing weight training and boluses with a 40 percent reduced dose of Humalog. If she needs a correction after working out, she also reduces that bolus by 40 percent. She reduces her overnight insulin dosing by 20 percent after heavy workouts and only 10 percent for lighter days.

When doing training with weights or kettlebells, Donny Swarmer of Cheswick, Pennsylvania, does not eat beforehand so he will not have to manage a peaking dose of insulin. If his blood glucose is stable and near normal, he changes nothing and simply goes off his pump and his normal basal rate while working out. If he is low or dropping, he drinks some juice.

Amy Coley from Decatur, Alabama, has to bolus 1 to 2 units while she is weight training because her blood glucose always goes up afterward. She always eats before any training to fuel her body for the activity.

## Other Effects to Consider

**Effect of Exercise Intensity.**  A resident of Brewer, Maine, Debbie Wright Theriault finds that many times she will go low if she is doing just cardio training, and many times she will go high if she is lifting weights. She takes a little extra insulin and does the weight lifting first, and then she finishes her workout by running a mile or two to lower her glucose.

Likewise, Molly McDermott of Ottawa, Canada, says that she rarely gets exercise-induced high blood glucose. However, when she does get high glucose, it occurs when she is exclusively lifting weights, and she may need a small dose of Humalog to bring her glucose back down after the workout.

Neil McLagan of Perth, Australia, has based his regimen changes on his planned workout. For weight and resistance training that ranges from light to moderate, he does not need any extra food or insulin before, during, or after the workout. However, if his training is heavy and intense and he starts with a normal starting blood glucose, he takes a 0.5-unit intramuscular injection 10 to 15 minutes before lifting to prevent a rise in his glucose.

**Effect of Time of Day.**  Vicky Hollingsworth of Newmarket, Canada, finds that bodyweight training will raise her blood glucose in the morning, but it will not do much in the afternoon unless she performs lots of burpees or mountain climbers. New Yorker Lauren Bongiorno also needs different changes based on the activity and time of day. She is very sensitive to cardio or circuit training in the late afternoon or evening; at these times, she has to eat a snack before and do a 20 percent lower temporary basal rate. If she does strength training in the morning, her blood glucose rises by about 40 to 60 mg/dL (2.2 to 3.3 mmol/L); during these sessions, she needs an increased basal (on average a 20 percent increase).

## YOGA AND STRETCHING

These activities are low level and require minimal muscular effort. Most stretches, especially in yoga, are static (involving no movement) and are held for a while. Because diabetes can often reduce your joint and muscle flexibility over time more than aging alone, stretching at least two or three times a week can be extremely beneficial. You should not need to do anything special to compensate because most yoga and stretching usually do not cause much change in blood glucose.

## Athlete Examples

Doing yoga, particularly in a hot environment, may require more adjustments than just practicing yoga or stretching on your own. However, even most yoga classes that last for an hour or more will use minimal amounts of blood glucose.

For example, Rachel Zinman from Australia does yoga as her main form of exercise, and she finds it has little effect on her blood glucose levels. Massachusetts resident Emily Marrama finds that if she starts with her blood glucose around 150 mg/dL (8.3 mmol/L), she does not have to make any changes for doing yoga either.

Likewise, Philadelphia resident Daniele Hargenrader finds that she does not have much trouble maintaining her blood glucose around doing yoga, and Courtney Duckworth of Washington, D.C., needs little to no change in her regimen for yoga. Neither does Heather Williams from Columbus, Ohio, who said she needs no real changes for stretching exercises or yoga because these low-impact activities do not tend to affect her blood glucose any more than a regular day.

But combining stretching with other exercises may have more of an impact. For instance, Brown from Laramie, Wyoming, says that she can stretch at any blood glucose level unless she has just finished running—in this case, her range has to be above 80 mg/dL (4.4 mmol/L) or she will go low before she finishes her stretching.

### Insulin Changes Alone

Californian Tian Walker tries different approaches for yoga. She is often surprised at how fast her blood glucose falls during yoga, even when it feels like a low level of exertion. She usually starts out with a normal basal rate and then decreases it as she starts to feel herself dropping. It takes 30 minutes for the decreased rate to kick in, but she typically feels her lows coming on within that time frame, so it works out for her.

### Diet Changes Alone

Daniel Schneider of Denver, Colorado, uses yoga typically just to warm up for his day, usually only 10 to 15 minutes in the morning, and he does not need to make any adjustments. He makes sure he has snacks nearby, though he usually does not need any.

### Combined Regimen Changes

Illinois resident Stetson Siler finds that for an easier exercise like yoga he can eat beforehand and take 75 percent of his wizard-recommended bolus over 60 or 90 minutes without going low. Unlike vigorous activities, he does not usually need an additional bolus at the end of being active.

As you can see from this chapter, fitness activities lead to varied responses in blood glucose levels, and athletes use a variety of approaches to keep their glucose in their target range. Whether you choose to work out in a gym, in a group environment, or at home alone does not matter nearly as much as simply staying active does. So keep up the great work, stay fit, and reap the benefits of better health that come from your lifestyle choices.

## Athlete Profile: **Christel Oerum**

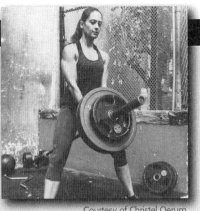

Courtesy of Christel Oerum.

*Hometown:* Santa Monica, California

*Diabetes history:* Type 1 diabetes diagnosed in 1997 (at age 19)

*Sport or activity:* Resistance training and bodybuilding. I'm into everything active, but my passion is resistance training. I competed in bodybuilding competitions (bikini division) in 2014 and 2016, but now I focus more on just having fun and being healthy rather than aesthetics.

*Greatest athletic achievement:* I competed and placed well in bodybuilding competitions in the NPC bikini division: NPC Gold Coast, March 2016, masters 1st place; NPC Gold Coast, March 2016, height group E, 2nd place; NPC North California, June 2016, masters 2nd place; and NPC North California, June 2016, height group E, 4th place.

*Current insulin and medication regimen:* I use insulin pens (Humalog and Levemir) and a Dexcom CGM. For fast-acting insulin, I use a durable pen so that I can take half-unit increments. I also use an app named RapidCalc that works as a bolus calculator and keeps track of my "insulin on board."

*Training tips:* Consistency and finding a type of exercise you enjoy is key and the best way to achieve real results. When it comes to diabetes management, the most important thing to do is take detailed notes, learn from your mistakes, and make sure you understand how to manage your diabetes tightly during your training. I do not recommend letting yourself run high (>200 mg/dL [>11.1 mmol/L]) to avoid lows, but rather reduce your insulin enough that you won't go low even if you start with blood glucose closer to 100 mg/dL (5.6 mmol/L).

I am also not a big fan of "carbing up" in order to exercise for less than 60 minutes (unless it is *very* intense training, you are hungry, or running low). It is typically better to reduce your insulin prior and potentially during your workout instead of consuming unnecessary carbohydrates (at least if you are trying to also control your calorie intake). However, if you find that you often go high during workouts (very common with anaerobic exercise), eating beforehand and taking a bolus can be very beneficial, not only from a blood glucose perspective but also from a performance perspective.

Don't be afraid to eat or adjust your insulin; just do it so that it makes sense for you and what you'd like to achieve. You will most likely find that you need significantly different diabetes management strategies depending on the type of training, time of day, time of month (for women), and so on.

*Typical daily and weekly training and diabetes regimen:* My training schedule depends greatly on whether I'm training with a certain goal in mind (like a fitness show) and how busy I am, but ideally I like to include a minimum of 5 resistance training days. My cardio training is often just hiking, biking, or other fun outside activities.

▶ *Monday:* Back (resistance exercises) and 20 to 40 minutes of cardio training.

▶ *Tuesday:* Legs (focused on hamstrings and glutes).

- ► *Wednesday:* Optional cardio workout.
- ► *Thursday:* Shoulders and abdominals.
- ► *Friday:* Chest and arms and 20 to 40 minutes of cardio training.
- ► *Saturday:* Legs (focused on quads and glutes).
- ► *Sunday:* Rest day–optional light hiking.

***Other hobbies and interests:*** My big passion project is my website, DiabetesStrong.com. I created it to share everything I have learned about diabetes, exercise, and healthy nutrition, and running the website is now what I do full time. I also love being outside with my husband and dog. Living in southern California has made it possible for me to go for hikes (wearing shorts and a T-shirt) pretty much year around.

***Good diabetes and exercise story:*** I often wear my Dexcom CGM on my upper arm, and I regularly test my blood glucose and inject insulin in the gym. I can't tell you how often that has started conversations about diabetes with other gym-goers. It has helped me dispel a lot of misconceptions about what people living with diabetes can do and what they can look like.

# 9

# Endurance Sports

Whether you want to run a marathon, cycle across the country, or compete in a full Ironman triathlon, you will be in good company. Even becoming an Olympian is entirely possible with diabetes. Consider the determination of Olympic cross-country skier Kris Freeman (see his athlete profile in chapter 6) to compete in events that would be grueling for any athlete while juggling his blood glucose and all his diabetes gear under harsh environmental conditions. Decades ago when I first started looking into athletes with diabetes, they were few and far between. Nowadays, they are coming out of the woodwork, and Team Novo Nordisk even consists of a group of over 100 professional athletes with type 1 diabetes who compete in myriad races and events around the world. Most of these athletes do workouts that are highly aerobic, but often with interspersed sprinting or harder intervals to build fitness. We would all do well to learn more about their training tips and diabetes management while they do highly aerobic and often physically and mentally demanding endurance training and events.

Endurance sports primarily rely on your aerobic energy system. Some aspects of the sports and activities included in this chapter, however, would also qualify as endurance–power sports (discussed in the next chapter), such as 50-meter sprints in swimming or sprint cycling. Whether you want to become the world's fastest swimmer or a top ultradistance runner, you will find that exercisers have taken on all these grueling events just to prove that they can do anything that they want to, despite having diabetes. Their examples, as well as others relevant to more modest exercisers, are included in this chapter, which covers activities like cross country running and skiing, cycling, marathons, running and jogging, swimming, triathlons, and ultraendurance events and training. Also, for adventure racing and other outdoor, less-traditional endurance activities, see chapter 12.

## GENERAL RECOMMENDATIONS FOR ENDURANCE SPORTS

Your body can use carbohydrate, fat, and protein to make adenosine triphosphate (ATP) to fuel your muscular activity over prolonged periods, but how intense and how long your workouts are largely determines the fuel mix, along with your diet. For example, during less intense activities like slow swimming, your body can use more fats (triglycerides and free fatty acids in the blood) along with some muscle glycogen and blood glucose. When you are working out harder, your muscles use less fat, relying more on carbohydrate instead—muscle glycogen and, to a lesser extent, blood glucose.

Typically, the total amount of glucose in your bloodstream is only about 5 grams of carbohydrate total—the equivalent of about 20 calories, or enough to run 0.2 miles (0.3 kilometers) or less—although your liver is constantly working to replenish and maintain that amount in your blood. Depleting your muscle glycogen changes the fuels that your body may be using, which will cause you to lessen your pace to be able to use more fat and often bump up your blood glucose use at the same time.

> *You can generally delay fatigue by taking in carbohydrates (and possibly protein and fat) during prolonged activities. Doing so can help prevent lows as your glycogen stores diminish. If your glycogen gets depleted, you will be forced to exercise at a slower pace.*

Intense efforts use carbohydrates as fuel almost exclusively, although fat starts to contribute more ATP as soon as you scale back your pace. You can also revert to temporarily relying more on your lactic acid system (fueled by muscle glycogen) whenever you increase your pace or start using faster muscle fibers, which happens as you run and cycle up hills or sprint for the finish line. Doing prolonged events can draw on your protein stores, too: up to 10 to 15 percent of your energy comes from breaking down protein during extremely long events, although for shorter ones lasting an hour or less, it is usually 5 percent or less. For a refresher on the energy systems and fuels for different types of exercise, refer to chapter 2.

When you are exercising long and either moderately or vigorously, you may need a combination of insulin reductions (bolus ones are shown in table 2.3) and carbohydrate increases (see table 2.2) to maintain your blood glucose levels. Exercising with minimal insulin on board helps prevent lows, but for extended events you can benefit from consuming adequate amounts of carbohydrates (and likely other fuels) during the activity, just as competitors without diabetes do. Although regular training increases your body's ability to use fat, you will likely have to reduce your overall insulin doses, both basally and for food intake, due to having enhanced insulin sensitivity. If you take oral doses of diabetes medications, check with your doctor about reducing how much you take if you are having more frequent lows with regular training. For more information about diabetes medications and those that increase your exercise-related hypoglycemia risk, refer to chapter 3.

# GENERAL ADJUSTMENTS BY DIABETES REGIMEN

Your performance may benefit from carbohydrate supplementation (up to as much as 75 grams per hour) or other food during prolonged activity, depending on how long and how hard you are working out. You will likely need more carbohydrates if you exercise during an insulin peak or if you do not sufficiently reduce your insulin

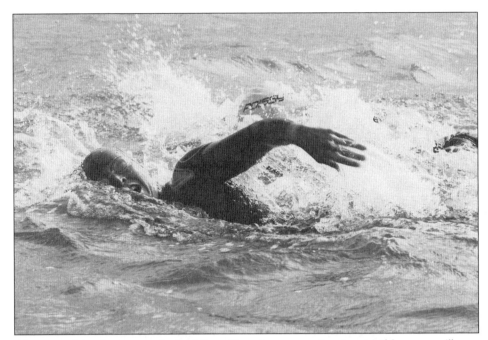

When exercising for long periods of time, like when competing in a triathlon, you will likely need to combine insulin reductions with greater food intake to maintain your blood glucose.

on board (basal and/or bolus). You may also need extra carbohydrate afterward and even at bedtime—along with some protein and fat—to prevent a drop in your blood glucose later as glycogen is being replaced over the next 24 to 48 hours (or longer). The best way to learn what works best for you is by checking your blood glucose responses during the exercise and afterward.

In general, your need for supplemental food is not as great during short, intense activities (see table 2.2). Although your body uses more glycogen as its primary fuel during such activities, their intensity causes a greater release of glucose-raising hormones such as adrenaline, which help maintain your blood glucose. Having minimal insulin on board also helps, although in some cases you may need some extra insulin after exercise.

One last point is that if you seriously overstress your body with an event or long-distance training, you may not be as insulin sensitive as you would expect to be for the next day or two. If you end up with delayed-onset muscle soreness (discussed in chapter 7), your body will not be able to replace glycogen until your muscles repair and rebuild themselves, and you may experience a greater level of insulin resistance while that process is going on.

*If you overwork your muscles so much during a long-distance event that you get really sore, expect to be more insulin resistant until your muscles repair themselves and your soreness diminishes. You cannot restore muscle glycogen fully until muscles are rebuilt.*

## Insulin Pump Users

As a pump user, you have the option of lowering your basal insulin during an activity by 0 to 100 percent, depending on its intensity and duration and how much carbohydrate or other foods you want to eat. In addition, you can reduce your meal boluses if you are exercising soon after the meal. Your blood glucose will generally be easier to maintain if you do not take any rapid-acting insulin within 2 to 3 hours of starting your event or workout. Afterward, you may need to reduce your meal boluses along with your basal rates for a while, possibly as long as 24 hours afterward in extreme cases, to prevent late-onset and overnight lows.

## Basal–Bolus Regimens

For endurance activities you can reduce your preworkout doses of bolus insulin by 25 to 100 percent, depending on how long and how hard you will be working, and increase your carbohydrate intake. You may also benefit from reducing your morning dose of basal insulin (if you take some then) before an extended activity. If you exercise when your insulin levels are lower, at least 2 to 3 hours after your last dose of rapid-acting insulin, then you will need fewer adjustments. After prolonged endurance exercise, you may have to reduce your meal insulin doses, lower your bedtime basal insulin to prevent nighttime lows, and consume extra carbohydrates, protein, and/or fat.

## Noninsulin and Oral Medication Users

If you do not use insulin, you probably are not any more likely to develop hypoglycemia during a prolonged event than an athlete without diabetes. You should still check your blood glucose to find out how your body responds. Ask your doctor about lowering your doses of medications if you start seeing significant drops in your glucose during or after your activities. You can still benefit from supplementing with carbohydrate during extended exercise, just as any other participant would do. If you use any medication that you feel is negatively affecting your ability to do endurance exercise, look into reducing your dose or adjusting the time of day when you take it.

## Other Effects to Consider

Many variables can affect your blood glucose responses to an endurance activity. How hard and how long you work have a significant effect. In general, more intense activities done for a shorter time will result in a smaller drop in your blood glucose compared with prolonged, slower activities. Exercising when your insulin levels are lower—either first thing in the morning or before meals—requires substantially fewer adjustments. Your starting blood glucose levels will affect your need for regimen changes, and you will need fewer changes when they start in a higher range. In addition, regular endurance training will likely enhance your insulin action, resulting in a need for less insulin, regardless of your type of diabetes or your medication regimen. You also need to consider factors such as your diet leading into a workout or event, the time of day you are active, the impact of mental stress if you are competing in an event, and environmental conditions if you are exercising outdoors.

*The environment (including heat, cold, humidity, wind, altitude, and even air pollution) itself can impact your exercise performance and your blood glucose responses on any given day. Learn as much as you can through research and practice about how to manage all those potential factors.*

## CROSS COUNTRY RUNNING

Competitive cross country running stresses endurance performance. Your body will primarily use muscle glycogen and blood glucose, and the harder you run, the more you use. To compensate, you need to alter your insulin doses, food intake, or both, depending on factors such as the time of day that you exercise, your starting blood glucose levels, and your insulin levels during your run. More intense running (such as during competitions) may temporarily raise your blood glucose, but doing it for long enough will often bring it down quickly—more so during practices than competitions because of the lesser anxiety associated with nonrace days. You will likely need lower overall insulin doses during the cross country season because of the heightened insulin action that you will experience from regular training, but if you are injured and have to take some time off, your insulin needs will go up.

## Athlete Examples

These athlete examples show that cross country running usually requires a combination of dietary and insulin adjustments to compensate.

### Combined Regimen Changes

Australian Ron C. usually takes off his insulin pump to participate in cross country races up to 10 kilometers (6.2 miles). Depending on his blood glucose level, he may eat something 15 to 30 minutes before the start of the race. He carries glucose gel and other fast-acting sugars as insurance.

A resident of Ashtabula, Ohio, Kayla Bertholf does competitive cross country and long-distance running. For these activities, she sets a temporary blood glucose target of 150 mg/dL (8.3 mmol/L) on her pump for 1 hour before and 2 hours after the run or competition. She consumes 20 grams of carbohydrates (usually as GU energy gel) before every run, but she eats more complex carbohydrates 3 to 4 hours before starting each competition or long run. These usually consist of about 25 grams of carbohydrates (toast with peanut butter and bananas or oatmeal) on competition mornings.

Janet G. from Scotland does cross country and road running and finds that her management depends on her starting blood glucose, the distance of the run, the weather, and the terrain. To manage her blood glucose, she usually reduces her basal rate to 60 percent 30 minutes before the start of exercise (if she does it any sooner, her blood glucose rises too high). If her starting blood glucose is in her target range, as monitored with continuous glucose monitoring (CGM), she often needs two glucose tablets per mile (8 grams of carbohydrates) and a carton of juice after 5 miles (8 kilometers). During competitions, adrenaline can make her blood glucose rise very high before the race, so sometimes she needs extra insulin to counteract that.

While running cross country or cycling, Bailey from Wachtberg, Germany, reduces his basal insulin rates down to about 50 percent. He also eats extra carbohydrates before and during the activity (30 grams for each 30 minutes of running or biking).

## CROSS-COUNTRY SKIING AND ROLLER SKIING

Cross-country skiing is one of the best overall aerobic exercises that you can do. Athletes who participate regularly in this activity are extremely fit aerobically. "Skiing" on a ski fitness machine (see chapter 9) can bestow similar benefits, although most people tend not to sustain the indoor activity for as long as they would ski outdoors. Those serious about training for cross-country skiing usually train during times of no snow (usually during the warmer months) by doing roller skiing, which uses short skis with wheels to replicate the movement of actual cross-country skiing. Changes in your diabetes regimen will depend mainly on how long you are skiing and the winter environmental conditions, including the temperature, windchill, and snow conditions. Roller skiing in warmer months can bring heat, humidity, high winds, or other environmental extremes for you to contend with.

The duration of your cross-country skiing is the most important factor affecting regimen changes. Skiing for longer periods uses more muscle glycogen and increases your risk of later-onset hypoglycemia. You will likely need to both reduce your insulin and to increase your food intake for skiing longer than 1 hour. Another factor is the skiing conditions on any given day. Your body will use more carbohydrates when it is cold or when you are working hard against a strong wind or stickier snow, or even against heat and humidity when roller skiing during the summer months. In all these extremes, you will likely need to adjust your diabetes regimen to compensate.

## Athlete Examples

The following real-life examples show that you need to make regimen changes to compensate for cross-country skiing. Also, see the profile of Olympic cross-country skier Kris Freeman in chapter 6.

### *Combined Regimen Changes*

For Daniel Schneider of Denver, Colorado, cross-country skiing, running, and cycling all involve carrying adequate food with him during activity. He aims to start with his blood glucose around 140 mg/dL (7.8 mmol/L) with no insulin on board, or at least with food in his stomach if there is insulin present. His glucose usually stays in the range of 140 to 180 mg/dL (7.8 to 10.0 mmol/L) for around the first 45 minutes of exercise. After that, he can eat 45 to 75 grams of carbohydrates per hour for the duration to stay balanced. He has pushed that out to 12 hours of endurance activity, and that formula remains fairly consistent as long as he gets more food in the middle of the activity (he tends to eat a peanut butter and jelly sandwich around the sixth hour of activity).

Tom Kalwitz of Madison, Wisconsin, uses a similar strategy for cross-country skiing or cycling for 1 to 3 hours at a time. At the start of an activity, he generally cuts back his basal rate by 30 to 75 percent, depending on what he is doing. He may, in some cases, cut it back an hour or an hour and a half beforehand, depending on his blood glucose level and the anticipated duration and difficulty of the activity. He also generally reduces his basal rate overnight by 25 to 50 percent, again depending on the length and difficulty of the course that he did earlier that day.

Excelsior, Minnesota, resident Bren Gauvin-Chadwick always decreases her basal rate by 85 percent for this activity, and she eats some carbohydrates if her blood glucose goes lower than 110 mg/dL (6.1 mmol/L) during cross-country skiing. She finds roller skiing a little more challenging because she must manage her blood glucose in the heat. She tries to start with a blood glucose of about 140 mg/dL (7.8 mmol/L), decreases her basal by 85 percent again, and closely monitors her glucose. This strategy works for about an hour, and then she may need a Clif Shot Blok or two or a GU energy gel to compensate if she keeps roller skiing.

## CYCLING

Cycling is generally aerobic in nature, although some cycling events involve sprinting and hill climbing, both of which rely on some anaerobic energy production using the lactic acid system. (See the profile of sprint cyclist Mandy Marquardt in chapter 2 as an example.) Prolonged, harder cycling uses mostly carbohydrate, both blood glucose and muscle glycogen, and requires more adjustments to keep your blood glucose in line. Less intense cycling allows for greater fat use, especially in fat-adapted and highly trained athletes.

Your cycling intensity and duration, timing of exercise, starting blood glucose levels, and usual diet will affect your blood glucose responses. For longer-duration cycling (2 hours or longer), you will likely need to eat more food and lower your insulin on board. Longer rides will also use up more of your muscle glycogen stores, thus increasing your risk for low blood glucose during the activity and later. If you cycle with lower insulin levels, either first thing in the morning or before meals, then your blood glucose may not drop as much. In some circumstances, you may need a small dose of rapid-acting insulin to counteract a rise in glucose from intense cycling or excess food intake during rides.

## Athlete Examples

Athletes decrease their insulin and increase their food intake to compensate for cycling. Prolonged cycling workouts invariably require greater regimen changes. For additional related examples, refer to the section on mountain biking in chapter 12.

### Insulin Changes Alone

Toronto, Canada, resident Mike Riddell tries to have little or no bolus insulin in his system when he does any aerobic training, including cycling and running. He cuts the basal rate on his pump by 50 percent starting 90 minutes before exercise and maintains this lower basal during exercise until he finishes his workout.

Philadelphia, Pennsylvania, resident Gary Scheiner reduces any bolus insulin doses by 50 percent before and during cycling. He also lowers his basal rate in advance by 70 percent, starting 1 hour before his ride.

Australian Warwick Sickling usually lowers his basal insulin a little for cycling but not by a huge amount. The farthest he has cycled is 110 kilometers (68.4 miles), and because he already cycles about 30 kilometers (18.6 miles) each day for commuting, the difference is not large enough to necessitate a huge change in his basal rates.

Anthony Mark of Philadelphia, Pennsylvania, skips his usual insulin dose for either breakfast or dinner to induce hyperglycemia before doing 1 hour on a bike (at a 17 miles-per-hour pace). His goal is to start with his blood glucose in the 220 to 240 mg/dL (12.2 to 13.3 mmol/L) range.

## Diet Changes Alone

American cyclist and athlete Jim Schuler makes decisions about his management based on trends and desired activity length. As in all management of diabetes, he says it depends! If he is dropping from a blood glucose of 300 to 150 mg/dL (16.7 down to 8.3 mmol/L) in 20 minutes, he eats a banana or glucose tablets. But if it is slowly rising from 80 to 100 mg/dL (4.4 to 5.6 mmol/L) in 20 minutes, he does not need to take any action. Generally, if his glucose is less than 100 mg/dL (5.6 mmol/L), he starts thinking about eating glucose tablets, an energy bar of some kind, or fruit. If he is less than 90 mg/dL (5.0 mmol/L) and falling, he definitely eats. But it also depends on when he is checking; for example, if he is at 80 mg/dL (4.4 mmol/L) with 10 minutes left in a scheduled run indoors (during the winter on a treadmill), he may just cut the run a little short and stop without treating it. If he is at 80 mg/dL (4.4 mmol/L) and is only 15 minutes into the run after starting at 120 mg/dL (6.7 mmol/L) and he wants to run another hour, he definitely eats. Sometimes, if he is within 20 minutes of a planned finish, he is much happier just ending a workout a bit early instead of having to fight to keep his blood glucose up.

For long rides, Sara Pomish of Farmington Hills, Michigan, only eats protein or fat for fuel during exercise, such as cheese sticks and a packet of peanut butter. But if her glucose is below 80 mg/dL (4.4 mmol/L), she may eat a jelly bean or two to bump up her glucose a tad, and she adds electrolytes to the water in her water bottle. Otherwise, she does not need to do anything different for this activity because her low-carbohydrate diet keeps her glucose extremely stable. She takes very little insulin, and she believes that insulin really is the wildcard in these scenarios.

St. Petersburg, Florida, resident Mark Christiansen keeps Skittles candy, fruit juice, and water handy while cycling. He has a mount on his handlebars for his CGM receiver/phone so he can view his blood glucose while riding.

## Combined Regimen Changes

The changes needed can vary greatly with how long and how hard you ride, but also your insulin regimen. See the examples that follow, organized in order of increasing duration of cycling training and events within each regimen section.

**Insulin Pump Users.**   Atlanta, Georgia, resident Greg Cashman eats 40 grams of carbohydrates before riding, along with 25 grams more every 30 minutes while cycling (usually around an hour). If he is at racing speed, he increases the amount of carbohydrates to 50 grams every 30 minutes. He likes eating Clif Shot Bloks the most during this activity because he can adjust the amount of carbohydrates by eating more or less of them (each one contains 8 grams of carbohydrates). In addition, 90 minutes before the event he reduces his basal rate by 25 percent and keeps it lowered while riding.

For cycling 1 to 1.5 hours at a time, Ron C. of Australia reduces his basal rate to 50 percent or less starting 30 minutes beforehand. He also eats 25 grams of carbohydrates to start (unless his blood glucose has risen over 234 mg/dL [13 mmol/L]), along with 20 to 25 grams of carbohydrates per hour. He may wait until 30 minutes into the ride if his glucose started out higher before he will start supplementing, though.

Biking is the first form of exercise where Tian Walker of Long Beach, California, says she has felt consistently in control of her blood glucose. She decreases her basal rate right when she begins, and her blood glucose stays stable. If she cycles more than 15 miles, sometimes she needs to eat a few Honey Stingers to compensate.

Stephanie Malmstrom of Salt Lake City, Utah, finds that typically when she is cycling for 1 to 3 hours, her blood glucose stays level. She monitors her levels throughout, and she eats 8 grams of carbohydrates (Clif Shot Bloks or GU energy gel) as needed, but she is more likely to go high if she eats too much. At the end of a ride, she either suspends her pump for an hour or sets a lower temporary rate so she does not bottom out 6 hours later. She mostly eats a low-carbohydrate diet (three meals of 15 grams of carbohydrates or less) with low-carbohydrate snacks in between. She tries to eat protein and fat before exercise and protein with a little carbohydrate afterward, and she only takes small bites of carbohydrate-based foods during long or strenuous workouts.

During cycling for 1.5 to 2 hours, Columbia, Maryland, resident Saul Zuckman treats his blood glucose when it drops below 100 mg/dL (5.6 mmol/L). (At rest he does not treat it until he reaches 80 mg/dL [4.4 mmol/L].) He uses fruit juice along with glucose tablets, followed by something with fat as well, such as half a power bar (along with 1 to 2 units of insulin). On a known hard day, he decreases his bolus injections, but generally he does not adjust the basal.

When North Carolina resident Michele Storr does vigorous workouts, she typically eats before exercising. She takes a bolus of 50 percent of what her pump wizard recommends and extends it over 90 minutes. She tends to need an additional bolus of 1 to 2 units at the end of hard exercise. If she is cycling for 2 to 3 hours, she usually eats a protein/carbohydrate bar midway through the ride.

For long weekend bike rides lasting 2.5 to 4 hours, Santa Barbara, California, resident Camille Andre eats a breakfast containing 40 to 50 grams of carbohydrates but decreases her bolus insulin by 75 percent to cover it. She also brings glucose with her on her ride and checks her CGM periodically. If she starts to drop below 100 mg/dL (5.6 mmol/L), she consumes another 20 grams of carbohydrates to compensate.

Andrew Angus from Aberdeen, Scotland, usually cycles for a couple of hours at a time. For his rides, he lowers the rate on his pump down to 15 percent (more or less, based on his route) and eats every 30 miles (Haribo gummies and High 5 energy gels). The more hills he rides, the less insulin he needs. Typically, he also keeps his basal rate lower for an hour after cycling.

For cycling 1 to 3 hours, Albert Nigro of Toronto, Canada, reduces his basal rate 1.5 hours before starting by 60 to 80 percent through his rides, although he often needs a bolus correction afterward. During exercise, if his glucose falls to 80 mg/dL (4.5 mmol/L), he has some glucose liquid or a regular gel. After exercise, if it is 72 mg/dL (4.0 mmol/L) or lower, he drinks orange juice and has a small snack.

For cycling 4 hours at a time, Scotland resident Jeff Foot reduces his basal rate of insulin by 90 percent from 1 hour before starting until 1 hour before finishing. He also eats 20 grams of carbohydrates without taking a bolus before starting and about every 45 minutes during his ride, depending on his CGM readings. He programs a temporary basal rate that is 150 percent of normal from 1 to 2 hours before finishing to prevent the rise in his blood glucose that he typically experiences as soon as he stops cycling.

When Heather Williams, a resident of Columbus, Ohio, bikes for long distances, she avoids injecting insulin or eating anything heavy in carbohydrates. For example, she has a regular breakfast (Atkins low-carbohydrate bar) and gives herself only half her usual insulin. If her blood glucose goes up during cycling, she knows that the activity will naturally bring it down. For lunch during long rides, she eats meat, vegetables, and some fruit, all without boluses (as long as her glucose stays under 250 mg/dL [13.9 mmol/L]). She eats a Tootsie Roll every time she is around 85 mg/dL (4.7 mmol/L) to ensure she does not drop further.

When he goes on a long ride, Derek Louquet from Missoula, Montana, drops his basal rate down to 40 to 50 percent of normal about 1.5 hours before starting, and he keeps it that much lower for about 8 to 12 hours after finishing to prevent lows. He fuels himself with balanced snacks throughout rides, just like any rider would. If he goes low, he treats it with a snack bar or gel, or sometimes with a glucose tablet for a quick spike.

**Basal–Bolus Injection Regimens.**    Indiana resident Troy Sandy has a similar approach to all activities, including cycling, running, and swimming for 1 to 4 hours. He makes sure it has been at least 1 hour since he last injected (or inhaled) any bolus insulin, and he keeps his injected basal insulin (Lantus or Basaglar) unchanged. He checks his blood glucose (he wants to be above 130 mg/dL [7.2 mmol/L]), and he takes 20 grams of carbohydrates if he is trending downward and goes below 100 mg/dL (5.6 mmol/L). His diet does not change too much based on his activity level; he tries to eat healthy foods at all times so his diet will not affect his overall energy levels.

Ireland native Jason O'Toole lowers both his basal (Lantus) and bolus (NovoRapid) insulins, depending on his cycling training schedule. He usually cuts back his bolus by 33 to 50 percent. If he is racing, he also cuts his Lantus dose in half. Races for him are typically 2.5 hours, and he may train by cycling for 1 to 5 hours, depending on the day. On the bike, he ingests sports drinks and gels, and he aims to keep his blood glucose between 126 and 180 mg/dL (7.0 and 10.0 mmol/L) to be on the safe side.

For Mark Robbins of Victor, New York, cycling is his go-to activity, and he usually rides for at least 2 to 3 hours at a time. In a recent year, he rode more than 7,000 miles (11,265.41 kilometers) in over 200 days. He typically checks his blood glucose before beginning a ride to ensure that he has a sufficient "carb cushion," starting with blood glucose of around 140 mg/dL (7.8 mmol/L). He always takes snack foods (often granola bars and peanut butter crackers) with him to eat, the amount depending on the heat and the duration, difficulty, and intensity of the ride. He used to get high blood glucose during intense exercise in the heat—perhaps from dehydration putting stress on his body—so now he is careful to hydrate adequately. He checks his glucose frequently and injects Humalog, as needed, to keep his blood glucose in a target range. In addition, he adjusts his Lantus dose between 15 and 20 units depending on his activity level on any given day.

Matthew Kearney of Cherry Valley, California, enjoys long runs of 20 miles or more (about 32 kilometers) and cycling events that are more than 100 miles (over 160 kilometers). He has different management strategies for his diabetes during extended, multihour events. Presently he eats a low-carbohydrate, high-fat diet, so he usually does not see the highs and lows that he used to experience while racing before he changed his diet. He also monitors his heart rate during training and racing events to keep himself in an aerobic energy range that uses more fat as fuel. Careful monitoring keeps his glucose stable, especially during the longer races when he has only his basal Tresiba insulin on board. When he ingests carbohydrates during an event, he takes glucose tablets. If he is doing a run, at around the 10-mile (16.1-kilometer) mark he eats a Greek yogurt along with a handful of macadamia nuts.

Lantus insulin user David Lozano, a resident of Barcelona, Spain, usually eats breakfast an hour before he begins a 4- to 5-hour ride. He eats his normal amount of carbohydrates (60 to 90 grams) without taking an insulin bolus. Once he is 1 hour and 45 minutes into his ride, he starts supplementing with about 40 to 60 grams of carbohydrates per hour until he finishes.

Declan Irvine, a resident of Raymond Terrace, Australia, plans ahead for next-day long rides. If he has a 5-hour ride planned for the next day, he lowers his Lantus basal insulin by 20 percent the night before, and he lowers his breakfast bolus doses by 20 percent as well to avoid having too much insulin on board during his extended ride.

Colorado resident Daniel Schneider cycles with adequate food available. He starts with his blood glucose around 140 mg/dL (7.8 mmol/L) with no bolus insulin on board, if possible. After the first 45 minutes of exercise, he eats 45 to 75 grams of carbohydrates per hour for up to 12 hours of endurance activity. He has been refining this protocol for over 15 years—as a previous member of Team Type 1 and a participant in the Race Across America, and during numerous endurance cycling and other races. He splits his Lantus dose and takes it twice daily, once in the morning and once at night. Taking Lantus twice daily allows him to adjust his basal insulin based on the activity, whereas he changes his Apidra (bolus) doses depending on time of day, dietary intake, and activity levels.

A Levemir user, Jim Yeoman of the United Kingdom always reduces the dose of his basal insulin in the morning before cycling workouts and lowers how much bolus insulin (Humalog) he takes for the carbohydrates he eats. Normally he eats about 40 grams of carbohydrates at breakfast (raised to 60 grams on weekends before long rides), 50 to 80 grams at lunch (increased to around 100 grams on weekends), and 60 to 100 grams in his evening meal. He also decreases his evening Levemir dose. While cycling and afterward, he monitors his blood glucose levels regularly and carries plenty of carbohydrates in his jersey pockets while out on the bike.

## Other Effects to Consider

**Effect of Insulin Levels.**   For Jonathan Mooney, a resident of Birmingham, Alabama, the biggest challenge is managing his blood glucose before being active to ensure he does not have a lot of active insulin in his body. Once he starts cycling or running for an hour, any remaining bolus insulin is ultra-effective and somewhat difficult to manage. He checks his blood glucose before exercise, takes in just enough snacks or GU energy gel while active to stay in range, and checks afterward to ensure his glucose did not spike.

**Effect of Competition.**   Jim Schuler finds that the adrenaline of races upends his blood glucose management because his responses are radically different from when he is training. He has to increase his insulin doses before the race, have higher basal rates, and more aggressively treat high blood glucose levels. This is also confounded by his preference to eat something during longer races (e.g., long bike races of 3 to 5 hours, half marathons, and marathons). He says dealing with the impact of competition stress is still a work in progress.

**Effect of Technology Use.**   Lawrence Phillips of Noblesville, Indiana, uses the latest diabetes technology to manage his blood glucose during moderate cycling for 30 to 45 minutes at a time. He sets his MiniMed 670G hybrid closed-loop system to exercise mode with a target blood glucose of 150 mg/dL (8.3 mmol/L). For him, it works like a charm.

## MARATHONS

Participation in marathons involves high-mileage training and the ability to cover the distance of 26.2 miles (42.2 kilometers) at race pace. Some athletes prefer the half-marathon distance, which is 13.2 miles (21.1 kilometers). Running either distance is almost purely aerobic in nature, resulting in significant depletion of muscle glycogen in many different muscles because of how long the marathon lasts. Your body will use a combination of carbohydrate and fat, but the harder you push yourself, the greater your carbohydrate use will be. Even nondiabetic athletes usually benefit from carbohydrate (or mixed food) intake during marathons to prevent early fatigue and hypoglycemia (and, yes, people without diabetes can also experience exercise-induced lows during marathons).

For athletes with diabetes, marathoning requires both extra fueling and minimal circulating insulin due to its prolonged nature. The actual changes that you make will depend on factors such as your race pace, how well trained you are, whether you are fat adapted (i.e., able to use more fat at a similar pace), and how low your insulin levels are during the race. The key to maintaining your blood glucose levels during a marathon is having minimal insulin in your system, which you potentially can accomplish by decreasing your basal insulin doses the evening before and the morning of the race, plus taking less or minimal insulin for anything you eat before you start. If your body can still make your insulin, you can keep your insulin levels lower by avoiding eating higher GI carbohydrates before racing.

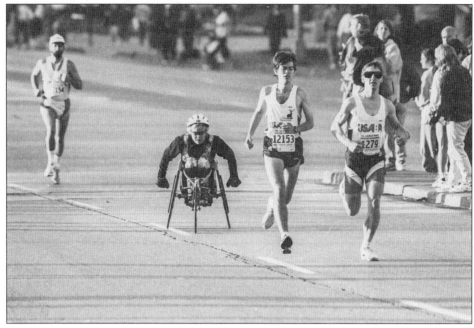

A marathon is almost purely aerobic in nature, resulting in significant depletion of glycogen in many muscles due to its long duration. Even athletes without diabetes usually benefit from food intake during the event to prevent fatigue and hypoglycemia.

## Athlete Examples

Marathoners and half marathoners with diabetes have tried a variety of strategies to maximize their performance. All their regimen changes involve decreases in insulin and increases in food intake. For additional examples, refer to the sections on running and jogging, triathlons, and ultraendurance events and training.

### Diet Changes Alone

Naomi from Spokane, Washington has a GU energy gel every 15 minutes for the first hour of running a half-marathon. During the second hour (of 2 hours), she does not need any more carbohydrates. She watches her glucose on her CGM closely. She finds she needs to have some insulin on board (at least basal insulin via her pump) during endurance activities like these or her performance suffers.

Before a long run, Pittsburgh, Pennsylvania, resident Melissa Donovan eats half a banana with peanut butter, a fried egg, and a slice of whole wheat toast, a meal that typically keeps her glucose steady. She takes a GU energy gel every hour but does not decrease her basal rate on her pump because she has had issues going into diabetic ketoacidosis (DKA) in the past after endurance events. She hydrates with water and Gatorade and drinks a few ounces every mile, as well as eating a peanut butter and jelly sandwich if she is running more than a few hours.

## *Combined Regimen Changes*

Coincidentally, almost all the athletes responding about marathoning for this book ended up being insulin pump users, and their examples follow first. But that is not to say that you cannot run a marathon or do similar training if you use injections. Check out additional examples of running using a basal–bolus injection regimen in the "Running and Jogging" activity section that follows this one.

**Insulin Pump Users.** New Jersey marathoner Aaron Kowalski wears his pump during races, turning the basal down at least 90 minutes before beginning. If his blood glucose is starting in range, he runs with a temporary basal rate of 40 percent of normal, taking in about 30 grams of carbohydrates per hour without any additional insulin, along with adequate water. His carbohydrates for running are often Swedish fish candies. Before the run, he often eats a low-GI meal, such as an English muffin with peanut butter. During exercise, he does adjust his carbohydrate intake based on his CGM tracing. At the end of the race, he often needs to bolus to avoid post-race glucose highs.

Stephen England, a resident of New York City, follows a specific regimen for running. For general training and up to marathon-distance racing, he reduces his basal during the activity by 50 percent. He tracks his blood glucose using CGM and finds he usually needs to take in 30 grams of carbohydrates per hour (usually as Honey Stinger gels). He only gets post-run overnight lows if he does not reduce his evening meal bolus enough.

On the day of a marathon, Dan Stone of Middletown, Pennsylvania, follows a set routine. He gets up at 4:00 a.m. to bolus and eat so that all bolus insulin is cleared out before the start of the race. He sets his basal rate at 0.1 units per hour 2 hours before and throughout the duration of the run and has a pre-race blood glucose target of 130 to 140 mg/dL (7.2 to 7.8 mmol/L). During the race, he consumes sports drinks whenever they are offered throughout the run, which normally keeps his glucose levels fairly stable.

Martin Draper, hailing from Bridgewater in Somerset, England, has run more than 270 marathons with type 1 diabetes. For any exercise, he reduces his basal rate by 80 percent beforehand and refrains from injecting boluses within 3 hours of activity so he has only a small amount of basal on board when active. During marathons, he eats some carbohydrates every 40 minutes or so. Afterward, he always eats more carbohydrates and boluses to avoid going too high. He has lots of other general advice, such as reducing basal insulin when you go running if it is for more than 15 minutes; getting a CGM, checking often, and looking for patterns in your readings; always carrying rapid-acting carbohydrates with you; and being careful in the 24 hours after an event because your blood glucose may not behave normally.

Emily Tiberio of Beaver, Pennsylvania, cuts her basal by 0 to 25 percent for running and long-distance rowing or cycling, depending on her starting blood glucose as well as the duration of the activity. Race day is a different story, especially for marathons: she needs to program a basal to cover the excitement of the starting line, the long distance, and the post-race stress. And then there are the 3 or 4 days afterward when she is recovering and not exercising like she normally would. She is trying to qualify for the Boston Marathon with an under 3:30 marathon finish this year, and she says she needs to cut 14 minutes off her best time from last year.

For marathons and associated training, Tristan Rice from Chico, California, sets a lower temporary basal during long runs (typically 20 percent lower), and he also ingests a GU energy gel packet every 45 minutes while running. On marathon race day, he reduces his basal rate by 30 percent and keeps it lower until 2 hours after the race ends.

Marathoner Bill King of Philadelphia, Pennsylvania, supplements with 10 to 20 grams of carbohydrate (e.g., Clif Shot Bloks Energy Chews, Sport Beans, and Elovate 15) every 20 to 30 minutes while running a marathon. He also lowers his basal rates. For him, wearing an insulin pump is the key to staying more tightly regulated during long training runs and marathons. Before races, he finds that nervous excitement makes his glucose go up, which he counters with a temporary increase in his basal rate long before the start. He then lowers it to 40 to 60 percent of normal, 60 to 90 minutes before a race or long run. As his conditioning improves with consistent training, his glucose may climb initially, but after 40 to 90 minutes into a longer, slower run, it starts to fall. So being able to adjust his basal rates on his pump is his key to matching his changing insulin sensitivity levels. With post-race excitement and the sudden stop of running, he often gives himself a small bolus and/or increases his basal rates before reaching the end of a marathon to avoid post-race highs. Also, he finds that high-intensity performance running over great distances can cause post-race insulin resistance for a day or two afterward.

**Basal–Bolus Injection Regimens.** For running long distances and marathons, Anita Harris from England eats porridge for breakfast at least 4 hours before to make sure her last bolus insulin is no longer working. She also reduces her morning dose of Levemir (basal) insulin. She eats a banana if she is lower than desired when starting her run, along with jelly babies after 5 miles and every mile thereafter and occasional gels if needed. Her target blood glucose during runs is 162 mg/dL (9.0 mmol/L).

For another great example of an athlete doing marathon (and triathlon) training using basal and bolus insulin injections, see the profile of Jay Hewitt at the end of this chapter. He has performed exceptionally well athletically and currently is using ultralong-acting Tresiba for basal dosing. And again, also see the other training examples under "Running and Jogging."

## *Other Effects to Consider*

**Effect of Technology Use.** A self-professed "marathon maniac," Karen Derrick from Columbia, Missouri, has run over 50 marathons (45 of those in the past 4 years) as a "casual" runner, with most of her finishing times between 5 and 5.5 hours. Having a CGM has been very helpful for regulating her carbohydrate intake during marathons and training. Her first marathon was in 1992 before she had an insulin pump; she was faster back then (finishing in 4 hours), but she still had to take a meter with her to check her blood glucose during the race. So she appreciates the ease of using a CGM instead, especially one coordinated with her insulin pump. However, she has had issues with her pump's auto mode during marathons. She tends to get a check glucose alarm due to not giving herself at least a minimal basal dose for an extended period while running. Another slight drawback she sees is having to wear the pump, along with carrying extra carbohydrates. She finds it challenging to get under the layers of her cold weather running gear to look at CGM readings or alarms. Plus, she has accidentally pulled off her CGM device during bathroom breaks.

Half-marathons are Paul Coker's self-proclaimed specialty, having run 40 in 1 year to celebrate having lived with type 1 diabetes that long. The Cardiff, Wales, native also follows a vegan diet. To prevent lows, he used to drop his basal rates by 20 percent for 36 hours during and after events. Currently, he is using a jerry-rigged hybrid closed-loop insulin pump system (using the Medtronic Paradigm 522, Dexcom G5, Riley Link, and Loop software running on his iPhone). His system makes constant basal adjustments for him and prevents most postexercise lows. He likes it except for its limitations around exercise. It does not lower elevated glucose levels quickly because the algorithms are all built around insulin sensitivity factors and carbohydrate-to-insulin ratios. When everything is running smoothly, he says the closed-loop works brilliantly, and it is fabulous overnight, keeping his blood glucose in range with no lows. However, he knows not to rely on it when preparing to run or during runs because it cannot accommodate the rapid increase in insulin sensitivity that he gets from a good run. When he is preparing to run for more than 20 to 30 minutes, he overrides the system completely, choosing instead to drop his basal by 80 percent 1 to 1.5 hours before a run and only return it to normal 30 minutes before he finishes running. At the finish line, he gives himself a half-unit bolus. Notably, on very hot days he needs even less insulin.

Pennsylvanian Emily Tiberio wears an Omnipod (tubeless) pump that she feels has been excellent for her running and cycling for marathon training. (She has had a little trouble with rowing because she usually wears her pump on her abdomen, but it has been manageable.) She gets some chafing during runs longer than 10 miles around the pump adhesive, but she says that is also manageable. On race days, she puts her pump on the back of her arm where she gets much less irritation from it. She additionally loves using her Dexcom CGM for long runs and cycling because without it she may confuse being tired with feeling low. She also enjoys being able to fuel throughout training by watching her blood glucose trends on the CGM.

## RUNNING AND JOGGING

Unless you are doing track events (covered in chapter 10) or all-out sprinting (chapter 11), running and jogging are both generally aerobic in nature. The main fuels that your body uses are carbohydrates and fat, and your reliance on blood glucose and muscle glycogen increases with running intensity. Thus, how hard you run affects your blood glucose, along with the duration of the run, the time of day, your insulin levels, your starting blood glucose, and your normal diet. Intense running releases more glucose-raising hormones, making it possible for your glucose to go up during intense 5K races or tough interval training. The longer you run, the more energy is depleted from your stores of muscle and liver glycogen, making it harder for you to maintain your blood glucose during long runs without eating, even if your fat use goes up. Using more muscle glycogen also increases your insulin sensitivity afterward and increases your risk for lows later on.

# Athlete Profile: **Cliff Scherb**

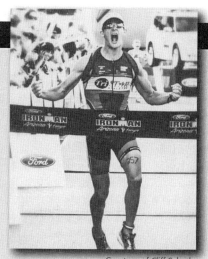

Courtesy of Cliff Scherb.

**Hometown:** Redondo Beach, California

**Diabetes history:** Type 1 diabetes diagnosed in 1988 (at age 9). Early on, with diabetes I was "crash and burn" as a kid, learning how to be active and live a normal life through the swings of blood glucose and insulin. In my 20s, I found triathlons, and I set out to be the best I could be at the sport. I logged many miles of training and nutrition with my type 1 diabetes, which eventually developed into the algorithms we use for Glucose Advisors (www.GlucoseAdvisors.com). My own personal diabetes learning has been enhanced and accelerated through the work I do with our diabetes patients and athletes. I have certainly benefited not only from my experiences in sport but also from being in the front seat of testing nutrition and insulin regimens on a wide range of people.

**Sport or activity:** Anything I can get my hands on. Most of my adult athletic career has been centered on swimming, biking, and running, but many early years of my life were spent playing basketball and soccer. I did intermittent weightlifting in college before finding triathlons.

**Greatest athletic achievement:** USA Team All-American 6 times, 19-time Ironman Triathlon finisher with a 9:07 Ironman personal record (second fastest ever for someone with type 1 diabetes) with a 56-minute swim, 4:48 bike, and 3:16 run. I also did a 4:16 Half Ironman, the fastest ever for an athlete with type 1 diabetes (at the Clearwater 70.3 World Championships). My Olympic distance triathlon personal record is 2:02. I raced the Ironman World Championships in Kona and the Half Ironman World Championships three times each. I have completed over 50 Half Ironman races, hundreds of triathlons, and many more running races.

**Current insulin and medication regimen:** I use a Dexcom CGM with Apple watch/iPhone combo and an Omnipod. I use Fiasp insulin, and at night I only wear a "do it yourself" legacy Medtronic 500g pump, closed loop in conjunction with a "Riley Link."

**Training tips:** I have many tips, but to distill them down, my number one tip would be to *always* monitor insulin on board before any activity and try to reduce it. This often means meal planning, typically 2 to 4 hours before, and lowering basal rates or Lantus doses.

**Typical daily and weekly training and diabetes regimen:** This will swing hugely for me depending on whether I am preparing for a major event or not. I will highlight the two scenarios because they are *very* different!

*Ultraendurance Training for Ironman*

**Total training hours:** ~17 to 35 per week on average, with ~4,000 to 7,000 calories per day (450 to 600 grams of carbohydrates)

*Total training stress (TSS):* 1,000 to 1,200 TSS: ~15,000 yards swimming per week, ~250 to 400 miles cycling per week, and ~60 to 80 miles running per week

- ▶ *Monday:* (a.m.) swim 4,000 yards, lift weights; (p.m.) easy spin on the bike for 45 minutes.
- ▶ *Tuesday:* 1-hour and 45-minute tempo intervals run (13 to 16 miles); 30-minute easy "shake out" swim.
- ▶ *Wednesday:* (a.m.) 3-hour moderate bike ride; (p.m.) 1- to 2-hour bike time trial, with 60-minute, 3,000-yard swim in between.
- ▶ *Thursday:* (a.m.) 45-minute swim, 2-hour bike ride; (p.m.) 80-minute run (10 miles) on dirt trails.
- ▶ *Friday:* 4,200-yard (60 minutes) Ironman swim; (p.m.) 1.5-hour interval bike ride with hills.
- ▶ *Saturday:* Long ride of 5 to 7 hours (90 to 130 miles) with 30-minute run after biking.
- ▶ *Sunday:* Long run of 19 to 23 miles (done in 2 hours and 30 minutes to 2:45); (p.m.) 90-minute to 2-hour swim.

*Non-Event Training Mode*

*Total training hours:* 7 to 12 (swimming, cycling, running, weights, and hiking), with 1,800 to 3,000 calories per day

*Total training stress:* 450 to 600 TSS

*Other hobbies and interests:* My hobby is my job . . . and my life's passion: to conquer insulin and activity management issues and consulting for others with type 1 diabetes. I help teach this decision support system to aspiring beginners—those trying to lose weight through healthy exercise and endurance training—via GlucoseAdvisors.com. In 2016 I created an app called Engine1 in my spare time to help others with type 1 diabetes who like to be active (although the app is no longer available). I still enjoy the one-on-one consulting and teaching of my decision support system to individuals struggling with diabetes.

My other interests are my supportive wife, Kimberly Scherb, and our two dogs Ralph and Cowboy, along with my mother (Bernice) and brother (Ryan Scherb), who have always supported my endeavors and at times crazy training regimen!

*Good diabetes and exercise story:* I live through the athletes I work for these days. Recently one of them completed his marathon personal record in 3 hours and 45 minutes, which is incredible for anyone. However, his average blood glucose for the race was 102 mg/dL (5.7 mmol/L). Even more incredible was the A1C of 5.0 that he had 2 weeks later through this training cycle. That's a win for him, for me, and for type 1 diabetes!

If you run when your insulin levels are lower (generally before meals or first thing in the morning), your workout will not cause your blood glucose to drop as much because you will have a more normal physiological response. Pump users can easily lower their insulin during exercise by suspending or reducing their basal rates. Your insulin levels are lower and your resistance greater early in the morning; therefore, if you run before breakfast (and before taking or releasing any insulin), you will have more stable blood glucose even without eating or drinking anything. In some instances, you may need a small insulin bolus to prevent a rise during morning workouts.

## Athlete Examples

Athletes with diabetes use various regimen changes to compensate for running. Their adjustments depend on a number of factors.

### *Insulin Changes Alone*

Salvador Martinez from Mexico disconnects from his pump for shorter runs. He only wears it during longer ones (more than 10 miles [16.1 kilometers]).

Scotland resident Connor Milton typically suspends his insulin delivery about 45 minutes before a run and keeps it that way until his blood glucose starts to rise. Sometimes he can run for 3 hours or more and not need any basal insulin. Either just before he stops running or right after, he does take a bolus to replace his missed basal insulin, typically 1 to 2 units for each hour that he had his pump disconnected.

Jason Sperry of Mannsville, New York, does not want any active bolus insulin on board during running. He sets a temporary basal rate of 40 to 60 percent starting 2 hours before exercise and extending throughout. Ideally, he starts at a blood glucose of 120 mg/dL (6.7 mmol/L) and likes to keep it between 80 and 120 mg/dL (4.4 to 6.7 mmol/L) while he is active.

For an hour and a half of running, Kris Maynard from Spokane, Washington, generally sets his pump at 30 percent of his usual basal rate starting 2 hours before the activity. This approach makes sure his insulin on board is low during the activity.

Stacey Mortenson-Spokes from Saskatoon, Saskatchewan, Canada, uses an Omnipod pump and eats a fairly low-carbohydrate diet. For running for over 1 hour at a time, which she usually does fasted, she has to take a tiny bit of insulin to avoid her glucose spiking from the activity.

### *Diet Changes Alone*

Rutger from the Netherlands, who uses Tresiba as his basal insulin and Novolog for boluses, make no changes for running up to an hour. For activities lasting longer than an hour, after the first 45 minutes he consumes 30 grams of carbohydrates, followed by the same amount every 30 minutes thereafter. He usually takes in gels, but during really long runs he prefers gummy bears and a bit of solid food to eat.

Patrick Bowyer in the United Kingdom rarely needs to take any glucose for running under 10 kilometers (6.2 miles). For runs of 15 kilometers or more (9.3 miles or longer) he may eat some jelly babies or a banana before starting his run. For 20 kilometers (12.4 miles) or longer, he has already increased his insulin sensitivity and lowered his insulin needs by doing more training in the weeks leading up to the event. This allows him to reduce the amount of insulin he needs to have on board, allowing him to exercise for hours with less chance of getting a low. He uses Lantus for basal insulin coverage and NovoRapid for meal boluses.

Fellow United Kingdom resident, and an Omnipod insulin pump user, Sarah always eats porridge with a banana 2 to 3 hours before a run. She likes to have her blood glucose between 144 and 180 mg/dL (8.0 to 10.0 mmol/L) before a run; if it is lower, she eats a small banana and has a few sips of orange juice before starting. During a long run, she takes two Clif Shot Bloks every 30 minutes; she finds them not too sweet, and they are easy on her stomach. After the run she drinks a glass of milk and has a slice of whole meal toast with peanut butter (with no added sugar).

Michela Belluta of San Diego, California, follows a low-carbohydrate (Dr. Bernstein) diet. She uses NovoLog at meals and for corrections, but she uses regular insulin for protein meals, along with Levemir for basal insulin coverage. Because of her low carbohydrate intake, before she runs 5 kilometers (3.1 miles) all she needs to do is take half a glucose tablet to avoid lows while running. Her blood glucose typically stays stable around 83 mg/dL (4.6 mmol/L).

## Combined Regimen Changes

Again, more of the runners surveyed are using insulin pumps than basal–bolus injection regimens. However, those on injections are using a variety of different basal options.

**Insulin Pump Users.**   Courtney Duckworth from Washington, D.C. (see her profile in chapter 10), has gone from figure skating to professional cheerleading to marathon running. She usually runs in the mornings when her circulating insulin is lower. Her protocol varies with the length of her activity: for long runs above 7 miles (11.3 kilometers), she sets a 15 percent temporary basal and takes 10 percent of her normal insulin bolus for breakfast without eating. While running, she may take 0.1 to 0.3 units for a GU energy gel or no insulin if she is below 100 mg/dL (5.6 mmol/L). After a long run, she covers her breakfast with her bolus plus 50 percent of the insulin missed during her temp basal run time. For runs below 7 miles, her basal setting (15 percent) and breakfast insulin plus 50 percent of lost insulin stay the same, and she may supplement with 15 to 20 grams of carbohydrates if necessary.

Avid marathoner Karen Derrick of Columbia, Missouri, has distinct plans for all levels of running and training. For runs of less than 40 minutes she makes sure her blood glucose is over 100 mg/dL (5.6 mmol/L), and she sets a temporary glucose target using her MiniMed 670G pump hours before that starts lowering her basal insulin delivery. During the run, she carries glucose tablets, just in case of a low. For longer runs or races (over 2 hours), she does all these things, along with taking a GU energy gel 45 minutes into her workout. Depending on her blood glucose level, she may also drink a sports drink at stops during races; around 16 to 18 miles (25.7 to 29.0 kilometers) in, she eats a Clif Bar. When marathoning, if her glucose starts dropping, she suspends her insulin pump until it starts increasing again.

Todd Daugherty from Carthage, Missouri, finds that for running it works best if he suspends his basal insulin an hour before he starts and during his run. He also eats 15 grams of carbohydrates every 3 miles (4.9 kilometers) when running a long distance.

When running longer distances, Ron C. from Australia reduces his basal insulin down to 20 to 50 percent of normal. He reduces it 30 minutes before starting a run, and he religiously eats 20 to 25 grams of carbohydrates every 30 minutes or 5 kilometers (3.1 miles) of running.

Stockport, United Kingdom, resident Andy Duckworth reduces his bolus insulin for meals before and after an hour of running by half. He aims for a starting blood glucose of 180 mg/dL (10.0 mmol/L), and he cuts his basal insulin by 50 percent during the activity. If he is doing a longer run or endurance activity, he drinks a bottle of Lucozade (30 to 60 grams of carbohydrates, depending on the flavor) every hour.

In India, Nupur Lalvani does marathons, ultramarathons, and running. If she does speedwork, she either follows it with a slower jog or takes a tiny bolus to counter the spike. For running, she reduces her basal to anywhere between 50 to 70 percent below normal. In rare cases, she suspends her pump. Because she is following a low-carbohydrate diet (via Dr. Bernstein), she eats her normal high-protein foods before and after running, but usually no food during runs. She used to do a lot of carbohydrate loading and supplementing with carbohydrates during exercise, but that is a thing of the past for her. She only refuels with salt, electrolytes, and water.

Rhet Hulbert from Boise, Idaho, turns down his basal rate by about 50 percent about 2 hours before exercise or a race. He monitors his blood glucose closely and tries to adjust about 30 minutes prior, if necessary. He wants to have very little insulin on board because once he starts moving at an endurance pace, his blood glucose can drop quickly, and he prefers not to have to eat at the beginning of the workout if possible. If he does have to eat something, he takes something small with lots of sugar in it to avoid having much in his stomach. During the event, he continues to monitor; during long events, he consumes 20 grams of carbohydrates per half hour to fuel the effort.

For running and marathons, Patty Mark of Norristown, Pennsylvania, sets her pump at 50 percent of normal for the amount of time before the exercise and during it. For instance, if she is exercising for 30 minutes, she sets her pump to 50 percent for an hour starting 30 minutes prior. If running for more than an hour, she only reduces the basal starting 1 hour beforehand. For a 3-hour run, her basal is lower for 4 hours total. She also snacks during longer runs.

Avon, Colorado, resident Kerry White has a similar approach to all long endurance activities lasting 4 or more hours. She generally lowers her basal (Lantus) insulin levels and frequently needs no bolus insulin during exercise, even when fueling. She fuels often but not in large quantities, such as half of a power bar, small amounts of Gatorade, 15 grams of candy, or fruit snacks for lows during running.

San Francisco, California, resident Holly Pepper reduces her basal rate to 60 percent 2 hours before workouts involving running, cycling, or swimming. She keeps it at that level until she is done working out. She may need to take in 15 to 25 grams of carbohydrates per hour if exercising more than 1.5 hours. After checking her glucose at the end of her workout, she gives herself a small bolus if she is over 150 mg/dL (8.3 mmol/L), as her blood glucose tends to rise after exercise.

Conor Smith from Fort Washington, Pennsylvania, also uses one approach to almost all endurance training (running, cycling, swimming, and triathlons). For activities less than 3 hours, he does not make many changes. He may take in about 15 grams of carbohydrates an hour. For 2 hours or more, he supplements with UCan (a slow-release, starch sports supplement). For 3 hours of exercise or longer, he also uses a temporary basal rate set at 25 percent of normal. He has also effectively used this protocol for Ironman triathlons of varying lengths.

Jay Handy, a resident of Madison, Wisconsin, agrees that most endurance activities can be handled with a similar approach. For him, whether he is running, swimming, cycling, or doing another endurance activity, he makes sure he has a flat or rising glucose trend, but most importantly he needs to see that it is not really low or trending down. He feels it is very important to have not even the tail end of a bolus on board, and his lasts at least 3 hours. If he does have too much insulin on board, it comes back to haunt him by causing a crash in his blood glucose. He believes that eating so that you can take small doses of insulin (the benefit of small numbers) helps immensely in not ending up with too much insulin during exercise.

Aline Verbeke, a resident of Brugge, Belgium, approaches all endurance training sessions, including running, similarly. She lowers her basal rate by 50 percent, starting 30 minutes before exercise and lasting throughout the training session. After a longer workout, she also keeps her basal lowered until 3:00 a.m. During sessions longer than an hour, she eats 12.5 grams of carbohydrates per hour.

Andrew M., a resident of Sydney, Australia, participates in middle-distance running (which includes events from 800 meters to 5 kilometers, including steeplechase). Training for this distance requires (among other things) endurance-based activities. Most of his training sessions for this activity last 75 minutes or less, so he does not take in any carbohydrates before or during them if his blood glucose is 74 mg/dL (4.1 mmol/L) or above. He rarely starts below 79 mg/dL (4.4 mmol/L) because he is on a keto diet and only experiences minor fluctuations in his daily blood glucose and he manages it in the hours before training.

Ron C., also from Australia, finds middle-distance running and training more difficult to manage than straight endurance running, as middle-distance training is not just sprinting or endurance training, but rather a combination of both.

**Basal–Bolus Injection Regimens.**　Claire T. from Alexandria, Virginia, usually runs moderately for 30 to 60 minutes at a time, 3 days per week. For this activity, she reduces her dose of Tresiba (basal) insulin by 25 percent on the days she exercises. She also tries to start her runs with a blood glucose of 180 mg/dL (10.0 mmol/L), and then she supplements with 5 to 10 grams of carbohydrates every 10 to 15 minutes when she runs for over half an hour. In addition, she needs to decrease her carbohydrate-to-insulin ratios by half for the meal immediately after her run and watches her CGM for the next 24 to 48 hours to catch unexpected lows or downward trends.

Paul Richards, a resident of Billericay, Essex, in the United Kingdom, reduces his basal insulin (Lantus taken once daily in the mornings) by 10 to 15 percent on days he is running. He also reduces his bolus insulin (Fiasp) doses by changing his insulin-to-carbohydrate ratio from 1:15 to 1:20 (1 unit per gram of carbohydrates) on those days. He closely monitors his blood glucose in the 12 hours after running and makes adjustments as necessary.

For running (or high-repetition kettlebell snatching), Christopher Gantz from the United States usually consumes at least half a glucose tab (2 grams of carbohydrates); depending on his glucose trends, he may need an additional 2 to 4 grams about every 20 minutes or so while active. He experiences heightened insulin sensitivity after exercise and reduces his bolus for his next meal by half or so (1.5 units regular, down from 3) because he eats a lot of protein and very few carbohydrates. He uses Levemir as his basal insulin, but does not adjust it for this activity.

Philadelphia, Pennsylvania, resident Anthony Mark forgoes his usual insulin dose for either breakfast or dinner to induce hyperglycemia to exercise. For a 6-mile run, he aims for 200 to 220 mg/dL (11.1 to 12.2 mmol/L). His routine for longer runs (or rides) is the same. Depending on his blood glucose response, he may need to eat a GU energy gel halfway through the activity. He makes no adjustments to his basal insulin (Levemir) for this training.

## Other Effects to Consider

**Effect of Environment.**  For Scotland native Janet G., both cross country and road running are affected by her starting blood glucose, the distance of the run, the weather, and the terrain. She usually reduces her temporary basal rate to 60 percent of normal, starting 30 minutes beforehand (any sooner and her blood glucose rises too high). She finds that she often needs about two glucose tablets per mile if she starts with her glucose in her target zone, followed by a juice carton after 5 miles. During racing events, she finds that the adrenaline from competing can make her blood glucose rise very high before races, so sometimes she needs extra insulin.

**Effect of Time of Day.**  Paris (France) resident Andrea Limbourg usually runs 5 to 10 kilometers (3.1 to 6.2 miles) in the morning, fasting if her blood glucose before the run is above 90 mg/dL (5.0 mmol/L) or after eating a few carbohydrates if lower than that. She often wakes up earlier and can adjust her basal rate if needed, but this is rare because a fasting run does not usually drop her glucose by much.

**Effect of Technology (and Nerves).**  Katherine Owen from Tallahassee, Florida, relies on her Medtronic MiniMed 670G system to help her regulate during running, cycling, and swimming. She uses a temporary target on her pump, fuels every 45 minutes with 10 to 15 grams of carbohydrates, hydrates well (sometimes with a Powerade/water mix), and occasionally needs a small dose of insulin if the pump auto mode is showing a predictive trend up. Although it has taken a lot of advance practice, planning, and training, she feels her Medtronic system has allowed her to lower her glucose variability, reduce hypoglycemia, manage during long endurance activities, and more. The only drawback of the technology is that her infusion set can become loose, so she must always have a backup plan involving extra sets or insulin pens. The CGM sensor she uses also can lose its connection to the pump when she is swimming.

San Francisco, California, resident Mary Alessandra Lucas is a self-proclaimed runner. For short runs, she does not fuel or do anything with her pump. If she is above 200 mg/dL (11.1 mmol/L), she gives herself a small bolus of insulin. She never starts running over 215 mg/dL (11.9 mmol/L) or under 100 mg/dL (5.6 mmol/L). For runs of 6 miles (∼ 10 kilometers) or more, she starts fueling with gels at mile 6, then again at miles 9, 12, and so on. Usually she does not need to take any insulin for the gels while she is running. She uses a hybrid, closed-loop insulin pump on auto mode to manage her blood glucose.

Oklahoma City, Oklahoma, resident Corianne Blotevogel finds that managing runs can sometimes be a wild goose chase, depending on her training status and running distance. She normally feels a bit anxious at the start of a race, so her blood glucose spikes 50 to 100 mg/dL (2.8 to 5.6 mmol/L). But she tries to manage that without bolusing to prevent lows during a run. Her pump's auto mode (Medtronic MiniMed 670G) has also helped her a lot on runs. Based on her trends, it determines what insulin she needs instead of a predetermined basal amount. She uses it for all running in general as well as for training runs and races.

## SWIMMING

Swimming is mainly aerobic in nature, especially when swimming long distances rather than competing in short races. Longer endurance swims use a mixture of fat and carbohydrate and, as with running, your reliance on blood glucose and muscle glycogen increases with your intensity. Short sprints or racing competitions (covering distances of 200 meters or less) use mainly anaerobic energy provided by your phosphagen and lactic acid systems, similar to the sports and activities found in chapter 11.

Your swimming intensity will affect the release of glucose-raising hormones; intense exercise, such as swim meets or other competitions involving short, intense efforts, may raise your blood glucose levels rather than lowering them as longer swims usually do. The more glycogen that you use, the greater your insulin action is afterward, so you will have to work to prevent later-onset lows if your glycogen use is significant. If you swim when your insulin levels are minimal (more than 2 to 3 hours after your last insulin dose or with lower basal rates), your blood glucose will not decrease as much. For longer swims (lasting an hour or more), you will likely need to eat extra to offset the glucose-lowering effect of using much of your muscle and liver glycogen. If you swim before breakfast, you will have more stable blood glucose levels, but you may need to supplement with insulin, particularly if you start out with higher glucose.

## Athlete Examples

The following examples show that the duration and intensity of your swimming, along with the time of day that you swim, largely determine the regimen changes that you will need to make to maintain your blood glucose.

### Insulin Changes Alone

Some insulin pumps can be worn while swimming (like Omnipod and the defunct Animas pumps), as Al Lewis (profiled in chapter 1) did for decades while doing masters swimming. However, John Mitchell of Maple Grove, Minnesota, disconnects his Medtronic MiniMed 670G pump and takes a manual bolus immediately afterward to address the lack of insulin caused by swimming without it on.

Likewise, for an hour-long swim, Jeff Foot of Scotland removes his pump for the duration (even though the Animas Vibe he uses is supposed to be waterproof). He only eats carbohydrates if he gets low.

John Boyer from Maryland also disconnects from his Medtronic pump (which is only watertight, not waterproof). He aims to keep his blood glucose in the range of 130 to 180 mg/dL (7.2 to 10.0 mmol/L) while off his basal insulin.

Colorado resident Jason D. cannot wear his Medtronic pump while swimming. His strategy is to get into the pool with his blood glucose around 180 mg/dL (10.0 mmol/L), which he accomplishes by lowering his basal insulin down to 25 to 50 percent of normal for at least an hour before the start of his swim.

## Diet Changes Alone

For vigorous lap swimming for 45 minutes to 1 hour, Greg Cutter of Norfolk, Virginia, cannot use his CGM in the water, so he adjusts his glucose higher than he does for his other exercise. He tries to start out around 200 mg/dL (11.1 mmol/L) to avoid hypoglycemia. Although he uses once-daily Tresiba as his basal insulin, he does not adjust that (or his bolus insulin) for swimming because it is a usual activity.

Estelle Grey from Cape Town, South Africa, has more trouble managing her blood glucose during swimming because she cannot check it during open water events. She aims to start her 3-kilometer (1.9-mile) swim with a stable blood glucose around 180 mg/dL (10.0 mmol/L) and then drinks half a liter of water before starting while she eats an energy snack.

Jessica Sherwood from Binghamton, New York, follows a very-low-carbohydrate diet for which she gives herself injections of regular insulin for meals while using Apidra in an insulin pump to cover her basal insulin needs. For her swims, she eats a small, high-protein meal beforehand. If she is downward trending during swims, she corrects with glucose tablets only.

## Combined Regimen Changes

Teenager Kayla Bertholf of Ashtabula, Ohio, sets a target of 150 mg/dL (8.3 mmol/L) on her Medtronic MiniMed 670G hybrid closed-loop pump (with integrated CGM) 2 hours before a swim practice and throughout entire swim meets. In addition, she has a 10- to 20-gram carbohydrate snack (such as GU energy gels, trail mix, granola bars, or pretzels) about every hour.

Before an hour of hard swimming after lunch, Sarah McManus of Pittsburgh, Pennsylvania, cuts her lunch bolus in half, eats about 35 grams of carbohydrates, and sets a temporary basal that is 50 percent lower about 1 to 1.5 hours before swimming. She typically checks her blood glucose every 20 minutes and turns her basal back up with 15 to 20 minutes left, depending on her glucose level. Her goal for swimming is to start at a blood glucose of 220 to 250 mg/dL (12.2 to 13.9 mmol/L) so that she does not go low or have to consume anything during her workout. She thinks that her Omnipod (tubeless and waterproof) pump works great for swimmers.

For lap swimming an hour at a moderate pace (2,400 meters, or 1.5 miles), Sheri Ochs of Santa Barbara, California, usually swims after lunch due to dealing with limited open-swim hours at her neighborhood pool and not liking to be hungry while working out. To manage this, she eats a small, low-GI lunch at least 1 or 2 hours before and takes half her usual lunch bolus. She seldom has any issues with going low during her swim (an activity that also includes biking 10 minutes each way along the beach to get to the pool), and she ends up with her blood glucose in a normal range. She is active every day, so she does not need to make any adjustments to her basal insulin (Lantus) to compensate.

Czech Republic resident Klara Pickova leaves her pump on during swimming and decreases her basal rate by half. If she cannot leave it on for some reason, she disconnects and gives herself a small bolus in advance to cover the basal she will be missing. After working out, she decreases her basal rate overnight by 20 percent to prevent lows.

When Jeanette Styles of Eugene, Oregon, swims moderately for 20 to 50 minutes, she either sets a temporary target blood glucose of 150 mg/dL (8.3 mmol/L) on her MiniMed 670G pump before swimming or cuts her basal rates by 50 to 75 percent. She also keeps Gatorade by the pool to sip if she starts to feel low.

United Kingdom resident Helen Cotton struggles with balancing her blood glucose for swimming for 60 to 90 minutes because her pump is not waterproof. But swimming is her main endurance exercise, so she tries to eat enough before she swims to avoid going low; usually she needs to bolus a little before her swims to cover the basal insulin she misses during the activity. She finds it easier to do other types of exercise for which she can lower her basal rate to avoid lows during and afterward without too much planning.

A resident of St. Thomas in the U.S. Virgin Islands, Steve Prosterman (profiled in chapter 12) always carries a glucose source with him when he is in the ocean swimming, scuba diving, snorkeling, or windsurfing. When he has fruit snacks, he has to change them out regularly as the packaging does not hold up in the salty ocean water for a long time. He also eats extra carbohydrates before an activity if his blood glucose is less than 140 to 150 mg/dL (7.8 to 8.3 mmol/L) when he is going to be working out for 1 hour or more. Being in an isolated exercise environment like the ocean can be dangerous if he is not prepared. After exercise, he checks and corrects then, if needed. He splits his Lantus dose (morning and evening), but usually does not adjust it for these activities, which are usual ones for him.

Western Australia native Bec Johnson is a long-distance swimmer. She completed the 19.7-kilometer (12.24-mile) Rottnest Channel Swim in 2018 and set a new goal to complete Australia's longest open-water swim (25 kilometers [15.5 miles]). She is a keto-adapted athlete who follows a low-carbohydrate diet. She always trains with a system clear of food and rapid-acting (or regular) insulin with only her basal (Levemir) on board to minimize the variables in play. Exercising before breakfast is ideal for her; but if she has training in the evening, she eats lunch early so there is no food or meal-related insulin on board before training. She finds that training under only basal conditions keeps things simple. Her blood glucose generally stays stable or possibly drops a little bit (if she trains longer than 1 hour) during swimming, cycling, and mountain biking. She manages with a low-carbohydrate, protein-rich snack like nuts, cheese, or a boiled egg at least 1 or 2 hours beforehand and finds that the slow protein spike keeps her steady. She also relies on caffeine if she is anticipating a drop during training, by having a coffee beforehand. If she is too late to eat the protein or have a coffee, she uses small, controlled amounts of glucose if her level is trending down.

When Plano, Texas, resident Don Muchow does open-water swims, he tries to fuel in advance for the distance he will be swimming before he gets in the water. Mostly he does this because he has not trained for feeding stops for swims longer than 3 miles. Plus, the farthest he has swum during training has been about 4 miles, so beyond that is unknown territory for him. He uses a Medtronic MiniMed 670G system, which determines his basal profiles and does microbolusing. Normally he gets about 30 to 35 units of insulin a day on a rest day and approximately 20 units a day on training days.

## Other Effects to Consider

**Effect of Exercise Intensity and Competition.**   Swim meets have a completely different effect compared with swim practices, as Kris Berg can attest. He tries to keep his blood glucose around 150 mg/dL (8.3 mmol/L) during meets, but the adrenaline release from the stress of competition and all-out sprinting during shorter events (50 or 100 meters) can easily make his glucose spike by 200 mg/dL (11.1 mmol/L) points or more. He finds that events of 200 meters or longer still cause an increase in his blood glucose, but not as much as shorter sprint distances.

**Effect of Time of Day.**   Although Californian Sheri Ochs usually swims after lunch, if she has to swim before breakfast instead she must take at least half a unit of Humalog beforehand. Without that small dose, her glucose can double during an hour of swimming, even without eating anything, because of her higher morning insulin resistance (even though she usually wakes up with her blood glucose in a normal range, thanks to her Lantus basal insulin that she unevenly splits into two daily doses).

Camille Andre, also a Californian, consumes about 30 grams of carbohydrates before doing an afternoon or evening workout, be it an hour swim or run or a longer bike ride. For the same activities in the morning, she never consumes carbohydrates beforehand without taking some insulin via a bolus from her insulin pump.

**Effect of Exercise Duration and Environment.**   Canadian Jen Alexander from Halifax, Nova Scotia, was the first swimmer ever to do a double crossing of the Northumberland Strait, which lies between Prince Edward Island and the southern and western shores of the Gulf of Saint Lawrence in eastern Canada. To cross the strait twice, Jen had to swim continuously for 19 hours and 17 minutes. During the swim, she consumed about 30 grams of carbohydrates every 30 minutes, mostly in the form of Kool-Aid and Gatorade, while adjusting the basal rate on her insulin pump to compensate. She had to increase her basal rate after about 2 hours until about 10 hours (25 to 75 percent above normal), after which she set it as much as 50 to 60 percent lower than normal. On several occasions when her glucose rose near the start and the end of her swim, she took small boluses to compensate. The latter increase was probably due to her suffering from hypothermia after swimming 18 hours in ocean water that averaged about 68 degrees Fahrenheit (20 degrees Celsius).

Texan Don Muchow has also had issues related to ocean conditions and going low during a particularly strenuous open-water swim. He has type 1 diabetes and his ultradistance swimming buddy has type 2. After a 3-mile swim in choppy ocean water to prepare for a relay swim around Key West, they both ran a bit low getting out of the water because they had had to work harder than anticipated. (They later learned the chop had been so severe that a marine wind advisory had been issued.)

## TRIATHLONS

Triathlons range in length from sprint and Olympic distance to half and full-length Ironman events. These prolonged activities use aerobic energy systems almost exclusively, regardless of their length (they can take anywhere from an hour to more than half a day to complete). Your body relies on both fat and carbohydrate, although you will use more carbohydrate the faster you go. Most events cause significant depletion of your glycogen stores, even if you are able to use a considerable amount of fat as a fuel. You can alter your insulin, diet, or both to compensate, but if you take insulin you will have to lower your doses to avoid hypoglycemia during and after longer triathlons.

The length of the triathlon will greatly affect your blood glucose responses. Sprint triathlons may be completed by doing an hour of intensive exercise. Sprint triathlons that result in a greater release of glucose-raising hormones may help keep your blood glucose higher throughout the event. Olympic, half, and full-length events, however, can last 3 to 12 or more hours, a duration that will have a more significant effect on your glycogen and blood glucose use. The more depleted your glycogen stores become, the more your body relies on your blood glucose. During longer events, you will have to take in extra carbohydrate throughout to prevent lows, along with lowering your insulin doses. Because of the muscle glycogen depletion, you must watch out for later-onset lows sneaking up on you after events of all lengths.

## Athlete Examples

The required regimen changes are largely determined by the length of the event. Longer triathlons require major insulin and food intake changes to prevent lows.

### Diet Changes Alone

When training for Ironman triathlons, pump user John Boyer of Mount Airy, Maryland, is constantly testing various nutritional strategies to reduce the risk of highs and lows and to optimize his performance. For him, higher protein and fat foods before workouts and during full-day cycling have proven most effective, but before swims a combination of simpler carbohydrates and protein has worked better. He also carries GU energy gel packets tucked in the sleeves of his wetsuit for long swims. For rides and runs lasting more than 1 hour, he alternates between water and sports drinks to help keep his blood glucose up. After the workout, he also needs an aggressive correction (20 percent greater than normal) to manage the glucose spikes that result from the volume of food he consumed during training.

### Combined Regimen Changes

United Kingdom resident Andy Kellar has a pretty simple regimen to deal with triathlons. He lowers the basal rate on his pump by 85 percent and consumes 20 grams of carbohydrates every 30 minutes, mostly in the form of sports drinks like Lucozade and jellies like Fruit Pastilles, both available in the United Kingdom.

Nigel Wilson, also from the United Kingdom, started out doing sprint triathlons and worked his way up to full Ironman lengths. He developed his current diabetes regimen through a lot of practice. He takes half his basal insulin (Tresiba) on the morning of the race. He used to cut his breakfast dose of Humalog in half as well, but after doing various races he found his glucose would go high due to anxiety and nerves and he would need a correction anyway. After those initial doses, he does not take any more insulin through the whole race. An hour and a half into the event, he begins to need about 80 grams of carbohydrates per hour, and he tries to sustain that intake over as much of the race as possible, along with adequate fluids. (By the end of the race, he says he cannot stomach too much.) Although Nigel starts out with his blood glucose higher than desired for full Ironman competitions, it averages 90 to 162 mg/dL (5.0 to 9.0 mmol/L) throughout the day. He admits he does not have the most scientific approach, but it has worked for him, and he has no gut problems during the race. His breakfast usually consists of a pear, a whole meal bagel with peanut butter and jam, and maybe a banana and sports drink while driving to the race, covered with about 1 unit per 10 grams of carbohydrates. Because he cannot stomach much on race mornings, he usually has to force breakfast down because he knows he needs to eat it. He has also found that eating it a few hours before the race starts is better, so as to have as little bolus insulin in his system as possible. However, he admits that even now, with all his experience racing, sometimes things can still go wrong!

Competing in triathlons of varying distances (lasting 1.5 to 15 hours) means that Scott Jozefowski of Seattle, Washington, needs different changes for each event. Usually, he eats at least an hour and a half before starting and boluses then. Depending on the length of the race, he may bolus and eat a glucose gel before the swim, and sometimes again after it. He eats and/or drinks every 35 minutes during the cycling portion. His CGM tells him where his glucose is during the run at the end, and he may consume some carbohydrates every couple of miles, depending on its readings. He also uses a descending temporary basal rate during the run, meaning that he has almost no basal insulin delivery during the last few miles, depending on the distance.

For marathons and triathlons (half-Ironman distance), Australian Warwick Sickling lowers his doses of his basal insulin (Lantus) as his training distances increase. He thinks Levemir is easier to make changes with, but he developed an allergy to it and can no longer use it. He also decreases his Humalog doses for the same carbohydrate content during training. Before the actual event he is participating in, he has to additionally lower his basal to avoid lows in the 12 hours before and during it. Afterward, he usually has at least one low in the next 24 hours, but he finds it too difficult to predict when it will happen in that period.

## Other Effects to Consider

### Effect of Insulin Levels and Technology.    John Mitchell of Maple Grove, Minnesota, finds that limiting his insulin on board is critical. Before Ironman events, he eats a full breakfast at least 3 hours before the start to get as much insulin out of his system as possible before he starts the event. Although he has a MiniMed 670G hybrid closed-loop system, as an athlete he chooses to use it only in manual mode instead of letting the system make basal insulin delivery decisions for him in auto

mode. He likes being able to see his glucose readings on his CGM during long training rides and his runs as an Ironman athlete (he is a two-time Wisconsin Ironman finisher). He says that using CGM makes diabetes a much more manageable disease, but it is never easy.

**Effect of Time Without Insulin.**   Elmhurst, Illinois, resident Patrick Kurtz finds that he can only go so long without insulin. For running and biking shorter distances, he leaves his pump off and carries extra carbohydrates, and the same goes for most races lasting 2 to 3 hours. For an Ironman event, he keeps his insulin pump off but carries an insulin pen with him just in case. He has randomly needed to bolus a few units during an Ironman race, but not during three other shorter races. (His Ironman time was 10 hours 30 minutes—too long for almost anyone to go completely without insulin.)

**Effect of Environment and Dehydration.**   Michel Cadieux from Austin, Texas, worries about staying hydrated. In fact, his best advice is to "Hydrate like mad!" He does Ironman triathlons and usually finishes off 10 full water bottles on long training rides, along with taking in some base salts. Without the hydration he gets painful muscle cramps in his legs during longer training in hot and humid conditions. (For another triathlon muscle cramping story, read about Jay Handy's first triathlon as detailed in chapter 6.)

## ULTRAENDURANCE EVENTS AND TRAINING

Ultraendurance activities often include multiple days of strenuous exercise (such as cycling, running, walking, or backpacking), as well as ultramarathons and other extremely long-distance events such as 50-mile (80.5-kilometer) races. Prolonged events use aerobic energy systems almost exclusively, with a mix of muscle glycogen and blood glucose, blood and intramuscular fats, and protein sources. Training for and competing in ultraendurance events can maximally stress the body's stores of energy, resulting in significant depletion. To participate effectively, you will need to lower your insulin (if you take it) and eat more during the event and for 24 to 48 hours afterward while your body is restoring what you used, particularly muscle and liver glycogen stores, along with repairing damaged muscles.

Your insulin sensitivity will generally be heightened during this time, and your risk for hypoglycemia will be greater. The only exception occurs when you have caused significant damage to your muscles, resulting in delayed-onset muscle soreness (see more on this in chapter 7). While your muscles remain somewhat damaged for a couple of days, you may be somewhat more insulin resistant (an effect that happens even in nondiabetic people) because glycogen cannot be restored until your muscles are repaired.

## Athlete Examples

These examples show the extreme regimen changes that are necessary for ultraendurance events and training. The type and length of the event or training determine your requisite changes, which usually include both insulin and food intake adjustments. For other relevant examples, refer to triathlons and marathons in this chapter and to adventure and trail running, backpacking, and mountaineering in chapter 12.

## Combined Regimen Changes

San Diego, California, resident Maggie Crawford competes in ultraendurance activities, most often 50-kilometer (31-mile) ultramarathons. For these races, she eats every 45 minutes (usually dried fruit) and does not dose with insulin during them. She does have her normal basal insulin (Lantus) on board during her runs, though.

Australian Neil McLagan is an ultraendurance road cyclist who rides for long distances that last more than 8 hours. He typically does not require bolus insulin (Humalog or regular) before or during the ride. As he starts each ride in the morning, he covers the food he eats during the ride with a reduced dose of injected Levemir, which he usually lowers by 50 to 70 percent of normal. All the foods he consumes before, during, and after are in accordance with the low-carbohydrate, moderate protein, and high-healthy-fat diet that he follows. He normally eats less than 30 grams of carbohydrates, 120 to 150 grams of protein, and 220 to 250 grams of fat daily. He divides his macronutrient profile among three daily meals, minimizing his intake of any processed or refined foods and sticking with whole food choices, typically from foods such as unprocessed meats, green leafy vegetables, macadamia nuts and avocados, and occasionally some cheese.

In the past 4 years, Navarre, Florida, resident Steven Rausch has run 11 50-mile (80.5-kilometer) races. During the events and training for this ultraendurance running, he may run for up to 10 hours. He likes to eat a large spaghetti meal the night before, which he covers with an appropriate amount of insulin. At the start, his blood glucose is usually around 150 mg/dL (8.3 mmol/L), which is a target he sets using his Medtronic MiniMed 670G pump with CGM system. During the race, he monitors using CGM and reacts with food. When his blood glucose starts dropping below 120 mg/dL (6.7 mmol/L) during the race, he begins eating about 25 to 35 grams of carbohydrates every 4 miles (6.4 kilometers). He carries trail mix, dried apricots, and energy bars, as well as consuming whatever is available at the event aid stations. If he has a low below 70 mg/dL (3.9 mmol/L), he stops running and eats until it comes up. For shorter runs, he often runs for up to 80 minutes without needing to eat anything.

Don Muchow from Plano, Texas, says that for marathons he has basal profiles on his pump for exercise days and nonexercise days. He also uses a Medtronic MiniMed 670G that determines basal profiles and gives microboluses. On full-day runs, he does not bolus extra for fuel stops (typically 25 to 30 grams of carbohydrates) every 5 miles or so, but during meal stops he does take half the amount his pump recommends to help replenish his glycogen stores. During ultraendurance runs, he keeps his basal rate at 100 percent of nonexercise days because he has found that his blood glucose rises due to the stress of running 40 to 70 miles a day.

During ultraendurance events, New Yorker Stephen England needs more calories and a higher carbohydrate intake (60 grams per hour) than during marathons. He lowers his basal rate on his pump down to 70 percent of normal during these events as well because his running is lower intensity and adjusts as needed throughout.

Sometimes he gets low during runs if he fails to take a gel before his blood glucose drops, which can happen if he is monitoring with CGM only and it loses its signal or gives him inaccurate readings.

For ultraendurance training and events (50-mile and 50-kilometer races), Kari from Galveston, Texas, has a fairly simple regimen. She takes half of her Lantus dose that morning. She takes 2 units of Humalog afterward to prevent a spike in her blood glucose, and she may need 2 units halfway through as well. She takes in some carbohydrates every 30 minutes as a fuel, along with salt tablets.

## Other Effects to Consider

**Effect of Physical Stress and Environment.**    Typically, when Don Muchow is under physical stress, his blood glucose goes higher. For example, he had persistent highs (in the 200s mg/dL [above 11.1 mmol/L]) during the last 40 miles of one 100-mile run because he was running on severely blistered feet for most of that distance. His crew had taped his feet so he was not feeling much discomfort, but after the overnight portion when temperatures climbed above 90 degrees Fahrenheit (above 32 degrees Celsius) for miles 85 to 95, the additional heat stress sent his blood glucose above 500 mg/dL (27.8 mmol/L). He and his crew had to decide whether he should finish the last 5 miles of the event. They opted to have him walk the rest of the distance and only sprint to the finish when he could see it.

**Effect of Bolus Insulin on Board.**    Regardless of the types of events he is training for, Peter Nerothin has one mantra: "Avoid having any fast-acting insulin in your system." He includes pump-delivered basal insulin in this as well (always a fast-acting insulin delivered with preprogrammed basal rates). He sees having any of this insulin on board as a huge drawback because he must chase it with food to prevent lows during training. He finds that his glucose is much more stable when he takes his basal insulin via injection (usually Levemir for him). He tries to do all his training at least 4 to 6 hours after his last dose of bolus insulin (Humalog). If he is using inhaled Afrezza, he can start exercising within 2 hours without any problems from it dropping his glucose too much because it is cleared from his body much more quickly than the other bolus insulins.

In this chapter, you hopefully gained many more ideas about how to handle endurance activities as an athlete with diabetes. Whether you choose to run a marathon or simply want to run, cycle, swim, or roller ski your way to better health and good diabetes management, you now have the tools you need for training as long and as hard as you desire. If you prefer team sports and other activities like tennis, you can find out much more about how athletes train for those in the next chapter.

## Athlete Profile: **Jay Hewitt**

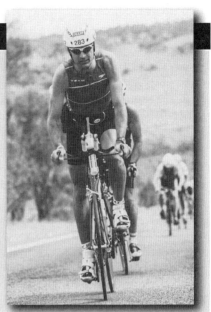

*Hometown:* Greenville, South Carolina

*Diabetes history:* Type 1 diabetes diagnosed in 1991 (at age 23)

*Sport or activity:* Ironman triathlon (2.4-mile swim + 112-mile bike + 26.2-mile run = 140.6 miles)

*Greatest athletic achievement:* I discuss all these in my book, *Finish Line Vision* (signed copies available on my website www.jayhewitt.com).

▶ Fourteen Ironman and ultradistance triathlons

▶ Twenty Half Ironman 70.3 triathlons (1.2-mile swim + 56-mile bike + 13.1-mile run = 70.3 miles)

▶ Eight individual marathons, including three Boston marathons

Courtesy of Jay Hewitt.

▶ Qualified and raced 3 years on the U.S. National Long Course Triathlon Team

▶ Raced for Team USA at the ITU Long Course Tri World Championships from 2004 to 2006 in Sweden, Denmark, and Australia

▶ Ironman triathlon personal best of 9:47

▶ Raced for Team Type 1 (now Team Novo Nordisk) cycling team, winning 2006 Race Across America by cycling 3,000 miles in 5 days, 16 hours, and 4 minutes.

*Current insulin and medication regimen:* I am not racing Ironman triathlons currently, but I still work out daily. I inject 20 units of Tresiba basal insulin and Novolog bolus insulin at meal-time and for correction boluses. During my racing career I used both insulin pumps and injection therapy. During Ironman races, I used only basal insulin and did not inject or dose any bolus insulin while consuming 60 to 80 grams of carbohydrates per hour because the basal insulin was sufficient to cover that. I also did not reduce my basal insulin on race day because (1) I wanted/needed to be motivated/obligated/free to fuel carbohydrates/calories consistently throughout the entire race; (2) I also needed the basal insulin to fight the adrenaline-elevated blood glucose that always plagued me in the first 3 hours of an Ironman race; and (3) I needed to keep sufficient basal insulin in me to prevent high blood glucose sluggishness, stomach upset, and dehydration over the 9 or 10 hours of a race.

▶ 2002–2003 Medtronic pump with Humalog insulin

▶ 2003–2005 Lantus basal insulin injection and Humalog pen bolus insulin

▶ 2006–2015 Omnipod insulin pump with Novolog insulin

▶ 2016–2018 Tresiba basal insulin and Novolog pen bolus insulin

*Training tips:* Experiment and develop a nutrition plan for training and race/competition days and then repeat what works for each. Training day nutrition and insulin dosing will probably be slightly different than race/competition days because of the different levels of stress, intensity, and duration. Don't expect the nutrition regimen to work perfectly every time, every workout, every day. You always should check your blood glucose and be prepared to adapt and adjust. Many unpredictable factors affect blood glucose that are not your nutrition (e.g., stress, anxiety, adrenaline, illness, and intensity). Experiment with pre-race and preworkout food and repeat what works 80 percent of the time. Always check to confirm and correct. I use high-carb drinks (e.g., a 20-ounce bottle of 80 grams of carbohydrates versus 40 grams of carbohydrates in 20-ounce typical sports drink) to correct or prevent lows by consuming only a few swallows rather than overloading my gut with large quantities of solid food or lower carbohydrate liquid before or during a workout or competition.

**Short workouts of 1 hour or less:** Eat before the workout (usually about 30 minutes before) such as a banana or smaller amount of carbohydrates to give you energy and glucose but not too much to spike your blood glucose. Do not bolus insulin within 1 hour of starting your workout unless you have to correct a severe high (over 200 mg/dL [11.1 mmol/L]), but even then reduce the amount of correction dose because your upcoming workout will help reduce your blood glucose as well. You should not need to eat anything during the workout, unless, of course, you go low. A sports gel with 20 grams of carbohydrates and 100 calories should be sufficient during an hour workout.

**Long workouts of 2 to 5 hours:** Before the workout, eat longer-lasting, low-glycemic carbohydrates like oatmeal to stick with you during your workout. Check your blood glucose about every hour, or continuously if you wear a CGM, to determine how many carbohydrates you need per hour. On long workouts I fuel with 60 to 80 grams of carbohydrates per hour from sports drinks and bars and gels. Also drink some plain water just for hydration—more in hot conditions.

**Post workout:** I bolus a small dose of insulin immediately after long workouts and consume a recovery drink of 50 to 70 grams of carbohydrates to replenish, recover, and prevent muscle soreness. Insulin is a recovery hormone that gets carbohydrates into cells, so use it to help your cells recover.

*Typical daily and weekly training and diabetes regimen:* The regimen depends on where I am in the race season: spring early season versus summer–fall midseason versus winter off-season. The following is a very general schedule for a midseason training week with an Ironman race coming up in about 6 weeks.

▶ *Monday:* Morning: swim 3,000 to 4,000 meters. Afternoon/evening: easy cycling for 30 miles for recovery from Sunday long run but with three or four 2-minute intervals.

▶ *Tuesday:* Morning/midday: track run workout with speed work including 800s and 400s for leg turnover. Evening: group cycling, speed work, 30 to 40 miles at an average speed of 25 to 28 mph; immediately after ride, do short brick run of 2 to 3 miles.

▶ *Wednesday:* Morning: swim 3,000 to 4,000 meters, including stroke and technique drills. Afternoon/evening: cycle 30 miles with hill intervals.

continued ➡

*Jay Hewitt continued*

- ▶ **Thursday:** Morning: run 8 to 10 miles, tempo run. Afternoon/evening: cycle 20 to 30 miles, including intervals.
- ▶ **Friday:** Morning: swim 3,000 to 4,000 meters consisting of speed work, with 100s, 200s, and 400s, timed and descending.
- ▶ **Saturday:** Long cycle ride of 70 to 100 miles, followed by a short brick run of 5 miles immediately after. Fuel with 60 to 80 grams of carbohydrates per hour during cycling without bolusing, and check blood glucose hourly. Give small bolus immediately after workout to consume recovery drink/shake with 60 to 80 grams carbohydrates for recovery.
- ▶ **Sunday:** Morning: long run of 12 to 20 miles. Evening: cycle 20 miles easy, recovery.

**Other hobbies and interests:** Tennis, basketball, hiking in national parks, public speaking, diabetes advocacy, and spending time with my wife and kids.

**Good diabetes and exercise story:** I have good and bad diabetes and exercise stories. A bad one is when I learned a valuable lesson about post-race and workout refueling early in my racing career. One week after I ran the Kona, Hawaii, marathon in June, I raced a 70-mile bike race in the mountains of North Carolina on July 4, a very hot, hilly, hard race. I finished the bike race and ate some food to refuel but not enough carbohydrates. Several hours later I was at home alone, asleep on my couch thinking I was just tired from the race—I was actually suffering very low blood glucose. I eventually woke up covered in sweat, and could not stand, talk, or control my body. It was the most severe episode of hypoglycemia I had ever experienced. I was able to get some glucose in my mouth and recovered, but it was terrifying.

A good story is about racing my 7th Ironman triathlon at Ironman Florida one year. Earlier that same year I had already raced three very poor Ironman races—at Ironman Coeur d'Alene, Idaho, Ironman Wisconsin, and the ITU Long Course Worlds in Sweden—caused by a mixture of dehydration, high blood glucose, and gastrointestinal problems. But preparing for Ironman Florida that November I changed my nutrition plan, kept my blood glucose managed well, and had the best race of my career, beating half of the professional field as an amateur. My discipline, dedication, and hard work paid off. The difficulties caused by diabetes made the success so much better.

# 10

# Endurance–Power Sports

**W**e have all heard of LeBron James, Tom Brady, and Tiger Woods because of the popularity of endurance–power sports. But have you heard of Chris Dudley, Adam Morrison, Jay Cutler, Patrick Peterson, Nick Boynton, Michelle McGann, and Scott Verplank? Although maybe not as well known, they are just a few of the many professional athletes with diabetes who are successfully competing in basketball, football, ice hockey, golf, and other such sports and activities.

In general, endurance–power sports require short, powerful bouts of movement that are repeated at frequent intervals. In basketball, the action may involve a jump and a dunk of the ball and then a sprint down the court; in tennis, it may be a serve and a short volley. Power activities may have no effect on your blood glucose or may raise it. But when the key movements are repeated many times over a prolonged period, they often have a cumulative effect on glycogen use and may require greater regimen changes to prevent your blood glucose levels from decreasing while you are doing them and later on, especially overnight.

Everyone can benefit in various ways from participating in team sports, either endurance or endurance–power sports. Participating in these sports can help children start to develop their coordination and skill, and help adults stay youthful and active. Check around your area for a local gym, recreation center, or sports league, and get the whole family involved in some of the sports covered in this chapter, including American football, rugby, basketball, field hockey, lacrosse, figure skating, flag football, ultimate Frisbee, golf, gymnastics, competitive horseback riding, ice hockey, soccer, tennis, water polo, and wrestling, among others. Maybe you can even take up golfing, get in on the new pickleball craze, or try out some high-intensity interval or CrossFit training options. Your options are many, and you can successfully engage in any of them that you choose to pursue (with the proper precautions, of course). If you are interested in purely power sports like baseball and bodybuilding, you will find more about those in the next chapter.

## GENERAL RECOMMENDATIONS FOR ENDURANCE–POWER SPORTS

Most of these sports require power performances that involve short, intense muscular activity. If the full activity lasts less than 10 seconds (like hitting a golf ball), your first energy system alone provides the energy. Children are particularly suited for these types of short-burst activities because their other two energy systems are less well developed before they reach adolescence (see chapter 2 for a review of these systems).

For any activity lasting up to 2 minutes (such as competitive cheerleading or gymnastics routines), your phosphagen system combines with the lactic acid one to provide muscular energy, adenosine triphosphate (ATP) and creatine phosphate supply the immediate energy, and glycogen is broken down to supply the remainder. When you are working less hard (such as walking between holes on the golf course) or recovering from these more powerful movements, your body uses aerobic energy derived from the metabolism of fat and carbohydrate. Participation in most of these activities requires you to work on both your muscular strength and your muscular endurance for that reason. Competing in and practicing for these activities can also emphasize your use of energy systems in quite different ways.

# GENERAL ADJUSTMENTS BY DIABETES REGIMEN

The sport or activity you engage in determines any diabetes regimen changes that you will need to make. Intense activities can decrease, increase, or have no effect on your blood glucose levels. Generally, though, power moves performed intermittently over an extended period, such as for a full basketball game, can have a cumulative effect, and you may need greater regimen changes to compensate both during and afterward. Keep in mind that competing in events can have quite a different impact on your diabetes management than team practices or training.

> *Powerful moves like hitting a golf ball or dunking a basketball do not use up much energy, but repeating these moves over an extended period of time can result in a greater use of muscle glycogen. Watch out for later-onset lows for this reason.*

## Insulin Pump Users

For participation in these activities, your insulin adjustments are sport specific. You may require no insulin or diet changes for easy or brief play. For prolonged team practices or games, you may need to reduce your insulin boluses before, as well as your basal insulin during the activity, depending on how long and how hard you are playing. Your insulin reductions, however, will generally be less than you would need for straight endurance sports because of the intense, brief nature of the power portion of these activities. In some cases, your blood glucose levels may increase due to a greater release of glucose-raising hormones, which may raise your need for insulin in the short run. For prolonged or intense participation, though, you may need extra carbohydrates and food, again depending on your insulin levels. You may also want to reduce your boluses after participating in certain sports, such as American football, basketball, soccer, and tennis; increase your carbohydrate (or other food) intake; and reduce your basal insulin after the activity and overnight.

## *Basal–Bolus Regimens*

For these types of sports, your insulin adjustments will depend on the sport. Short or easy play may require you to make no insulin or diet changes. Before longer practices or games, you may need to reduce your premeal insulin doses. You will probably have to cut back less than you do for endurance sports, given the intense, brief nature of the power part of these activities. In some cases, your blood glucose levels may increase from the high intensity of the activity, necessitating an increase in your insulin rather than a decrease. For prolonged or intense participation, you may need to eat more carbohydrates or food, depending on your reductions in insulin and the timing of your last bolus dose. After certain sports, you may want to reduce your bedtime basal insulin doses, along with possibly eating a bedtime snack to prevent overnight lows when you have depleted a significant amount of muscle glycogen during the activity.

## *Noninsulin and Oral Medication Users*

The power portion of these activities can raise your blood glucose (albeit temporarily), unless you do them for a long enough time. Doing an aerobic cool-down after these activities will help you counter any rise in your blood glucose. Later on, your blood glucose is likely to be better controlled, especially if you used up more muscle glycogen by doing the activity for longer. The heightened insulin action that follows these activities can persist for 24 to 48 hours, so be on the lookout for lows if you are taking certain medications like sulfonylureas (e.g., Diabinese, DiaBeta, Micronase, or Glynase). Refer back to chapter 3 for more information about the exercise effects of these and other glucose-lowering medications.

## *Other Effects to Consider*

How long, how hard, which sport, and how you play it (recreationally or competitively) can affect your blood glucose responses. Another factor to consider is what position you are playing. For instance, in soccer, midfielders may run significantly more during a game than defenders, and goalies even less so. Being more active overall (and thus depleting more glycogen with repeated, powerful movements) can reduce your blood glucose levels more dramatically. Moreover, recreational play and practices are usually less intense—but often more prolonged—than competitive matches or games. A short, intense competition like a wrestling match may cause your blood glucose levels to rise because of its intensity and brevity, whereas recreational softball may have no discernible effect on your blood glucose in the short run. Basketball matches, due to the stress of competition, may keep blood glucose up, whereas less intense (and longer) practices can lower it instead. Playing 2 hours of basketball at any level may cause a substantial decrease in your blood glucose during and afterward, and even overnight due to a greater use of muscle glycogen from longer play.

> *There is a big difference between practices and competitions when it comes to blood glucose responses: the former usually lowers glucose, whereas the latter can raise it.*

## AMERICAN FOOTBALL AND RUGBY

Both of these sports are extremely anaerobic in nature. Most football plays last only 10 to 20 seconds and involve power moves, such as pushing with full force on the offensive or defensive line, throwing the ball, sprinting into position, running powerfully with the ball, or tackling an opponent. Rugby is essentially the same as playing football without wearing all the protective pads and helmets.

Many factors affect your blood glucose responses to these activities. Whether you are involved in a practice or a game will determine some of the differences. During practices, you will likely run more than during competitive games when the plays are more intense and shorter and offensive and defensive units take turns on the field. Players in football positions that require more running overall (e.g., wide receiver, running back, defensive back) may use muscle glycogen at different rates than those in "brute force" positions (offensive and defensive linemen) who just block or try to shed blocks and do anaerobic work during plays. All players will end up using a great deal of muscle glycogen by the end of a game (unless your usual position is benchwarmer), for which you will likely need to eat more and take less insulin after the activity.

In addition, preseason practices, especially twice-a-day sessions, will significantly increase your insulin action and require greater regimen changes compared with doing shorter, easier practices during the regular season, especially before upcoming games. For recreational play in these sports, you will likely run more and work less hard, which means that your blood glucose is more likely to drop at some point during the activity. See an example of playing flag football listed separately in that section later in this chapter.

## Athlete Examples

These examples show that recreational football or rugby requires quite different regimen changes than more competitive games.

### *Insulin Changes Alone*

Cooper J. from Goleta, California, disconnects his MiniMed 670G pump while playing contact sports like football. He finds it helps if he can reconnect at least hourly and take the dose of insulin he missed, or else his blood glucose tends to go high during this activity due to its intensity and the lack of basal insulin during it. For him, exercise-induced highs continue to be a daily struggle.

Cameron, North Carolina, resident Patrick Peele tends to have higher blood glucose during football, so he checks and corrects more with small boluses during practice and games. His target range during this sport is 150 to 200 mg/dL (8.3 to 11.1 mmol/L). He sees wearing an Omnipod during exercise as a big benefit because he does not have to disconnect from it, and he can also decrease his basal rate if he sees his blood glucose dropping at any point.

### *Combined Regimen Changes*

Alexandria, Virginia, resident Simon Smith serves as a referee for rugby matches. He wears his continuous glucose monitor (CGM) while refereeing, but also does a blood glucose check at the start and again at halftime. He corrects with insulin or food as needed. He uses the CGM as a predictor and then considers the type of game he is refereeing, either easy or intense, and also whether it is slower paced or fast. In his case, there is as much mental effort as physical involved. To manage his diabetes, if his glucose is trending down, he eats glucose tablets, gummy candy, or a banana. If it is creeping up, he does not do anything. For steep climbs, he treats with insulin (Humalog) and extra water to stay hydrated. His basal insulin, Tresiba, remains unchanged for this activity.

## BALLET

Unlike more recreational forms of dancing, ballet requires years of practice to get really good, countless hours spent performing physical work of varying intensities, and amazing muscle strength, endurance, and flexibility. The intensity of performances is high, but the hours of practice tend to lower blood glucose due to muscle glycogen use.

## Athlete Examples

The intensity of ballet performances is likely greater than most of the activity during practice sessions, but the duration is shorter. In either case, management likely requires both lower insulin levels and taking in extra food to compensate.

### Diet Changes Alone

For 90-minute ballet or jazz classes, Juliana Kotsifakis of Ocean City, Maryland, eats enough beforehand to get her blood glucose into the 150 to 200 mg/dL (8.3 to 11.1 mmol/L) range. Usually her blood glucose level is around 70 mg/dL (3.9 mmol/L) when she finishes.

### Combined Regimen Changes

Former professional ballerina and soloist for the New York City Ballet, Zippora Karz (author of *The Sugarless Plum: A Memoir* and *Ballerina Dreams: A Book for Children With Diabetes*), who is now a resident of Los Angeles, California, performed for years without the benefit of newer technologies like CGM to help her manage her blood glucose. Here are some of her insights looking back on her experience.

"It took me years to learn the best way to approach my performances as a ballerina with New York City Ballet. I learned it was best not to eat carbohydrates before I went on stage. While all foods eventually turn to glucose and require insulin, protein, fats, and nonstarchy vegetables require the least amount of insulin. By minimizing my intake of carbohydrates before performances or practices, I was less likely to go too low because I had less circulating insulin in my system. My snacks included protein, like chicken or turkey (I prefer organic), avocado, nuts and seeds, and vegetables like cucumber, broccoli, or cauliflower, for example, and those are the foods I carried with me as snacks before performances. In time I learned that eating lower carbohydrate foods, even as a teacher of ballet and more, keeps me more balanced with fewer highs and lows. Nowadays there are many recipes to help people find variety and pleasure from a low-carbohydrate diet (Paleo and ketogenic diets are mainstream now).

For my occasional low, I carried dates in my dance bag. It was far easier to put a date in my mouth in between entrances than to stop and drink juice. Just know how much it will raise you, so you do not overeat the food raising your glucose, bringing it too high. For my diabetic feet, I used Epsom salt baths and soaks often for sore and achy muscles, and for occasional blisters and corns between my toes. I also changed my socks frequently, and dried my toes out with tinactin powder."

Jillian Wiseman of Tarzana, California, dances for 3 to 8 hours daily, for which she makes changes in both insulin and food. She lowers her bolus doses (taking almost none during long days of dancing) and eats more carbohydrates and protein before workouts. Her biggest challenge is dealing with lows during the night after evening ballet practice, but she is often on the high side after dancing because of how hard she works. Her primary strategy for preventing such lows is to cut back dramatically on her dose of basal insulin (Lantus), which she takes in the evening, by 33 to 50 percent.

## BASKETBALL AND NETBALL

These court activities involve many stop-and-start movements and quick, powerful moves like shooting, passing, and dribbling. As a result, they are more anaerobic than aerobic. But when you play for an hour or more continuously, you will use up a lot of muscle glycogen and blood glucose. Both also have an aerobic component when you run up and down the court at a moderate pace or stand in place during passing moves. You may need changes in your insulin and food intake to prevent a drop in your blood glucose levels during or after a game or practice.

How long you play and how much insulin you have on board are the factors that affect your blood glucose the most. If you can exercise with minimal insulin (i.e., 2 to 3 hours after bolus insulin, early in the morning, or with lowered basal amounts), you will maintain your blood glucose levels more effectively while taking in less food. If you play for a long time, your use of muscle glycogen will cause lower blood glucose later that you can prevent with increased food intake and possibly lower doses of insulin.

## Athlete Examples

These real-life examples demonstrate that diet, insulin, or both can be modified to maintain your blood glucose control during and after basketball play. No athletes surveyed reported playing netball, although it is popular around the world.

### *Insulin Changes Alone*

Gary Scheiner of Philadelphia, Pennsylvania, finds that his response to basketball is unique. He plays for about 2 hours at a time, for which he gives his usual meal bolus beforehand, but reduces his basal insulin rate on his pump by 50 percent starting an hour before playing and lasting until he is done. The main time his glucose may go up is if the game he is playing becomes heated or intense (that is, more competitive).

Joshua Reese of Knoxville, Tennessee, does not change his diet when he plays basketball. He does disconnect his pump, however, because it is a contact sport. He wears his CGM and monitors during breaks from play. Kris Maynard from Mead, Washington, also disconnects his pump for basketball and wears his CGM.

West Allis, Wisconsin, resident Jack Borck has different basal insulin profiles set on his pump for a variety of activities, including basketball, baseball, football, track, and weight training. In general, he reduces his basal 1 hour before, with how much depending on his blood glucose at the time. Right before the activity, he will lower his basal rate further, up to an 80 percent decrease. He leaves the basal rate lowered 25 to 50 percent for 2 hours, again depending on his blood glucose levels.

Toronto, Canada, resident Mike Riddell used to have to take his pump off to play a contact sport like basketball for 2 hours, and he would have elevated blood glucose after playing, He has resolved that issue by switching to a tubeless (Omnipod) pump when playing basketball so that he can have some insulin on board to counter

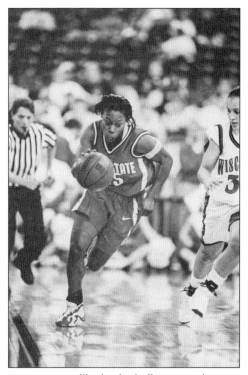

Power sports like basketball may not have much of an immediate effect on blood glucose, but over an extended period, such as for a full basketball game, they can have a cumulative effect, and you may need greater regimen changes to compensate.

the rise in his glucose. He tends to keep his basal rate at 100 percent during intensive mixed activities like basketball. If his blood glucose increases above target, he gives a correction bolus at 100 percent of recommended based on his own insulin sensitivity factor and targets set up on his insulin pump (typically about one-half to 1 unit if his glucose rises to 200 mg/dL [11.1 mmol/L]).

## *Diet Changes Alone*

Aaron Seward of Parks, Louisiana, just tries to eat enough carbohydrates before playing basketball to keep from going low. As a growing teenager, he usually eats 60 grams of carbohydrates per meal, along with two 20-gram carbohydrate snacks during the day. He covers his meals with Humalog and takes Lantus at night to cover his basal needs.

Illinois resident Dwain Chapman stopped playing league basketball a few years ago at about age 50. While he was still playing, he checked his blood glucose, gave a bolus if needed, removed his pump, and played. Afterward he would reattach the pump and check and bolus or eat carbohydrates (such as glucose tablets or Gatorade) as needed. If he had a rare low while playing, he treated it with glucose tablets or a sweet drink. Before he had a pump or easy access to a blood glucose meter, he just used to eat a lot before playing, and it was always just a guess.

Australia native Warwick Sickling finds that if his blood glucose is at a good level before playing basketball, he usually does not need any additional carbohydrates or insulin beforehand. Occasionally, he may have a low during the game or finish the game a bit on the high side, but as long as he does not have much bolus insulin on board, his blood glucose stays around the same level from pregame to postgame.

The time Matt from Royersford, Pennsylvania, is most likely to get low is when he does more activity than he was planning, such as when his son asks him (spontaneously) to play basketball. In those cases, he tries to eat something before he starts and during playing to keep his blood glucose from dropping.

### *Combined Regimen Changes*

Patrick Peele, of Cameron, North Carolina, finds that his blood glucose drops more during basketball than football. His biggest challenge as a starting center on the basketball team is to keep his blood glucose in control to help his team win. He looks at his CGM often to make sure he is on track and manages it, if needed. The CGM also helps prevent lows by giving him alerts while he is playing, which allows him to continue playing instead of having to come out of the game for several minutes. If he is low, he drinks apple juice, but if his glucose gets down to 130 mg/dL (7.2 mmol/L) during play, he eats a snack or protein bar. Ideally, he aims to stay closer to 185 to 220 mg/dL (10.3 to 12.2 mmol/L) while active. Because his pump (Omnipod) is tubeless, he wears it during games and can also lower his basal rate when getting low. If he plays two or three basketball games in 1 day, his glucose drops during the night, so he uses his CGM to try to catch his lows early and to prevent them overnight.

Ottawa, Canada, resident Molly McDermott plays basketball three times a week (along with doing spin classes twice a week, boot camp workouts on Saturdays, and boxing on Tuesdays). She is constantly checking her CGM to prevent lows, but she also always eats breakfast (some of her classes or workouts are during the lunch hour) and checks her blood glucose immediately before and after exercise. Within 20 minutes of exercising, she tries to eat a snack of 20 to 30 grams of carbohydrates and sometimes also some protein (chicken or cheese and crackers). On days she plays basketball in particular, she has to reduce her second dose of Lantus in the evening by close to half, as she often goes low overnight otherwise.

## COMPETITIVE CHEERLEADING AND DRILL TEAM

Most cheerleading or drill team routines last for only a couple of minutes, but they can involve powerful moves like jumps, kicks, and explosive arm movements. Moreover, both professional and competitive cheerleading also include aspects of gymnastics that require powerful moves (e.g., back flips and cartwheels). Because practices can last for 1 to 2 hours, this sport is considered an endurance–power one. Although practices are more likely to cause your blood glucose to drop than doing short routines during competitions or athletic games, the amount of glycogen that you use will determine which adjustments you will need to make afterward to prevent later-onset lows.

## Athlete Examples

These examples show that competitive cheerleading and drill team practices and competitions usually require food and insulin adjustments to compensate. Also see the profile of former professional cheerleader, Courtney Duckworth, later in this chapter.

### Combined Regimen Changes

Maggie Hudson of Glen Allen, Virginia, has 7 hours of competitive cheerleading practices a week, which also involve working out on the trampoline and practicing her gymnastics. To compensate, she frequently checks her blood glucose and sets lower basal rates on her pump or eats snacks, as needed. In addition, she sometimes has to take her pump off, but reconnects to give a correction bolus if her glucose starts to rise after a while.

For cheerleading, Kelsey McGill of Bear, Delaware, takes her pump off but checks her blood glucose every 30 minutes to adjust her food or reconnect to bolus. Sometimes she keeps it on but lowers her basal rates. Before this activity, she tries to eat a healthy, light snack to keep her blood glucose stable.

A Memphis, Tennessee, resident, Lindsey O'Hare was the captain of her high school drill team. Their activities varied greatly from day to day, sometimes involving only stretching but on other days including 2 hours of high kicks. She kept her blood glucose meter nearby and paid close attention to how she was feeling. During intense workouts, she often reduced her basal rate by 20 to 50 percent, occasionally keeping it lower for 60 to 90 minutes afterward. Before morning practices, she often ate a small breakfast (toast and an orange) without bolusing.

## CROSSFIT TRAINING AND GAMES

A trademarked fitness trend that started in the United States in 2000, CrossFit is a strength and conditioning program mix of aerobic exercise, body weight exercises, and Olympic weightlifting. The goal is to improve your fitness across a broad spectrum of modalities, including endurance, strength, flexibility, power, speed, coordination, agility, balance, and accuracy, but training must be done with proper form to prevent injuries or "rhabdo" from occurring (see more on this topic in chapter 7).

CrossFit training on any given day in most gyms typically lasts an hour (the so-called "WOD," or workout of the day). In a usual workout, the first 10 minutes are spent warming up, followed by 20 minutes of strength training and another 20 minutes of an intense workout. The other 10 minutes serve as a transition time between activities and explanation. Although the intensity varies within each workout itself, most are similar from one day to the next, which may make anticipating your blood glucose responses easier. CrossFit Games have been held every summer since 2007.

## Athlete Examples

The intensity of this activity can vary somewhat between training sessions, but having a set length (1 hour) makes regimen changes somewhat easier to predict. Its intensity may cause your blood glucose levels to rise or stay more stable than purely aerobic workouts.

### Insulin Changes Alone

John Mitchell of Maple Grove, Minnesota, does CrossFit 2 or 3 times a week and usually disconnects his pump while doing these workouts because they are so incredibly intense. He often must take an increased manual bolus afterward to offset the adrenaline rush.

Because Illinois resident Gin Carlin takes her pump off when doing CrossFit workouts (because it gets in her way), she typically has an elevated blood glucose about an hour after finishing. To correct that, she typically boluses to cover the next 1.5 hours of missed basal before working out.

Lantus user Cindy Ski from Canada is fat-adapted and does not take in many carbohydrates. To prevent a spike in her blood glucose for either CrossFit or high-intensity interval training, she boluses with 2 units of Humalog before working out. Then she just monitors her glucose with her CGM throughout.

### Diet Changes Alone

Kari from Galveston, Texas, does CrossFit 3 days a week. On those mornings, she has some toast and coffee and eats a banana halfway through the class to prevent lows. Teenager Aaron Seward from Louisiana also does it 3 times weekly and simply ensures that he eats a meal (with 60 grams of carbohydrates) beforehand to manage his blood glucose levels.

Missoula, Montana, exerciser Derek Louquet does not need to drop any basal rates for CrossFit workouts as his blood glucose actually goes higher during short or intense workouts. He has to give a correction bolus after a workout, and then he has a meal afterward to recover best.

### Combined Regimen Changes

Danielle Okuly from Seattle, Washington, does CrossFit workouts early in the morning 6 days a week. She boluses 0.5 units for 10 grams of carbohydrates before leaving her house for the gym, adding a correction to the bolus if her blood glucose is elevated to start. Her hybrid closed-loop system auto-adjusts based on her blood glucose and delivers anything from 0.3 to 0.7 units per hour during the activity. She never eats before these workouts and checks her CGM at least once during it. She eats a breakfast of veggies (usually tomato soup) after the workout, and then eats something with more protein like eggs or a sandwich 2 hours later. She finds that CrossFit and hot yoga are the only activities for which she finds blood glucose management easy, saying that perhaps it is because they both have a set duration and level of intensity that makes it easy for her to predict what her blood glucose is going to do.

To participate in CrossFit workouts, Syosset, New York, resident Allison Caggia takes a unit of rapid-acting insulin as she walks in the door to exercise to prevent a rise in her blood glucose.

Some wise words of advice about managing your blood glucose during CrossFit workouts come from the personal experience of Diabetes Daily blogger, Allison Caggia: "Before starting CrossFit, I would hear horror stories about people spiking like crazy during the strength portion and WOD (workout of the day). I was very reluctant to try it out because I do like to keep my blood sugars under tight control. But by playing around for the first few months, I was able to figure out a system that worked for me. I would wake up and take my long-lasting insulin along with a bolus for my natural morning rise in blood sugars and factor in my high-protein, no-carbohydrate breakfast. I would usually get to the gym between 100 to 140 mg/dL (5.6 to 7.8 mmol/L). I would wait until right before walking into the gym to take one unit more. My reasoning is that both weightlifting and HIIT (high-intensity interval training) can spike people, so this would minimize it. I wait until right before I walk in so that it starts working toward the end instead of midway through."

## FIELD HOCKEY AND LACROSSE

Depending on the position you play, field hockey and lacrosse involve a combination of stop-and-start movements and longer sustained runs that involve both anaerobic and aerobic components, although lacrosse players may use their arms a bit more (holding their sticks up and handling and throwing the ball) than field hockey players. Both are similar to soccer play in comparison with other endurance–power team sports, and playing them can cause you to use a great deal of your muscle glycogen and blood glucose.

The position you play will greatly affect your overall activity level (e.g., goalies will run a lot less than the field players do), so you will need to make adjustments based on what position you play and how much time you play during the games. Its intermittent nature is better for maintaining (and potentially raising) blood glucose than continuous aerobic activities. In general, playing longer may require more regimen adjustments before, during, and after playing. During practices, the activity levels among positions may be more similar if all team members do continuous running, throwing, or shooting drills. During the playing season, you will generally need to decrease your basal insulin doses compared with what you do in the off-season.

## Athlete Examples

These examples show that insulin and food adjustments may be necessary, both for playing field hockey and lacrosse and for maintaining blood glucose levels during the season.

### *Insulin Changes Alone*

Virginia resident Michael Blackwell seldom needs to lower his basal rates during lacrosse games due to his limited individual playing time. If running on the low side during practices, though, he may reduce his basal rate up to 80 percent for an hour starting 30 minutes before practice.

### Combined Regimen Changes

New Yorker Joe Fiorucci lowers his overall basal insulin (Lantus) doses during the lacrosse season and eats during practices and matches to prevent lows. He avoids running on the high side at all beforehand as it negatively impacts his performance.

Victoria Thorn of Melbourne, Australia, finds that field hockey has a large effect on her blood glucose. Although her blood glucose often goes up during strenuous play, it comes down afterward, and she needs to eat immediately after games to prevent lows. If her glucose is on the lower side before games, she may drink some Gatorade during them to compensate. After a game of full-field play, she is much more insulin sensitive and must lower the basal rate on her pump to compensate.

Virginian Riley McCullen turns off his basal insulin when he starts to go low during lacrosse practices and games. He eats enough to raise his blood glucose above 100 mg/dL (5.6 mmol/L) before playing, and he treats any lows with candy or juice.

## FIGURE SKATING

This activity involves periods of quick jumps, holding positions, and completing routines lasting 2 to 5 minutes, much like gymnastics, and thus has elements of both power and endurance. Blood glucose will likely respond differently to hours-long practice sessions and actual performances and competitions. The first two energy systems supply most of the energy for performances because of their high intensity and short duration, but aerobic energy will fuel the recovery between routines and during the slower parts of practices. Prolonged practices will likely lower your blood glucose levels, but performances and competitions may have little effect on your blood glucose or even raise it (particularly with the mental stress of competition added). Long practices will lower your blood glucose because of your greater use of muscle glycogen over time.

## Athlete Examples

Due to the differences between intensity and duration for skating practice and competitions, insulin and food adjustments will vary widely. The amount of time spent in a colder environment can also have an impact.

### Combined Regimen Changes

Cara Gabriel from Green Bay, Wisconsin, is a synchronized figure skater who competes on a team in Michigan representing Team USA. She trains about 6 days a week on ice for 3 to 5 hours, along with practicing ballet, stretching, resistance training, and more 3 days a week for about an hour. She admits that she is struggling with maintaining a good glucose level with activity because it is an intense team sport, and she gets more highs than lows. Competing is also very stressful, so she ends up with sustained highs afterward that usually result in her blood glucose crashing later. During competitions, she has to check frequently to find out the effects of the adrenaline from mental stress and whether it will keep her blood glucose up. Her coach holds fruit snacks for her just in case of lows. She says that she once competed in an air-pressurized rink with her pump (when she still wore one) and did not know that the air pressure change can cause insulin to be absorbed more quickly, and she kept having extreme lows. She ate 10 rolls of Skittles (about 60 grams of glucose) before stepping on the ice with a blood glucose around 50 mg/dL (2.8 mmol/L) because she did not want to let her team down.

For an example of another skater, one who is a competitive figure skater, see the athlete profile that follows for teenager Arianna Domenech from Switzerland.

## Athlete Profile: **Arianna Domenech**

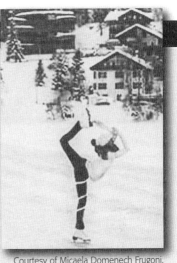
Courtesy of Micaela Domenech Frugoni.

**Hometown:** Bever, Switzerland

**Diabetes history:** Type 1 diabetes diagnosed in 2015 (at age 11)

**Sport or activity:** Figure skating

**Greatest athletic achievement:** Came in second place in a Swiss Cup competition and third place in a small international figure skating competition

**Current insulin and medication regimen:** NPH (twice daily), regular insulin at breakfast, and NovoRapid for corrections and sometimes for dinner (or regular)

**Training tips:** Check blood glucose before and after training or competition. If I'm in range (70 to 120 mg/dL [3.9 to 6.7 mmol/L]), I eat a little snack like berries, dark chocolate, or nuts (more if I'm on the low end of my range). If I'm low, I treat it with fruit juice or candies. If my blood glucose is more than 140 mg/dL (7.8 mmol/L), I take a correction dose of insulin.

During training sessions, I take in water or tea and sometimes fruit juice. There are also two other things that I really have to pay attention to and use tips when I train: (1) time of training and (2) weather conditions. If my training coincides with or is near lunch or takes place immediately after breakfast, I am more prone to going low, so I try to eat a little more carbohydrate, mixed with some protein to keep my blood glucose more stable. As for the outside temperature, I live in the mountains, and my ice skating training is always outside. In the winter, at times I have to skate with the temperature around −10 to −20 degrees Celsius (14 to −4 degrees Fahrenheit), and I have seen that extreme cold causes me some stress. On those days, I may end up with my blood glucose a little high. I know that I don't need to eat anything before skating then. But in the spring and summer with the sun out and it being much warmer, I have the opposite problem and have to eat a little more.

continued➡

Normally, when I skate for 1 to 2 hours, there isn't a big impact on my blood glucose values, but when practice is 3 to 4 hours, I am prone to getting low hours later after dinner or overnight. I usually have to take less insulin in the evening on those days, but it is not always predictable.

***Typical daily and weekly training and diabetes regimen:*** Regular and NPH in the morning, regular or NovoRapid for dinner, NPH at bedtime, and NovoRapid for corrections.

- ▶ ***Monday:*** 1 hour of fitness dancing.
- ▶ ***Tuesday:*** 1 hour of figure skating and another hour of conditioning training.
- ▶ ***Wednesday:*** 3 hours of skating practice.
- ▶ ***Thursday:*** 2 hours of skating practice.
- ▶ ***Friday:*** 1 hour of skating practice and 1 hour of stretching.
- ▶ ***Saturday:*** 1 hour of skating jump practice.
- ▶ ***Sunday:*** 1 hour of skating.

When I have school vacations, I normally have 3 to 4 hours of training Monday through Friday and 1 hour of jump training on Saturday.

***Other hobbies and interests:*** Riding on my horse, skiing, walking with my dog, listening to music, watching films, and spending time with friends.

***Good diabetes and exercise story:*** In an ice skating show on Easter this past year, I knew that my diabetes management during the day was going to be really difficult. I was scheduled to participate in the season-ending show taking place around 3:00 p.m., where I was going to skate dance my choreographed routine lasting around 3 minutes and do a later final dance with the rest of my dance team. Now that I am an adolescent, I am more prone to running high (180 to 216 mg/dL [10 to 12 mmol/L]) when I have to do skating competitions or shows. It may be due to my stress hormones from concentrating so hard on doing well or the short duration of my intense routine, but I know I need enough insulin and not to eat much beforehand if I want to be in a good blood glucose range (80 to 100 mg/dL [4.5 to 5.6 mmol/L]).

So I had no choice but to take my full morning dose of NPH and regular to prevent later highs, but I followed that with 2 hours of training in the morning before lunch and another hour right before the 3:00 show. It was stressful because I wanted to eat lunch and not go too high, and I knew I wouldn't have much time to correct my blood glucose if it did rise because I had to do my hair and makeup after lunch and before my second practice session. I'm proud that I was able to pull it off and with great control. About 20 minutes before the show started, my blood glucose was at 76 mg/dL (4.2 mmol/L). I knew my NPH was still working but from experience I also knew that taking in 10 grams of carbohydrates would be too much, so I just ate a few strawberries (around 4 grams of carbohydrates), and after the show I was at a perfect 120 mg/dL (6.7 mmol/L), even with the adrenaline rush!

(It needs mentioning again that this young figure skater accomplished this diabetes management feat at only 13 years of age!)

## FLAG FOOTBALL

Just as rugby is similar to American football without all the protective pads and helmets and slightly different rules, flag football is another version of football. In this case, the basic rules stay the same, but the play is different. American football is "tackle football." In the flag version, the defensive team must remove a flag or flag belt from the ball carrier instead of tackling him or her to end the play, and absolutely no contact is supposed to occur between players. No tackling means that there is more running and fewer power moves involved, but plays can still be relatively short.

Again, many factors may impact your blood glucose response to flag football. Most people play games instead of doing practices. The position that you play can still influence your response, particularly if you are in a position that requires more running overall. You are likely to use up quite a bit of muscle glycogen if you play most or all of the game, and you may need to adjust your insulin down and your food intake up to compensate after games. The time of day you are playing can also influence the adjustments you need to make.

## Athlete Example

Fatima Shahzad of Cambridge, Massachusetts, plays flag football once or twice a week. Most of her games are scheduled late in the day. When she plays in the evening, she tries to eat a low-carbohydrate meal if it is closer to game time to manage her glucose by the time the game starts. If the games are earlier, she has to balance eating low carbohydrate later to be able to keep her glucose stable overnight. She often does not know how to eat (how many carbohydrates) after games because it is hard to predict the impact of her exercise on her glucose. Football is interesting in that she may run 20 percent of the time one game and 90 percent in another, which adds to the unpredictability of her responses. She tries to keep her blood glucose between 90 and 140 mg/dL (5.0 and 7.8 mmol/L) during games. She finds that sports like this one that require high-intensity bursts and sprints often give her glucose highs. She corrects with insulin dosing and monitors her CGM as much as possible while playing.

## FRISBEE (ULTIMATE)

This activity involves periods of sprinting, running, and standing and is considered an endurance–power sport, much like other team sports played on a field (e.g., soccer, field hockey, and lacrosse). Recreational games of Frisbee may not require many changes in your diabetes regimen. but competitive games are more likely to make you alter your diet or your insulin regimen. The more you run and the longer you run, the less insulin and the more food your body may need to prevent hypoglycemia. After particularly long or intense play, you may need an extra snack at bedtime and less basal insulin overnight.

# Athlete Examples

How intensely you play Frisbee will affect your required regimen changes. Just throwing a Frisbee around may not require many adjustments, compared with playing a game of ultimate Frisbee.

## Diet Changes Alone

For playing 2 to 3 hours of ultimate Frisbee, Canadian Nina Horvath tries to eat 1.5 to 2 hours in advance. During playing, she checks her blood glucose and may eat small snacks between games (after 1.5 hours of play) and afterward. She uses Lantus as her basal insulin, but does not usually adjust it for playing.

## Combined Regimen Changes

Virginia resident Margaret S. Urfer decreases the basal rate on her pump before playing ultimate Frisbee for 2.5 hours. She tries to eat lower-GI carbohydrates beforehand and keeps snacks on hand such as granola bars, protein bars, and chocolate.

## GOLF

This activity requires short bursts of energy for hitting, driving, and putting, which are anaerobic in nature and mainly use the first energy (phosphagen) system. Walking the golf course is aerobic in nature, and carrying your own golf clubs increases the work that you are doing. Of course, driving a golf cart does not require much work at all. The amount of walking you do has the greatest effect on your blood glucose, and walking the entire course requires you to make greater regimen changes, especially if you play 18 holes instead of just 9. Playing in hot and humid conditions lowers your blood glucose more because your body must use more glucose to cool itself.

# Athlete Examples

The amount of walking you do, the air temperature and humidity, and the duration of your play affect what adjustments you will need to make. It also depends on your regimen and your diet.

## No Changes Necessary

Pumper Aline Verbeke from Belgium does not need to adjust anything during golfing for about 4 hours. Fellow pumper Ginny Barndollar of Pennsylvania also does not need to make changes, but she rides in a golf cart rather than walking the course while she is playing. Others do have to make multiple adjustments.

## Insulin Changes Alone

When Spencer Band of Stittsville, Ontario, Canada plays golf, he either suspends his pump or lowers his basal rate during 9 or 18 holes. Which one he does depends on what his starting blood glucose is and when and how much insulin he took in his last bolus.

## Combined Regimen Changes

If he is planning on golfing 18 holes, Matt from Pennsylvania makes sure he has not had any bolus insulin within 2 hours of when he starts. If he is golfing less than 2 hours after bolusing, he eats or drinks more (often Gatorade) before and during golfing to compensate. He does not adjust his bedtime dose of Lantus, though.

Aaron Kowalski of Somerville, New Jersey, finds that he needs to reduce his basal rate and eat almost as many carbohydrates for golf (30 grams per hour) as he does for running. For him, having a CGM is mission critical when exercising; having the ability to monitor trends can make all the difference as far as staying in his target range and minimizing glucose highs and lows.

For golfing, Rose Pisano of Chicago, Illinois, lowers her basal rate on her insulin pump by 50 to 75 percent for 2 hours before starting and during the activity. In addition, she eats 15 grams of carbohydrates when she starts playing if her blood glucose level is 120 mg/dL (6.7 mmol/L) or lower.

Michigan resident Christopher Pentescu plays golf four or five times a week, during which he tests his blood glucose every three holes when walking the course. He eats small, frequent snacks with carbohydrates and protein during the activity and decreases his overnight basal rate after play.

When golfing for 4 hours, Adelaide Lindahl of Minnesota usually reduces her basal rate to 0.5 units for the first 3 hours of play but then returns it to normal during the last hour or so. During long rounds of golf, she often has a 20-gram carbohydrate snack (like a granola bar) and takes little or no bolus for it.

Julie Heverly of Richmond, Virginia, reduces her basal rate by 50 percent before golfing. She also eats before playing without making any insulin adjustments.

## Other Effects to Consider

**Effect of Environment.** Rose Pisano walks when golfing, usually carrying her clubs but sometimes pulling a cart. If the course is hilly, her glucose goes lower than when it is flat; if it is hot and humid, her glucose usually comes down faster than normal as well.

## GYMNASTICS

Doing gymnastics requires mainly short, powerful movements both during practices and competitions to complete routines of 2 minutes or shorter on various pieces of equipment. The first two energy systems supply most of the energy because of the intensity and duration of the activity. Prolonged practices can result in drops in your blood glucose, but gymnastics routines themselves may require minimal changes in your diabetes regimen because of their intense nature. Doing several short routines during a meet may have little effect on your blood glucose or even raise it, but 2 or 3 hours of practice will likely have more of a glucose-lowering effect as you use more muscle glycogen over time.

## Athlete Examples

The required changes vary with the length and intensity of the gymnastics or other related activity, as well as whether you are involved in a practice or a competition.

### Diet Changes Alone

For gymnastics classes lasting 1.5 hours, Maryland resident Juliana Kotsifakis tries to eat enough before class to raise her blood glucose to 150 to 200 mg/dL (8.3 to 11.1 mmol/L). If all goes well, her blood glucose level is around 70 mg/dL (3.9 mmol/L) when she finishes the class.

### Combined Regimen Changes

During gymnastics classes that last 90 minutes, Kelsey McGill of Delaware takes her pump off but checks her blood glucose every 30 minutes to make adjustments in food or to reconnect to bolus. She eats a light snack beforehand to help keep her blood glucose stable.

Maggie Hudson of Virginia frequently disconnects from her pump during gymnastics practices and meets. If she keeps it off for several hours, her blood glucose starts to rise. To counter this, she takes small injections with an insulin pen while her pump stays off. She also snacks before starting practices.

Meredith Bussett from Oklahoma does 3 hours of gymnastics most days of the week, during which she disconnects from her pump. She checks frequently during the activity and reconnects to give boluses as necessary, and she eats 15 grams of carbohydrates before practice.

Wisconsin resident Shannon Triller participates in 9 hours of gymnastics training a week year-round. Before practices, she makes sure to eat well but decreases her boluses to take much less insulin to cover her food. In addition, after practices she does not correct her elevated glucose because it comes down naturally over time.

Delaine Wright of Rhode Island participates in training for trapeze and aerial fabric work. For this activity, she takes her pump off during workouts because it hinders her performance. After checking her glucose every 30 minutes, she reconnects to her pump to bolus as needed. Unlike when she does treadmill running, she needs more insulin during trapeze and aerial fabric work due to the greater anaerobic and strength components they require. She also does quite a bit of trampolining, which she finds drops her glucose quite rapidly and requires a lower basal rate if she jumps with her pump on.

### Other Effects to Consider

**Effect of Competition.** Even without eating anything, Shannon Triller often experiences large increases in her blood glucose during gymnastics competitions because of the mental stress of competing, along with the intense, short routines that she does. She tends to run low in the morning on the day after meets, though.

## HIGH-INTENSITY INTERVAL TRAINING (HIIT)

Doing workouts or training that includes high-intensity intervals is not a new concept—competitive athletes have long been integrating interval workouts into their weekly training to compete at the top of their sports. What is new about it is the amount of research that has been done on it recently in more average exercisers (even in people with diabetes), showing it to be safe for most individuals and superior for implementing fitness gains and promoting fat weight loss. Interval training can be done in a number of ways, with variations in the length of training intervals (from seconds to minutes), intensity, and total duration of training. Adding faster intervals into any type of training you are doing can improve your fitness faster.

Due to their ability to cause a greater release of glucose-raising hormones, most HIIT workouts are likely to either raise your blood glucose temporarily or make it more stable during the activity, but be on the lookout for later-onset hypoglycemia due to a greater use of muscle glycogen from both the aerobic and anaerobic components of such workouts.

## Athlete Examples

The intensity of this activity is likely to either raise your blood glucose or make it easier to maintain during workouts. Watch out for lows later on, though, as the muscle glycogen use during harder intervals can be quite dramatic, resulting in heightened insulin sensitivity later on and overnight after HIIT training.

### *No Changes Necessary*

Like many athletes, Rachel Rylands from Liverpool in the United Kingdom finds that HIIT always raises her blood glucose, at least temporarily. On the flip side, although HIIT prompts a jump in her blood glucose during exercise, Chris Creelman from New Jersey finds her glucose comes down once she finishes the workout, and she tends to get low for about 12 to 16 hours after doing HIIT. Scotland native Becs Badger also experiences a rise in blood glucose from doing HIIT or very intensive (maximal) running sessions that she does not treat because she knows it will come down on its own in due course. Even Charles R. Clark from Rule, Texas, who uses Levemir insulin only to manage his type 2 diabetes, finds that his blood glucose comes down on its own 1 to 2 hours after he finishes this type of training.

### *Insulin Changes Alone*

Hailing from Canada, Elizabeth Drabble usually needs to take a half-unit bolus of insulin immediately before she starts exercising in the morning. She does 5 minutes on the elliptical to warm up, followed by strength training, and then 15 to 20 minutes more on the elliptical doing HIIT, followed by 5 minutes of an easier cooldown and stretching.

A resident of Santa Monica, California, Christel Oerum has a similar need for a corrective dose of insulin. When she does HIIT later in the day, she gives herself a half-unit bolus to prevent a rise in her blood glucose as well.

Similarly, Jenna Blaza from the United Kingdom finds that she needs a bolus correction of a few units of insulin 30 minutes before she starts 45 minutes of vigorous HIIT exercise. Without it, this activity causes her blood glucose to rise. She covers her basal insulin needs with Levemir, taken twice daily, but she does not adjust this basal insulin for HIIT.

Cindy Ski from Canada is on a low-carbohydrate diet regimen and uses Lantus as her basal insulin. To prevent a spike in her blood glucose when doing HIIT, she has to bolus with 2 units before working out.

Philippines resident Sally Clark finds that all high-intensity workouts, including HIIT, have a glucose-raising effect on her. She exercises in the mornings and has to take a bolus of 1 to 2 units of Humalog before working out. She sometimes but only rarely corrects her exercise-induced high glucose. Her glucose tends to come down pretty quickly on its own when her exercising is over.

Canadian Nina Horvath always takes HIIT classes in the morning. To manage those, she does not eat anything before, but she takes 2 units of NovoRapid to counter the glucose spike it causes afterward, followed immediately by a post-workout breakfast. She takes one nightly dose of Lantus insulin, which she does not adjust for this type of training.

### Combined Regimen Changes

For Tammy Miller of Churchville, Virginia, her main exercise classes are HIIT, which includes many different activities and workouts of the day. To manage these, she mainly keeps an eye on her CGM glucose numbers; if her range is trending upward, she only treats it with glucose tablets, as needed. Also, if her glucose is trending low at any time, she disconnects her pump for the duration of the workout.

## HORSEBACK RIDING, COMPETITIVE

This activity is usually of high intensity and short duration, especially during competitions. You contract your postural muscles to keep yourself atop the horse while it is moving through the competitive course. The faster the horse is moving, the more energy you will have to use to stay on. The physical stress of this event, combined with the mental stress of competition, may cause your blood glucose to rise. While practicing for such events, you will repeat these movements many times, resulting in a glucose-lowering effect for which you may need to increase your food intake slightly or lower your insulin doses. For recommendations for recreational horseback riding, see chapter 12.

## Athlete Examples

For competitive riding and shows, you may need to make adjustments to compensate, depending on the length and intensity of the activity. The changes needed for riding practice may vary from competition-day adjustments.

### Insulin Changes Alone

While riding dressage, Delaine Wright of Rhode Island usually experiences a slight rise (50 mg/dL [2.8 mmol/L]) in her blood glucose levels, which she tries to prevent with a slightly higher basal rate. She always feels better not having food in her stomach during short-duration exercise, so she avoids eating beforehand.

### Combined Regimen Changes

To ride her pony competitively during shows, Juliana Kotsifakis of Maryland eats snacks to increase her blood glucose to 130 to 150 mg/dL (7.2 to 8.3 mmol/L), and she then takes less insulin during the day if she is active and outdoors all day. For

90-minute lessons or riding on her own, she tries to start out a bit higher, between 150 and 200 mg/dL (8.3 and 11.1 mmol/L).

For competitive horseback riding (jumping), Maggie Drysch of Coto de Caza, California, usually takes more insulin in the morning when she is competing and mentally stressed, but after she has been riding for a while, her blood glucose starts to come down. If she drops below 100 mg/dL (5.6 mmol/L), she eats a snack. If she takes her pump off, she gives a small bolus before disconnecting to cover the basal insulin she will miss, or else her glucose will rise after a couple of hours. Overall, she needs less insulin for practices than for competitions.

## ICE HOCKEY

Ice hockey involves short, power moves like shooting the puck and skating quickly to another position. The activity can be intense, however, resulting in significant use of muscle glycogen and blood glucose when you play for an extended time. Depending on how long and how hard you play, you may need to make some regimen changes. Practices may require more changes because of their prolonged, less intense nature compared with games. A confounding variable is that ice hockey competitions and practices often occur at unusual times (e.g., early morning practices, late-evening games). Early morning practices when your insulin levels are low may require you to make fewer adjustments. At other times of day (especially during evening games) or when you play for longer periods, you may need to increase your food intake and take less insulin for meals before exercise.

## Athlete Examples

These real-life scenarios show that ice hockey participation usually requires at least insulin changes, but sometimes a combination of diabetes-related adjustments to compensate.

### *Insulin Changes Alone*

Canadian Sarah McGaugh does not change her insulin regimen during hockey. However, she typically has to give a bolus of insulin afterward to correct high blood glucose (due to the high intensity and intermittent nature of the sport).

When playing a power sport like ice hockey, Beaver, Pennsylvania, resident Emily Tiberio usually has to take between 1 and 3 units of bolus insulin about 30 minutes before games to combat the adrenaline rush as much as possible. She also increases her basal rate about 2 hours beforehand to at least 150 if not 200 percent of her normal rate.

### *Combined Regimen Changes*

Teenager Spencer Band of Canada takes off his insulin pump when he plays hockey because of the physical contact that playing entails. He usually removes it 30 to 45 minutes before his hour-long games start. On the bench, he has Gatorade during the games. He tends to experience a delayed effect from the activity, and his glucose often drops overnight.

To play travel team ice hockey, Michael Blackwell of Virginia has to adjust for the games by setting a temporary basal rate on his pump that is 20 percent of his normal, starting 30 minutes before his games or practices and continuing for an hour. He tries to avoid eating really high-carbohydrate snacks afterward (such as french fries) because his glucose tends to be higher right afterward. Because of his tendency to drop about 4 hours later, he does not give any insulin for his post-hockey elevations. He also plays roller hockey, an activity that makes regulating his glucose a bit harder because there is no ice to cool him off.

Aaron Kowalski of New Jersey takes off his pump when playing ice hockey, but he does not usually need to make many modifications to his insulin delivery and carbohydrate intake. He has Gatorade around in case his CGM glucose levels trend downward too much and he needs to bring them back up.

For hockey games played once a week in an adult league, Brian Witschen of Alberta, Canada, lowers his bolus insulin by 20 percent of his dinner dose. He also drinks a juice box halfway through to prevent lows.

## INDOOR RACKET SPORTS (BADMINTON, HANDBALL, RACQUETBALL, SQUASH, AND TABLE TENNIS)

Racket sports involve quick, powerful moves, such as hitting or throwing the ball and moving into position, that are mostly anaerobic in nature. How hard and how long you play, along with your skill level, largely determine what changes you need to make for these activities. Playing longer will have more of a glucose-reducing effect, even if you are playing intensely, simply because you are doing more total activity. In addition, better players are more skilled at ball placement and may not have to run and move as much as their less-skilled opponents. Well-placed, point-winning serves may also result in more waiting time and less active playing time.

## Athlete Examples

These examples show that court sports are intense enough to require some regimen changes to prevent hypoglycemia. Prolonged play has more of an aerobic effect as well.

### Diet Changes Alone

Javad Ramezani from Iran does not change his insulin or diet for most exercise, including indoor racket sports. He keeps his blood glucose from dropping by exercising at least 3 to 4 hours after his last meal. During exercise or right after, if he feels that his blood glucose is a little low, he eats a chocolate.

### Combined Regimen Changes

Janet G. from Scotland finds that both badminton and table tennis bring her blood glucose down quickly. She has to reduce her pump basal rate by 75 percent and have snacks handy for topping off as necessary.

When Susan Greenback of Australia plays squash for an hour, she takes her insulin pump off 30 minutes before she begins and keeps it off until she is done playing. If she eats within 2 hours of playing, she does not bolus for less than 20 grams of carbohydrates; otherwise, she reduces her premeal bolus as well.

United Kingdom resident Chris Bartlett plays badminton at a high club level for 1 to 2 hours at a time, once or twice a week. He removes his pump (for comfort), but checks his blood glucose levels throughout so he can easily adjust. He plays in the evening and tries to eat a light or medium-sized meal at least 2 hours before in hopes that his glucose levels off before exercising. Due to the anaerobic nature of this activity, his glucose normally does not drop, but he may need to reduce his basal rate by 10 to 20 percent overnight to avoid lows then.

## PICKLEBALL

The oddly named sport of pickleball is played on a (half-size) tennis court with a solid, oversized table tennis paddle and a plastic ball that is similar to a whiffle ball. Its movements are analogous to playing table tennis but are done while technically standing on the "table." It does not require overhand serving like tennis does, so it is growing in popularity among American seniors in particular. Given that movements and steps are limited, this activity may not have much of an impact on your blood glucose levels. No pickleball players answered the survey for this book, but for similar athlete examples, refer to the section on indoor racquet sports or tennis.

## RACE CAR DRIVING, ON- AND OFF-ROAD

A variety of types of race cars and venues are involved with automobile sports. The most well-known in the United States are the IndyCar and National Association for Stock Car Auto Racing (NASCAR) series, along with the Lucas Oil Off-Road Racing short course series. Events like the Indy 500 involve 2.5 to 3.0 hours of intense driving in specially modified race cars around a 2.5-mile (4-kilometer) track 200 times, covering 500 miles (almost 805 kilometers), usually at average speeds of more than 200 miles (322 kilometers) per hour. Not only do these events require muscle endurance and strength, but driving safely at high speeds on variable tracks while striving for a competitive position generates mental stress; all this leads to possible elevations in blood glucose followed by a later (postevent) glucose drop. Training for these events may be less stressful, but may involve other types of physical workouts such as resistance training.

Because driving race cars is an intense sport, both physically and mentally, it can raise blood glucose. Most races last hours, and your blood glucose potentially may drop over that span of time. When even a minor alteration in your judgment or reflexes could result in accidents or injuries, possibly even death, for yourself or others, effective blood glucose management is truly essential to racing survival.

## Athlete Examples

For an example of how to compete at such a level, see the athlete profile of IndyCar race car driver Charlie Kimball, found in chapter 3. Ryan Reed, another driver with type 1 diabetes, competes in NASCAR races. Trevor Briska of Perris, California, is a top-ranked driver competing in the Lucas Oil Off-Road Racing series in the Pro Buggy class (named Rookie of the Year in 2017). Track conditions, performance issues, breakage, reaction time, and mental agility all play a role in his success competing on dirt tracks at high speeds and with occasional 125-foot drops. To race, he keeps his basal and bolus insulin doses unchanged, but he supplements with Pedialyte (with electrolytes and some glucose) every time he gets on the track—whether for practices, qualifying runs, or a main event. Race day adrenaline can spike his levels, but heat and extreme driving can lead to lows. He aims to keep his blood glucose around 150 mg/dL (8.3 mmol/L) by checking it regularly to avoid lows at all costs.

## ROLLER DERBY

An American-invented contact sport, roller derby takes place on a circular track onto which two teams send five players at a time: three blockers, one pivot, and one jammer (the only scorer). The contest involves three 20-minute periods that include 2 minutes of intense activity at a time (called jams), during which the teams attempt to score points. Players at certain positions (i.e., jammers) will generally work harder (and use up more glycogen) because they alone can attempt to pass the pack during the jams and lap around the track as many times as possible. The other players on each team bunch together in a pack and skate at a slower speed. Because of the mix of anaerobic and aerobic work involved, this sport requires changes in food intake and insulin doses to prevent lows. The intensity of this sport can vary greatly during games and competitions, making regimen changes harder to predict. The stress of competing can also impact your blood glucose.

## Athlete Example

To participate in roller derby practices and competitions, Abigail Tinker of Somerville, Massachusetts, eats about 30 grams of carbohydrates without bolusing. She may also reduce her basal rate on her pump by 50 percent starting an hour before exercise and throughout the activity. She finds that in this sport the intensity of activity is not constant, so the effect on her blood glucose is hard to predict. Her biggest challenge is dealing with spikes in her blood glucose from the stress of competing. To compensate for all these variables, she checks her blood glucose levels often and consumes glucose if it has dropped below 120 mg/dL (6.7 mmol/L).

## ROWING (CREW)

Also called "crew," outdoor rowing involves rhythmic, intense, full-body workouts over the length of a course or race on the water. Teams generally have one, two, four, or eight rowers per boat, and races usually consist of 5 to 8 minutes of all-out rowing for a standard-length event, which is 2,000 meters for the Olympics and 1,500 meters for U.S. high school races. But race distances can vary from 500-meter sprints to marathon or ultramarathon lengths.

Regimen changes depend on the intensity and duration of your practices and events. Longer, less-intense crew practices may require greater regimen changes to maintain blood glucose levels. Wind conditions can increase the intensity of rowing because stronger winds will increase resistance. In addition, crew regattas (races on open water) may be more intense and have a larger anaerobic component, which can make your blood glucose more stable or even elevated.

## Athlete Examples

These examples show that the intensity and duration of rowing activities have the biggest effect in determining what regimen changes you will need to make.

### Combined Regimen Changes

For collegiate crew team member Sam Kukler from Atlanta, Georgia, rowing lowers his blood glucose significantly. He always goes into his 2.5-hour-long practices with his blood glucose at least at 120 mg/dL (6.3 mmol/L) with no insulin on board. He finds that even the most intense practices usually cause his blood glucose to drop at some point due to their long duration. He monitors himself with his CGM only about half the time because he finds it does not hold up well during exercise. But he finds it invaluable when it actually stays on his body for longer than 3 days. He has an intense practice and competition schedule: 2.5 hours of training 5 afternoons a week, along with 3 hours on Saturday mornings. For practices, he tries to stop eating long enough in advance to leave minimal extra insulin in his body, and he carries glucose tablets with him in the boat. He felt it was harder for him to manage his diabetes in a previous competition year when he was rowing as a lightweight (under 150 pounds [68.2 kilograms]). Cutting up to 20 pounds before racing to make his weight class forced him to do fasts of 3 days or longer. During those periods, he had to cut his Lantus basal insulin dose by half, and there were times when he did not take Humalog doses for an entire week. Because he does not have to cut weight anymore, he treats his race days about the same as his normal practices; the main difference has been that he takes in about 400 milligrams of caffeine before races, which sometimes leads to an intense low about an hour after he has finished his crew race.

A resident of Cape Town, South Africa, Estelle Grey finds that rowing is the only endurance exercise in which stopping to check her blood glucose is not ideal. She sets a goal of rowing 5 kilometers (3.1 miles), and she covers that distance before letting herself stop to check. However, she has found that she has never gone low while rowing. She used to wear a pump, but now she uses Levemir twice daily to cover her basal insulin needs. On a lower-carbohydrate diet, she tries to not eat more than 60 grams daily, but she seldom needs to cover her exercise with any carbohydrates or food. If she does, though, she eats dark chocolate or drinks some Powerade or a nonfizzy energy drink; she has a gel if her glucose drops as low as

63 mg/dL (3.5 mmol/L). As she is more likely to get low 3 hours after training, she usually eats a snack after working out.

Canadian Olympic rower Chris Jarvis watches his glucose trends and pays attention to how much insulin he has on board, his carbohydrate intake, how hard his workouts are, and the stress of competition, all of which can affect his blood glucose. He may practice more than once a day, but for morning practices he reduces his bolus for anything he eats beforehand as well as his basal rate. During warm-ups, he may lower his basal further and eat gels to prevent lows. When he has 30 minutes of practice to go, he raises his basal rate back to normal. After practice, he usually boluses with 1 to 3 units, waits for the bolus to start working, and then eats breakfast.

## SOCCER (NON-AMERICAN FOOTBALL)

Depending on the position you play, soccer is a combination of stop-and-start movements, power moves such as kicking or throwing the ball, and long runs. Midfielders and strikers may do sustained running, whereas fullbacks and goalkeepers may do only short bursts of intermittent activity. During practices, almost all team members may do continuous running or shooting drills.

You will likely need changes in both insulin and food intake for most soccer play, but the adjustments will vary with your position and the duration of your play. You may need extra carbohydrates or food, depending on your insulin levels, your intensity, and the duration of play. Longer practices or more playing time during games will cause greater use of your muscle glycogen stores and blood glucose, thus requiring more food and less insulin before and possibly after playing. During the soccer season, you will probably need to reduce your basal insulin doses as well, especially if you are less active during the off-season.

## Athlete Examples

These examples show that combined insulin and diet changes are often, but not always, necessary to compensate for soccer play.

### Diet Changes Alone

Robin Leysen of Belgium tries to have his blood glucose in the range of 100 to 160 mg/dL (5.6 to 8.9 mmol/L) when he starts playing soccer because he knows his glucose can drop quickly at certain moments. To keep it at that level, he mostly eats slow carbohydrates or drinks a sugary beverage. He used to use a sugar shake in his water bottle, but he stopped this strategy because his blood glucose would often be high at the end of a game and stay elevated for a couple of hours.

### Combined Regimen Changes

While playing soccer for 1 to 1.5 hours once weekly, Chris Bartlett of the United Kingdom removes his pump so as not to risk damaging the pump, himself, or others. He says it is less about what level his glucose is and more about whether it is falling or heading toward a low. He is usually happy to keep his blood glucose around

90 mg/dL (5.0 mmol/L) during soccer because he knows this sport usually only causes his level to fluctuate, not to drop. If he knows it is falling, though, he will take some glucose tablets at 108 to 126 mg/dL (6.0 to 7.0 mmol/L). An active adult with young kids, he often finds himself paying less attention to his diabetes than he should. Accordingly, he has learned that doing sports when his glucose is very high is difficult. In the past, when it has been inconvenient to stop during a game of soccer to check his level, he has found his glucose has often gone higher than 252 mg/dL (14 mmol/L). In a couple of matches, he felt incredibly tired and slow and checked to find his blood glucose was nearly 360 mg/dL (20 mmol/L). He has overcome these issues by working hard to manage his glucose before playing, which he has accomplished with more frequent glucose checks and investing in a CGM.

Ontario, Canada, resident Sarah McGaugh reduces her basal insulin by 50 percent before starting a soccer game. She finds that her glucose usually stays stable for the entire game, and sometimes she has to take in some glucose at half-time to prevent lows late in the game.

Ireland resident Stephen Bailie has the same approach to most activities, including playing soccer. He takes only half of his usual meal bolus for the meal before training or games. If he is getting low (below 72 mg/dL [4.0 mmol/L]), he eats some glucose or jelly babies to raise his blood glucose. He uses Levemir as his basal insulin (twice daily), and he does not change this regimen for activities.

To play high school soccer, Ethan Wehrly of Dayton, Ohio, usually needs to drink Gatorade during practices and games, and he eats a high-protein snack beforehand. Although he is often on the high side afterward, his sugars drop later, requiring him to cut back on his Lantus dose at bedtime and give himself a smaller amount of NovoLog for his bedtime snack on days when he plays games or has long practices.

To play competitive, year-round soccer on a travel team, Jake Sheldon of Maryland reduces his meal bolus by 20 to 25 percent and then takes off his pump during the activity when he has practices right after dinner. If he has a game scheduled midmorning or midafternoon, he eats a snack with protein and carbohydrates 30 minutes before starting and removes his pump during the game. After this activity, he only uses half-corrections for highs because he is likely to drop later. He then prevents lows by cutting back his basal rates by 50 percent for up to 8 hours after a practice or game.

For United Kingdom resident Joel Quinn, playing football (soccer in the United States) requires him to set a temporary basal rate that is 80 percent lower than normal starting 40 to 60 minutes before the activity. In addition, he eats a cereal bar with 15 grams of carbohydrates or a banana beforehand, and he may consume up to a bottle of Lucozade (sports energy drink) while playing.

A resident of New Jersey, Michael Luzzi tries to have his blood glucose around 150 mg/dL (8.3 mmol/L) before soccer games. After games, he takes only half of his usual bolus but does not adjust his bedtime Lantus. He eats his usual meal before practices, and before games he consumes about 15 grams of carbohydrates.

Jenny Vandevelde of San Diego, California, plays indoor, beach, and regular soccer in several adult leagues. She takes her insulin pump off during all soccer play. Because beach soccer is extremely strenuous, she eats 30 to 40 grams of carbohydrates before she plays.

For playing soccer, youngster Andrew Steckel from Pennsylvania cuts back on his premeal bolus by half a unit and eats a snack after the game if he plays soon after a meal. For practices or games at other times, he drinks a juice box halfway through. He does not adjust his bedtime Lantus dose, though.

### Other Effects to Consider

**Effect of Position.**   Kirsteen Mitchell of Virginia finds that not wearing her pump works well when she plays forward, a position that requires a lot of running. When she ends up playing a defensive position, she has a much harder time keeping her blood sugars under control without any basal insulin.

**Effect of Competition.**   For Florida resident Mike Joyce, playing soccer leads to unpredictable blood glucose levels due to his emotions and nerves on game days. Having glucose and access to the inhaled insulin Afrezza helps him quickly correct his glucose in either direction. He tries to keep his blood glucose in a tight range (90 to 130 mg/dL [5.0 to 7.2 mmol/L]) to keep his performance up. Having a CGM makes him unafraid to exercise because he can see the direction of his glucose trends.

## SPEED SKATING

An Olympic sport since 1924, speed skating is a competitive form of ice skating. Competitors race on skates around an ice track (standard lap length of 400 meters) in events of varying distances, including short track, long track, and marathon skating. Short-track speed skating takes place on a smaller rink, normally the size of an ice hockey rink. The distances are shorter than in long-track racing, and the longest Olympic individual race is 1,500 meters. All events are short enough to rely heavily on the first two energy systems, with only some of the longer track and marathon skating events moving more heavily into being fueled by aerobic energy sources. So the duration of your races will impact your blood glucose responses, as will the skating speed (intensity) and effects of competition stress. Practices may be less intense and more prolonged and have more of a glucose-lowering effect. The most similar sport to check for athlete examples is track events from 400 to 1,600 meters in length (found later in this chapter).

## TENNIS

Playing tennis involves short, powerful moves such as serving, returning serves, moving into position, and hitting the ball, but extended periods of waiting occur between actions. Because of its stop-and-start nature, tennis is a mix of anaerobic and aerobic activity. The intensity also depends on whether you are playing singles or doubles: playing alone on your side of the court will usually force you to run farther and more overall, compared with playing with a partner. Both how long and how hard you play will affect your blood glucose responses and the adjustments that you will need to make, and substantial differences are likely to be present between playing competitive and recreational tennis. Longer tennis games or practices will generally have more of a glucose-reducing effect than shorter ones. The skill level of the players can affect exercise intensity because being more skilled may mean that you end up running less often as well. High-level serving can additionally result in more waiting and less active playing time.

## Athlete Examples

The following examples show that you can make many regimen changes for tennis, depending on the length and type of tennis play.

### No Changes Needed

Texas resident Tom Seabourne has no issues with his control when playing tennis. He has found that playing tennis may increase his blood glucose for a short time, but it will come back to normal on its own. He only uses Lantus insulin, and he follows a very-low-carbohydrate

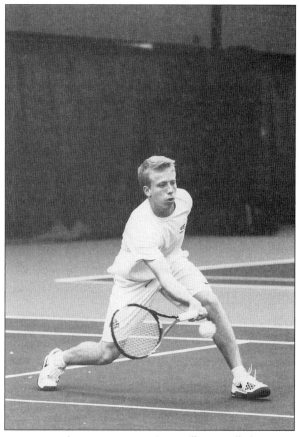

Longer tennis games or practices will generally have more of a glucose-reducing effect than shorter ones.

diet that he says has made managing his glucose easier for all the activities that he does because his insulin on board is low.

### Diet Changes Alone

For playing tennis, Moraga, California, resident Marialice Kern just makes sure that her glucose is a little higher than normal (above 150 mg/dL [8.3 mmol/L]) before starting. She always has a Quest Bar and glucose tablets handy in case of lows.

### Combined Regimen Changes

Susan Greenback of Australia usually plays tennis for 1 hour for singles or 2 hours for doubles. When playing an hour, she takes her insulin pump off 30 minutes before her exercise; for doubles, which last twice as long, she simply reduces her basal rate to 25 percent of normal 30 minutes beforehand and keeps it there during play. If she eats within 2 hours of playing, she does not bolus for less than 20 grams of carbohydrates, or she reduces it for more.

A resident of Arizona, Carter Gillespie participates in tennis practices and tournaments. His practices are after dinner for 2 hours, so at that meal he reduces his boluses for the carbohydrates he eats. About an hour into practices, he drinks a bottle of Gatorade. Tournaments are generally more intense for him, so he does not have to consume as much. He adjusts only his bolus doses for exercise, not his basal Lantus.

Alan Kent Teffeteller from Tennessee is a wheelchair athlete who adjusts for playing tennis by lowering his basal rate and giving smaller insulin boluses for carbohydrates taken in before he plays. He also eats Extend bars if he needs to during games.

## TRACK EVENTS (400 TO 1,600 METERS)

Most track events are short, lasting from 45 seconds to 5 minutes or so and requiring a near-maximal effort. (Sprinting for fewer than 45 seconds is covered in the next chapter.) These types of events rely primarily on anaerobic energy sources. Longer track events such as 800-meter runs require more energy production from the lactic acid system but are still primarily anaerobic. Runs lasting longer than 2 minutes start to use a greater proportion of aerobic sources of energy, and track practices that involve running longer distances or repeated intervals are more aerobic in nature than the track meets during which athletes run only shorter distances.

The regimen changes you need to make are determined more by the duration of aerobic activities and are less affected by anaerobic events. Your blood glucose will tend to decrease more after track practices or meets when muscle glycogen is being restored than during the activity itself, when you are releasing glucose-raising hormones that keep your blood glucose higher. You may need more regimen changes to maintain your blood glucose both during and after practices when you are running longer to build endurance (compared with meets when you run intensely for a shorter period of time).

### Athlete Examples

Even marathoner Bill King from Philadelphia agrees that track racing and speed-work require more insulin on board due to the explosive, anaerobic nature of these activities. The following examples demonstrate the usual types of regimen changes required for track practices and competitive meets.

#### Combined Regimen Changes

For track running, Janet G. of Scotland has not fully sorted out any general pattern for her glucose, but she finds it depends a lot on the distance—200 meters, 800 meters, or 1,500 meters—that she runs, the number of repetitions, and whether she is training or competing. For all distances and situations, she just checks her blood glucose frequently and adjusts with temporary basal rates and fast-acting glucose as necessary.

Alistair McDonald, hailing from Melbourne, Australia, normally likes to have his blood glucose above 90 mg/dL (5 mmol/L) to begin running. In shorter track races and 400-meter or 1-kilometer repeats, the intensity causes his glucose to rise into the double digits (180 mg/dL [10 mmol/L] and higher). It normally takes a long cool-down to bring it back into a more normal range. He then has a normal meal with insulin to cover it.

Andrew M., from Sydney, Australia, does middle-distance running, which requires power and endurance in competitive racing because it includes events from 800 meters to 5 kilometers in length, including steeplechase. Because most of his training sessions are 75 minutes or less, he does not take any carbohydrates before or during sessions if his glucose is 74 mg/dL (4.1 mmol/L) or above. He finds it is rare that he would start out below 79 mg/dL (4.4 mmol/L) because he manages his glucose in the hours before that with basal rate changes. Generally, due to being fat adapted (eating no more than 20 grams of carbohydrates, even on harder exercise days), he experiences relatively limited variability in his blood glucose. Even high-intensity workouts rarely increase his blood glucose by more than 36 to 54 mg/dL (2.0 to 3.0 mmol/L).

## WATER POLO

Water polo involves a combination of aerobic activity and anaerobic sprints, especially during competitions. Overall, this sport is primarily aerobic because it involves constant motion in the water to stay afloat by using an eggbeater motion with your legs. You will encounter the anaerobic component when you have to do a sprint when the play shifts from one end of the pool to the other or when you throw the ball. Training for water polo involves doing some distance swimming as well as shorter sprints.

The duration and intensity of water polo play usually requires adjustments to both food intake and insulin doses to compensate. For a comparable sport, refer to the section on swimming in chapter 9 and focus on the more intensive swimming recommendations and athlete examples.

## Athlete Example

Given that his water polo practices involve 2 hours of nonstop treading water and some swimming, Jake Adams of Carlsbad, California, disconnects from his pump during the sessions. He checks his blood glucose before practice; if it is over 150 mg/dL (8.3 mmol/L), he boluses with 0.1 unit before disconnecting. After practices, he gives himself another 0.3 unit after reconnecting. If his blood glucose before practice is under 100 mg/dL (5.6 mmol/L), he usually eats a snack with 15 grams of carbohydrates.

## WRESTLING

Wrestling involves short, powerful muscle contractions and is largely anaerobic in nature. A wrestling meet may require few regimen changes to maintain your blood glucose because the matches are brief and intense. On the other hand, wrestling practices may lower your blood glucose levels because of the cumulative effects of repeated bouts of activity.

## Athlete Examples

Wrestling is a short-duration, intense sport that can be effectively compensated for in different ways.

### Diet Changes Alone

High school wrestling was hard for Dan Stone of Middletown, Pennsylvania, due to the adrenaline (and, at that time about 20 years ago, his lack of knowledge), which led him to have high blood glucose before competitions. In college, he overcame stress-related highs by warming up through jumping rope for 45 to 60 minutes before events; he also ate fewer carbohydrates before matches and learned how to focus and manage his competition anxiety.

### Combined Regimen Changes

For wrestling, Donny Swarmer, a resident of Cheswick, Pennsylvania, takes 50 percent of his basal as Lantus and runs his insulin pump at a 50 percent lower temporary basal for 24 hours. He disconnects from his pump for as long as needed shortly before starting wrestling. Right afterward, he boluses to knock down the spikes from adrenaline. If he happens to go low or his glucose is dropping, he has some juice. He also does not eat or bolus any insulin before wrestling, unless he needs a correction—but he reduces his prewrestling bolus by around 50 percent.

In this chapter, you have learned that it is entirely possible for athletes with diabetes to also compete and train effectively in sports and activities that are not just aerobic in nature. Whether you want to row crew, play tennis, shoot some hoops at basketball, be a cheerleader, or do CrossFit training, you can do it. In the chapter that follows, you will find out more about the pure power sports that you can engage in as well, with a few adjustments.

## Athlete Profile: **Courtney Duckworth**

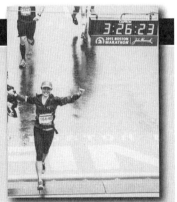

Courtesy of Courtney Duckworth.

**Hometown:** Woodville, Virginia

**Diabetes history:** Type 1 diabetes diagnosed in 2003 (at age 10)

**Sport or activity:** I grew up as a competitive figure skater, started running marathons in college, and have cheered professionally since graduating from college.

**Greatest athletic achievement:** Qualifier and competitor, 2015 and 2018 Boston Marathon, Washington Capitals Red Rockers Cheerleader (2016–2018), Gold Medalist in United States Figure Skating Moves in the Field, Silver Medalist in United States Figure Skating Ice Dancing

**Current insulin and medication regimen:** Medtronic MiniMed insulin pump; basal ranges from 0.55 to 0.65 units per hour; insulin/carbohydrate ratios ranging from 1:13 to 1:15; correction ratio of ~1:70; average daily insulin dose ~25 units.

*Training tips:* Every experience is a tool that helps us learn which strategies work well for particular types of activities. Logging and collecting as much data as possible (through testing blood glucose levels more often or using a CGM) helps us to learn faster.

When forming strategies for exercise, I've found it helpful to do the following:

▶ Tweak one component of care at a time while leaving the others consistent. With marathon training, I will usually eat the same thing, run at the same time in the morning, and change the percentage of recommended insulin dosage.

▶ When making changes, be conservative.

▶ Carry twice the amount of low food you think you may need.

▶ Wear a medical ID–*always*, but especially during exercise. I've found RoadID to work well.

▶ Time your exercise so that it coincides with lower levels of circulating insulin, such as the morning or more than 4 hours after a meal.

More on these tips can be found in my recent book, *The Marathon We Live: Training for a Personal Best in Life With Type 1 Diabetes.*

***Typical daily and weekly training and diabetes regimen:*** While balancing professional cheerleading with training for the 2018 Boston Marathon, my training regimen was the following:

▶ *Monday:* Speed work in the mornings (5 to 6 miles) followed by 30 minutes of strength training and stretching exercises.

▶ *Tuesday:* Long run in the morning (10 to 20 miles) with 15 minutes of stretching, followed by cheer practice (2 to 3 hours) at night. These days were hard.

▶ *Wednesday:* Circuit training.

▶ *Thursday:* Game day or independent cheer practice and easy shakeout run (3 to 4 miles).

▶ *Friday:* Speed work in the mornings (5 to 6 miles) followed by 30 minutes of strength training and stretching exercises.

▶ *Saturday:* Semi-long run in the morning (7 to 9 miles) followed by 15 minutes of stretching.

▶ *Sunday:* Yoga.

My diabetes regimen changes and is varied by the day and activity.

▶ **Runs <7 miles and circuit training:** No changes to basal, supplement with 15 to 20 grams of carbohydrates with no bolus with starting blood glucose in range, no extra carbohydrates if blood glucose is above 180 mg/dL (10.0 mmol/L).

▶ **Runs > 7 miles:** Set 15 percent temporary basal 30 minutes before the run and throughout the run until the last 4 miles (about 30 minutes before meal time); 20 minutes before the run, eat plain bagel (50 carbohydrates) and take 10 to 15 percent of recommended bolus. Every 6 miles, eat GU gel (20 carbohydrates) and take 0.1 to 0.3 units, depending on CGM reading and trend.

▶ **Cheer practice and games:** Disconnect pump during practice (see the cheer story below for a humorous clarification), supplement with 15 to 20 grams of carbohydrates with no bolus if starting

continued ➡

*Courtney Duckworth continued*

blood glucose in range, no extra carbohydrates if blood glucose is above 180 mg/dL (10.0 mmol/L). Monitor with CGM for longer practices, and take small bolus for basal every hour. The bolus will be slightly more or less than the missed basal based on my CGM reading and trend.

▶ **Yoga:** No changes in regimen.

*Other hobbies and interests:* I am attending medical school (starting in fall 2018) with interests in sports medicine, preventive care, and endocrinology. I love writing–I wrote the book I've mentioned, and I also love writing old-fashioned letters to friends. Very few things beat a good podcast or book.

*Good diabetes and exercise story:* I have two good stories, one about marathon running and the other about cheerleading.

**Marathon running:** When I first started training for marathons at 19 years old, I had absolutely no strategy. I learned the hard way that amazing athletic feats with type 1 diabetes are not done through random guesses in care. This is an excerpt from my book that details that story.

When I would finish a long run in range, it was 90 percent luck and 10 percent of what I happened to remember from past runs. I was wasting valuable clues to which combinations of insulin, food, and timing worked best. The pinnacle of my experimentation came about 2 months into training on a Saturday morning around 6:30. Thomas and I usually did long runs together so he could hold my extra glucose. Up to that point, I had never needed to use it and figured I would be just fine going solo. Per usual, I didn't pay too much attention to food or bolus insulin. I ate, reduced my insulin by a random amount that seemed right, and decided to try something new: take my long-acting basal insulin before the run instead of after. Why I tried something new the day I was running alone is beyond me . . . not a smart move (please don't try this at home!).

The run started down Colonial Parkway leading to a spot every student called "Jamestown Beach." It's a really pretty run and not too much traffic. But about 4 miles in, I started feeling lightheaded and tested: 53 mg/dL (2.9 mmol/L). I ate a whole roll of glucose tablets, waited 20 minutes: 45 mg/dL (2.5 mmol/L). I had another roll. I waited another 20 minutes, and I was down to 35 mg/dL (1.9 mmol/L) and officially out of glucose. I needed help, but no cars had passed by all morning, and there was not a soul in sight. I tried calling all my close friends, but of course no one was up that early on a Saturday in college. My last and only resort was 9-1-1.

"9-1-1, what's your emergency?"

Through tears (I was also new at the whole 9-1-1 thing), I said, "Hi, my name is Courtney Duckworth. I am 19 years old, and have type 1 diabetes. My blood glucose is low and dropping, and I ran out of glucose. I'm sitting on the side of the road by Jamestown Beach."

"Do you see a ferry?"

"There are no ferries here."

"Then you are not at Jamestown Beach."

"I took a right down Colonial Parkway and ran 4 miles from the William and Mary campus. Where does that put me?"

"I don't know, but we can't send a dispatch team until we know your exact location."

I started to panic. My emergency help was no help at all or didn't know how to operate GPS (either way, she was in the wrong profession). I wasn't wearing a medical ID, so even if someone were to find me, they would have no idea how to treat my emergency. I was convinced I would die at what was apparently not Jamestown Beach.

While I still on the phone with 9-1-1, a car parked on the side of the road. A dad with two young sons and a kite got out. It was a miracle. With all my uncoordinated, low-blood-glucose effort, I ran over and asked for a ride back to campus. My dispatcher was beside herself.

"What are you doing?"

"Getting REAL help. Bye!" I replied, hanging up.

Like any good dad to young kids, the man had juice boxes and snacks in his car. They probably saved my life. That incident was a huge wake-up call. I needed a better system. From that day on, I kept a log of what I tried and the results. Item 1: Do *not* take full basal dose right before a run. From there, things got a little more detailed: time of day, mileage, carbohydrates, insulin, and starting and ending blood glucose.

Pretty soon, I started finding strategies that worked and wasn't just getting by on luck. I could be more certain that what I did was safe and effective. Why? Because it had been done before. As I got more confident that I would have stable blood glucose, that loud, nagging voice in my head started to quiet down. Just like skating had been, running became a sort of escape from everyday life and type 1 diabetes. With running came freedom. And when I started to improve and complete progressively longer runs, I got really addicted. I had no idea how fast I was, but I could run without stopping for a long time and loved it. It felt like I was proving myself wrong and even other people who tried to convince me after the Jamestown Beach incident that running a marathon with type 1 diabetes would be too dangerous.

**Cheerleading:** At the beginning of my rookie season, I was figuring out where to wear my insulin pump in my uniform. Every home game, we had a special dance routine that was performed in front of the arena and aired on the JumboTron. Only about 12 out of 20 girls were able to perform the routine—each practice was a tryout for the next game. The first time I was selected to perform, my insulin pump came out of my sports bra when I was coming up from a move low to the ground. With the tubing connected, it hit me square in the nose! In front of ~20,000 people. My nose started bleeding, and I ran out of line of the camera. Luckily it wasn't aired over the JumboTron, or even worse, ESPN. After that incident, I decided to disconnect the pump during games and reconnect every hour or so to bolus for the missed basal insulin.

# 11

# Power Sports

**P**ower sports require you to perform short, powerful bouts of activity. In baseball, the activity may involve hitting the ball and sprinting to first base. In field events, it may be the high jump or discus throw. Recently, athletes with diabetes have excelled at playing baseball professionally, along with other power sports like cricket and beach volleyball. They have even done well in bodybuilding and power-lifting events, including winning Mr. Universe and other titles without using steroids or other performance-enhancing drugs.

And by now most people have heard about power athletes like Gary Hall Jr., formerly one of the fastest swimmers in U.S. history and worldwide. He is a three-time Olympian, 10-time Olympic medalist (winning five gold, three silver, and two bronze medals by 2004), and a former American record holder in 50-meter freestyle (swum in about 21 seconds). Diagnosed with type 1 diabetes between his first and second Olympic Games, he still won an individual gold medal in 50-meter freestyle in two Olympic Games in a row with type 1 diabetes and was inducted into the U.S. Olympic Hall of Fame in 2012. Yes, gold medal dreams are possible even if you have diabetes.

This chapter discusses some of these power sports and activities, including baseball and softball, bodybuilding, fencing, field events, power lifting and Olympic weightlifting, various types of sprinting, and volleyball (indoor and beach), and the athletes who participate in them.

## GENERAL RECOMMENDATIONS FOR POWER SPORTS

For most power sports, the requisite bursts of activity last less than 10 seconds, which means that your phosphagen system, composed of adenosine triphosphate (ATP) and creatine phosphate (CP), alone provides the energy that your muscles need to contract. If the activities last longer (from 10 seconds up to 2 minutes), you will also be getting some of the ATP through your lactic acid system, which you know is working hard when you start to feel the burn in your muscles. (Both of these energy systems are discussed fully in chapter 2.) The burning sensation results mainly from the breakdown of glycogen and the buildup of metabolic acids as a byproduct. The resulting drop in pH in your muscles causes the discomfort.

# GENERAL ADJUSTMENTS BY DIABETES REGIMEN

The power sport or activity that you do determines the changes you need to make in your regimen. Various power activities can decrease, increase, or have no immediate effect on your blood glucose. However, these activities' potential use of glycogen can cause a lowering of your blood glucose later on, particularly when you do these activities over an extended period. For example, the occasional hits, sprints, and throws required to play baseball or softball can have a cumulative effect on glycogen use, and you may need to watch out for later-onset lows when all that glycogen is being restored.

> *The most common response to doing power sports is an immediate increase in your blood glucose. Their intensity causes an exaggerated release of glucose-raising hormones like adrenaline and glucagon, but their duration is too short to let your muscles use up the new glucose.*

## Insulin Pump Users

For doing power sports recreationally, your insulin adjustments must be sport specific. You may require no changes for easy or brief play. But for prolonged play like team practices you may need to reduce your rapid-acting insulin boluses and your basal rates during the activity, depending on the intensity and duration of your workout. You will need to reduce your insulin less than for endurance sports because of the intense, brief nature of power activities. If they cause a great enough release of glucose-raising hormones, your blood glucose may increase, and you may need more insulin to compensate. If you participate in these sports and activities for an hour or more, you may have to consume more food, depending on your insulin changes. You may also have to reduce your insulin boluses or basal rates after participation in certain sports as well as eat more to prevent lows.

## Basal–Bolus Regimens

For power sports, your insulin adjustments will depend on the sport. If you are doing short or easy activities, you may not need to adjust anything in your regimen. Working out for longer, such as when you are involved in team practices for an hour or more, may require that you reduce your preactivity boluses. If you do cut back on your insulin, you will need a smaller reduction than you use for more aerobic sports because the brevity and intensity of power activities often cause your blood glucose to go up temporarily instead of down (meaning that you may need some insulin to bring your glucose back down). For prolonged participation, you may need to eat more, depending on how much you reduce your rapid-acting insulin and how much insulin is in your system. After certain activities, you may choose to reduce your bedtime doses of basal insulin and have a bedtime snack to prevent lows when you have depleted a substantial amount of muscle glycogen.

## *Noninsulin and Oral Medication Users*

The powerful nature of these activities is likely to raise your blood glucose (albeit temporarily), which happens even in athletes without diabetes. If you do these activities intermittently over an extended period, however, your blood glucose should come back down. As with the endurance–power sports, doing an aerobic cool-down of any length afterward will bring down elevations more quickly. In the day or so after these activities, your blood glucose may tend to stay lower while your body is using glucose to restore the muscle glycogen that you used up. You may be more insulin sensitive for 24 to 48 hours afterward. If you take certain oral medications (i.e., Diabinese, DiaBeta, Micronase, or Glynase), check your blood glucose if you ever start to feel any symptoms that you associate with getting low. (Refer back to medication effects on exercise in chapter 3.)

> *Be on the lookout for later-onset lows due to the amount of muscle glycogen that most power activities use. Though each motion is short in duration, the repetition of movements during practices or competition can result in significant muscle glycogen depletion.*

## *Other Effects to Consider*

The type, duration, and level of effort of the power sport (recreational or competitive) that you do will have the biggest impact on your blood glucose. Recreational activities and practices are usually less intense but more prolonged than competitive play. Being more active overall, and thus depleting more muscle glycogen from repeated, powerful movements, can reduce your blood glucose, whereas an intense competition like throwing a shot put (a field event) may cause it to rise from the release of glucose-raising hormones. On the other hand, recreational softball may have no effect on it at all. But if you play for 2 or more hours, even recreational play can eventually cause a decrease, and doing repeated power activities can cause your glucose to be lower after the activity and overnight.

> *Low-carbohydrate eating can potentially be detrimental to your performance in power events, but all recovery from exercise is fueled by fat and will improve after you adapt to such diets. Just watch out during the events themselves for potential performance issues if your muscle glycogen levels are low for any reason.*

## BASEBALL AND SOFTBALL

These activities usually require only short bursts of movement like sprinting, hitting, throwing, and catching, so they are anaerobic in nature. As a result, you may not use much energy doing them or need to make many adjustments. How hard you are playing and at what level (i.e., recreational or competitive) will affect your blood glucose responses. For example, in baseball or softball, the catcher and pitcher

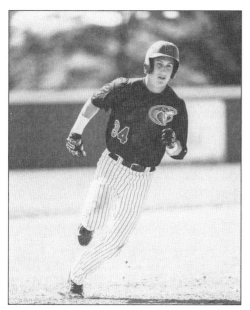

The occasional hits, sprints, and throws required to play baseball can have a cumulative effect on glycogen use, making it necessary to watch out for later-onset hypoglycemia while glycogen is being restored.

are more active than the other fielders because they are involved in almost every play. A recreational softball game can be quite sedentary because only one player at a time is up to bat for half the inning; during the other half, most players are not directly involved with every play. Doing conditioning drills during practices will increase the potential glucose-lowering effects of these activities, as will doing any drills more continuously.

## Athlete Examples

The following examples show that recreational play may require minimal changes but that longer, more intense practices can reduce your blood glucose to a greater degree.

### Insulin Changes Alone

Jack Borck from Wisconsin uses different basal insulin profiles on his pump for baseball, basketball, and other sports. In general, he reduces his basal rates 1 hour before playing; how much depends on his blood glucose at the time. Right before the activity, he lowers his basal rate further, up to an 80 percent decrease. He leaves it reduced 25 to 50 percent for 2 hours after playing.

To compensate for baseball, Jake Sheldon of Maryland reduces his before-practice insulin boluses by 10 to 15 percent. If he needs to, he may set a lower basal rate for a while after a game or practice.

While playing baseball, J.P. Delisio of Virginia keeps his pump on without adjusting anything except when he is up at bat. If he gets low, he treats it by drinking small juice boxes.

Baylee Glass of New Mexico plays softball. On game or practice days, she decreases her basal Lantus dose by 1 unit (down from her usual 12). Her blood glucose is typically stable until 2 to 5 hours after playing, but after that point it is more likely to drop.

Kaylee Swanson of Long Beach, California, pitches fast-pitch softball, and during practice and games she usually leaves her insulin pump on. Sometimes she disconnects it and gives her hourly basal amount as a bolus beforehand.

### Diet Changes Alone

North Carolina resident John Elwood plays baseball at the middle-school level. For this activity, he leaves his pump on and does not adjust his insulin doses unless he sees a pattern of lows. Normally, he simply eats more carbohydrates to compensate for the activity.

## Combined Regimen Changes

Minnesota resident Aaron Gretz travels and plays baseball for the Sioux Falls Canaries. During the season, he plays games 6 nights a week. During that time, he does less weight and endurance training (lifting twice a week and doing cardio training once) compared with his off-season. Most of this training takes place after games (typically at 10:00 p.m.). In general, he eats a higher carbohydrate diet during baseball season because of food availability while traveling and because he is active for longer periods of time throughout the day (6 hours daily). He uses more Humalog during the season due to eating more carbohydrates. (His diet is pretty low-carbohydrate during the off-season.) However, he decreases his Basaglar (basal insulin) to prevent lows in the middle of the night after so much activity.

Kate Zender of Washington State plays fast-pitch softball, for which she usually lowers her basal rate by 50 percent. Occasionally, she takes her pump off during games when she is extremely active. She also makes sure to have some carbohydrates and protein before starting to play, and she may drink some Gatorade to prevent lows during games.

Phoenix, Arizona, resident Debbie Shisler plays softball at her university. She finds that she does not have to take much NovoLog to cover her food during the softball season because she is a pitcher and practices a lot. To prevent lows when pitching, she consumes Oreos and orange juice. She usually takes Lantus in the morning and the evening, but she may take less of an evening dose on days when she has been very active.

Brandon Hunter of West Plains, Missouri, usually disconnects from his pump during baseball practices and games. He generally eats a snack with about 15 grams of carbohydrates before playing and often eats extra during games. When he can, he monitors his blood glucose; if it starts to rise during 2-hour games, he reconnects his pump and gives himself a small bolus to counter it.

New York City resident Gayle Brosnan always turns off her insulin pump an hour before she starts playing softball during the spring and summer months. She likes her blood glucose levels to be at least 160 mg/dL (8.9 mmol/L) when she starts playing, and she will take in carbohydrate if it drops down to 130 mg/dL (7.2 mmol/L) or below.

## BODYBUILDING

This activity depends on anaerobic energy sources for the muscle-building portion but also includes a more aerobic component than activities like power lifting or weight training. Bodybuilding competitions themselves, depending on which division you have entered, may have little effect on your blood glucose other than from mental stress. The more prolonged training for these events is similar to high-resistance weight training, and the resulting increases in muscle mass can greatly increase your overall insulin sensitivity, causing you to need less insulin. Aerobic workouts undertaken to lower your body fat levels are entirely different and may always cause reductions in your insulin needs and blood glucose levels.

Heavy weight training causes a large release of glucose-raising hormones, and your blood glucose may rise rather than fall during this activity. A prolonged weight-training session can use up a lot of muscle glycogen, thus increasing your risk of later-onset lows. For specific regimen changes for higher-intensity workouts, refer to the sections on weight training in chapter 8 and high-intensity interval training (HIIT) in chapter 10. Combining weight workouts with some cardio training can effectively lower your blood glucose. For the cardio portion, your regimen changes will depend primarily on the intensity and duration of your workout. Refer to chapter 8 for recommendations for working out on specific aerobic conditioning machines.

## Athlete Examples

The following examples show that training for bodybuilding can have different effects than those that occur in competition.

### Insulin Changes Alone

Christel Oerum of Santa Monica, California (profiled in chapter 8), finds that for bodybuilding workouts she needs to have sufficient insulin on board to avoid going too high from training. She has to take a bolus of at least half a unit before training (or possibly more, depending on whether she eats anything).

Maine resident Debbie Wright Theriault finds that heavy weightlifting raises her glucose. Her remedy is to usually run a mile or two afterward with a small amount of insulin on board to lower her glucose level.

Because she follows a strict high-protein bodybuilding diet, Lisa Harlan of Ohio mainly adjusts for bodybuilding with her insulin regimen. She exercises consistently by lifting weights regularly and intensely, and by doing 1 hour of cardio work a day. Because her routine is set, she only has to lower her insulin by 0.5 to 1 unit when doing a draining workout. For her, the posing part of competitive bodybuilding is extremely difficult, although her cardio training is more likely to cause her blood glucose to drop.

### Combined Regimen Changes

Missouri resident Kim Seeley finds that high-intensity lifting makes her blood glucose rise, whereas cardio training lowers it. When she is dieting down (eating "clean") over 9 to 12 weeks for a show, her body fat gets extremely low, and her overall insulin requirements drop by at least 30 percent. But she also has to watch how many calories she is eating to continue losing fat. When she is getting ready for a competition, she switches to using Lantus and Humalog instead of a pump because when her body fat gets low, she does not have any suitable places to insert her pump infusion sets. The only time that she has to increase her Humalog instead of lowering it is on leg workout days and during competitions, when her stress levels cause her blood glucose to rise.

Former Mr. Universe (Natural, Tall) title holder Doug Burns from California finds that his training schedule differs drastically when he is just training to stay healthy compared with preparing for a show. He adjusts his insulin doses slightly based on his body weight and body fat levels. He also finds that the leaner he becomes, the less insulin he needs to take. He alters his diet when he is trying to get lean for a show, which also affects his insulin needs.

A resident of New Zealand, Nev Raynes finds that when he does hard weight training and bodybuilding workouts, he has to lower his boluses by about 25 percent to prevent lows. Unless he has some insulin on board when he trains, his blood glucose rises. To prevent lows, he occasionally sips fruit juice throughout his workouts or training sessions. To prevent overnight lows, he lowers his bedtime basal insulin on days he was more active.

## CRICKET

The game of cricket was born in England centuries ago and involves batters, pitchers, and short sprints. It is England's national summer sport and is played throughout the world, particularly in Australia, India, Pakistan, the West Indies, and the British Isles. Played with a bat and ball, it involves two competing sides, or teams, of 11 players. The field is oval with a rectangular area in the middle, known as the pitch, that is 22 yards (20.12 meters) by 10 feet (3.04 meters) wide. Wickets (two sets of three sticks) are set in the ground at each end of the pitch with horizontal pieces called bails across their tops. The sides take turns at batting and bowling (pitching); each turn is an "innings" (plural). Both sides have one or two innings each, and the object is to score the most runs.

This sport is most analogous to playing baseball or softball and other activities that require only short bursts of powerful movements, making them anaerobic in nature. As a result, playing cricket may not require many immediate adjustments to maintain blood glucose, but it can result in significant muscle glycogen depletion and increase the risk for later-onset lows. How hard you are playing and at what level (i.e., recreational or competitive) will affect your blood glucose responses. Doing conditioning drills during practices will increase the potential glucose-lowering effects of these activities, as will playing more continuously. For other comparable (but not entirely relevant) examples, see baseball and softball earlier in this chapter.

## Athlete Examples

To play cricket in the United Kingdom, Joel Quinn of Somerset sets a temporary basal rate on his pump that is 50 percent lower, starting 40 to 60 minutes before the activity. He also usually eats a cereal bar with 15 grams of carbohydrates or a banana beforehand, along with drinking Lucozade (about one bottle) while playing for 2 hours.

Wasim Akram, a well-known Pakistani cricket player with type 1 diabetes, is a fast bowler and considered one of the greatest players in the history of cricket. After his diagnosis at the age of 31 at the peak of his career, he captured another 250 wickets, which is apparently a staggering achievement.

## FENCING

One of only four sports featured at every modern Olympic Games, fencing involves short, powerful thrusts and jabs and quick movements, as well as constant leg movement during a given round of competition. Training for this activity involves a combination of power and endurance movements. Doing well in fencing requires a good level of general fitness, which can be achieved through a combination of yoga, weight training, and other cardio and endurance workouts—even jump rope training and plyometrics. The effect on your blood glucose will vary most with the duration and intensity of your training. Working harder for longer produces the greatest chance of lowering it. When you are competing, your blood glucose may go up instead of down because of the intensity of the match and stress of competition.

## Athlete Examples

Due to its brief but extremely intense periods of activity followed by lengthy down times, this activity can be compensated for in a variety of ways.

### Combined Regimen Changes

A teenager from Beverly, Massachusetts, Jackson Burke aims to start his fencing practice with his glucose around 150 mg/dL (8.3 mmol/L) but his fencing tournaments at 120 mg/dL (6.7 mmol/L) because it goes up due to competition stress. Fencing practices require him to reduce his basal insulin delivery by 50 percent. He eats dinner 2 hours before (to limit the impact of the last bolus) or else has 0 carbohydrates (and no bolus) for dinner. If his glucose happens to be above 200 mg/dL (11.1 mmol/L) at the start of practice, he does not reduce his basal. If it is below 150 mg/dL (8.3 mmol/L), he takes 15 grams of fast-acting carbohydrates, followed by a protein-based food like cheese or jerky. His practices typically last for 90 to 120 minutes and consist of warm-ups, drills, jogging, and then fencing bouts.

Adrian Connard of Victoria, Australia, takes half his usual meal bolus if he eats within 2 hours of the start of a fencing bout but otherwise makes no adjustments to his insulin doses (bolus or basal). He substitutes sports drinks for water during a competition because he finds that he cannot eat anything while competing.

## FIELD EVENTS

Most field events (at track and field competitions) are short and intense, requiring either a near-maximal muscular contraction (like throwing a shot put or throwing a discus) or near-maximal full-body effort (e.g., long jump and pole vault). These types of events use anaerobic energy sources almost exclusively. The intensity and brevity of events during competitions should make your blood glucose levels easy to maintain, although they may decrease more when your muscle glycogen is being restored afterward. You may need more regimen changes to maintain your blood glucose levels both during and after practices (compared with meets) because of the more prolonged activity. As one track and field athlete commented, "If I am doing long, slow efforts, I need very little insulin in my body. But for shorter, intense events and training, I need insulin on board to counteract the glucose spikes those cause."

## POWER LIFTING AND OLYMPIC WEIGHTLIFTING

These activities rely on short-term energy sources like ATP and CP to fuel maximal lifts lasting no more than 10 seconds. But power lifting and Olympic weightlifting competitions are different sports; power lifting involves doing maximal lifts in the squat, bench press, and dead lift, whereas Olympic weightlifting consists of only two lifts, the snatch and the clean and jerk. Both activities may initially cause a rise in your blood glucose because of their intensity, but your blood glucose may drop later. Doing prolonged training for these events is similar in many ways to high-resistance weight training. Increases in your muscle mass resulting from this training, however, can greatly increase your overall insulin sensitivity and lower your insulin needs. For specific regimen changes for higher-intensity weight workouts, refer to the section on weight training in chapter 8.

## Athlete Examples

Depending on how intense your training is and how long you train, you may have to make various adjustments to manage your blood glucose effectively with these activities.

### Insulin Changes Alone

When doing this type of lifting or bodybuilding, Christopher Gantz from the United States finds that his insulin needs are greatly reduced. Although it is rare that he boluses before any type of resistance workouts, if his glucose does go up, he usually chooses to finish his workout with a cardio activity to lower it naturally. He needs much less insulin for food after working out. He follows a very-low-carbohydrate, high-protein (Dr. Bernstein) eating plan, covers food with regular insulin, and takes Levemir for basal insulin coverage.

For intense weightlifting workouts, Fresno, California, resident Dalton Merryman increases the basal insulin setting on his pump by 50 percent starting 15 minutes before beginning. Heavy lifting often otherwise makes his blood glucose spike to 140 mg/dL (7.8 mmol/L) or above.

On dead-lift training days, American Shelby T. eats a high-protein, moderate-carbohydrate, low-fat diet before her workout 1 hour before lifting. For that, she takes a bolus reduced by 40 percent. If she needs a correction after her workout, she also reduces that by the same amount. In addition, she reduces her overnight basal afterward by 20 percent to prevent nighttime lows.

### Diet Changes Alone

For intense Olympic lifting training, Guy Hornsby of West Virginia makes few changes unless his glucose drops, in which case he treats it with glucose tablets or regular sodas. He finds that exercise lows are rare, but he may get them 6 to 8 hours after workouts. He uses Basaglar (twice daily) as his basal insulin and does not adjust it or his bolus insulin (Novolog) for this activity.

Because Rosalind Sutch from Pennsylvania lifts almost every day, she changes her regimen only on days she does not train. She usually has a snack before lifting, eats a meal afterward that is high in protein and moderate in carbohydrates, and takes in most of her daily carbohydrates around workouts.

## Combined Regimen Changes

North Carolina resident Stephanie Winter eats lots of protein in the form of eggs, meat, and cheese for bodybuilding. She also takes creatine supplements when regularly lifting. She works out with only basal insulin on board (via her pump) and takes some glucose if she gets low. She does not correct her weightlifting high blood glucose with insulin, choosing instead to just dance or walk it back down to a normal level.

Seattle, Washington, resident Danielle Okuly does Olympic lifting once a week. For this activity, she boluses for 10 grams of carbohydrates before leaving home and adds extra to cover any blood glucose elevations. She does not eat before exercise, but does drink coffee between sets. She checks her continuous glucose monitor (CGM) readings once during lifting. She eats a breakfast of eggs, bacon, and potatoes afterward; if she is hungry or feeling low energy during her workouts, she eats an Rxbar.

Rob Mansfield from Brisbane, Australia, uses a NovoMix30 (with 70 percent basal and 30 percent bolus insulin) twice daily and trains for power lifting. He tries to eat a lot of protein because he is on a low-carbohydrate regimen, but he may eat more carbohydrates on a training day after the workout. Although his workouts can cause his blood glucose to rise a lot, on his insulin regimen he finds it also comes down quickly, and he needs to reduce his insulin dose to around 10 to 12 units afterward (down from his usual 14 to 20) or else he gets low later on.

## SPRINTS AND SPRINT TRAINING

Although a true power sprint would be running at your maximal speed until you cannot keep up the pace any longer (usually for 5 to 10 seconds), sprinting can be done for different lengths and intervals. For example, 800-meter runs require more energy production from the lactic acid system and are still primarily anaerobic, whereas runs lasting longer than 2 minutes will begin to use a greater proportion of aerobic sources of energy and are less of a true sprint for that reason (you have to slow down some). When you practice doing longer distance or repeated intervals, your recovery is mainly aerobic, although the actual sprint or faster intervals is usually more anaerobic. If you do a single sprint, your blood glucose may go up (you can do this to keep it higher at the end of an aerobic workout, as discussed in chapter 2). If you do repeated sprints, the immediate effect will likely be a rise in your blood glucose, followed by a drop later when your body is restoring glycogen that your body used. When sprinting multiple times (such as during sprint interval training), focus on preventing later-onset lows after training.

## Athlete Examples

These examples show that the primary effect of sprinting—whether you do sprint training for running, cycling, swimming, or some other activity—is an increase in your blood glucose rather than a decrease, at least while you are working out.

### No Changes Necessary

Wales native Martin Berkeley always does a 10-second sprint at the end of a longer run. He finds this helps prevent lows by releasing adrenaline that raises his blood glucose, and he can clearly see the effect on his CGM.

Greg Cashman of Atlanta, Georgia, finds that he is most likely to experience elevations in his blood glucose caused by exercise when he does high-intensity cycling sprints. Normally when he rides for longer periods, his blood glucose starts dropping, and he has to cut back on his basal insulin and eat more. This is not the case for bike sprints, though.

A Pennsylvania resident, David Walton finds that sprinting at the end of a long run raises his blood glucose. For example, during a 3-mile (4.8-kilometer) run that he did at a fast pace, when he practically sprinted the entire last half-mile his blood glucose rose by 30 mg/dL (1.7 mmol/L), although it would have dropped had he not done the all-out pace at the end.

### Insulin Changes Alone

Hailing from western Australia, Bec Johnson tries to exercise when she has little insulin or food on board, such as before breakfast, to minimize the variables in play. When she does sprint sessions of swimming, she has to have more insulin on board based on the fact that it makes her heart rate go over 170 beats per minute. She may take 0.5 to 1 units (depending on her starting glucose) 30 to 40 minutes before working out to avoid spikes.

When Felix Kasza of Redmond, Washington, does maximal sprints, he finds that he needs to give himself about 1 to 1.5 extra units of insulin per hour. Likewise, Fatima Shahzad of Cambridge, Massachusetts, finds that sports that require high-intensity bursts or sprints often give her postexercise high blood glucose levels. These require her to take a correction bolus afterward, and she monitors her CGM during play to make sure her glucose does not get too high.

## VOLLEYBALL AND BEACH VOLLEYBALL

These activities involve short, powerful moves (jumping at the net, diving for the ball, serving, or hitting the ball) and are generally anaerobic in nature. Your overall energy expenditure may be relatively low, depending on how long and hard you play, but beach volleyball may expend more energy because you walk, run, and jump on loose sand. Generally, volleyball practices require more energy than games, simply because practices usually last longer. Moving to and hitting the ball require only short bursts of activity, and you will need to make fewer changes for volleyball than you do for more active court sports like basketball, but it also depends on how many people play on each team. For example, many beach volleyball matches have only two players per side, meaning that you have to be involved in every other hit on your side while the ball remains in play and in your possession. If you play volleyball or the beach variety recreationally, you may not need to make many adjustments to your diabetes regimen because the intensity may be low and you may not be actively involved in every play. Higher-level play may initially raise your blood glucose. Whenever you play hard or long, be on the lookout for later-onset lows.

## Athlete Examples

The following examples demonstrate that the intensity of play has the greatest effects on your blood glucose response to volleyball, as well as the mental stress of competition in some cases. In addition, see the profile of beach volleyball player Paul Madau at the end of this section for strategies for intense training.

### No Changes Necessary (in the Short Run)

New York resident Paul Madau finds that prematch jitters raise his blood glucose. At least in the short run, he does not correct for these because he knows his blood glucose will come down on its own once he gets into the groove of playing a 2-person per team beach volleyball match. He notes that his glucose also drops after the match is completed.

### Insulin Changes Alone

Californian Dalton Merryman takes a small bolus and disconnects from his pump while playing volleyball. He checks his glucose and corrects highs with mini-boluses between games. If he is not able to do that, he may inject some (slower-acting) regular insulin instead to mimic his usual basal delivery of Humalog, especially during athletic events that require long times without his pump connected.

Jenny Vandevelde from California lowers her basal rate on her insulin pump to 20 percent of normal when she plays volleyball, and she treats lows with gummy bears. Similarly, Julie Majurin of Indiana decreases her basal rate to 25 percent of her normal rate when playing volleyball. California resident Richard Feifer reduces his basal to 10 percent of normal starting 30 minutes before playing, until 30 minutes before he stops.

Canadian Tania Knappich disconnects her pump when she plays, as does Leannne Lauzonis of New Mexico. Leanne usually plays for 1 or 2 hours and then has problems with her blood glucose dropping afterward.

### Combined Regimen Changes

To play high school varsity volleyball, Virginia resident Taylor Thornton decreases the bolus doses she takes for food on days when she does extreme amounts of exercise, but she does not adjust her Lantus doses. She also drinks Gatorade while playing to prevent lows.

Christa from California plays year-round volleyball. When she eats a meal before playing, she cuts back on her bolus by 1 unit or 2, and she may take 1 unit less later after playing. If she starts to feel low while playing, she eats a strawberry Zone bar because they have carbohydrate and protein in them.

Not as many people routinely do these power sports as some of the other sports covered in this book, but your body can benefit from doing many of them. I walk by the beach near my house every day and see people practicing their beach volleyball skills (just like Paul Madau in the profile that follows). Some high-intensity interval training is actually more like sprint interval training, and sometimes you can even use sprints to raise your blood glucose if dropping low during more moderate activities. Even if you did not find as many sports and activities in this chapter to your liking, you are sure to find an outdoor activity that you enjoy in the next one. Get started doing one today.

## Athlete Profile: **Paul Madau**

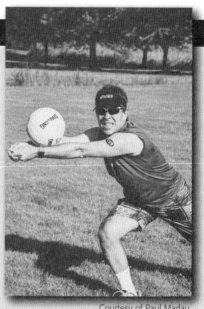

Courtesy of Paul Madau.
Photographer: Stephanie Morrow.

**Hometown:** Rochester, New York

**Diabetes history:** Type 1 diabetes diagnosed in 2014 (at age 44). I had gone the 2 years prior undiagnosed and was treated for everything from vertigo to having a parasite, due to extreme weight loss and muscular atrophy. I was then misdiagnosed as having type 2 diabetes in June 2014 before being referred to an endocrinologist who took one look at me and sent me to the emergency room for proper testing and care. I was properly diagnosed with type 1 diabetes the next morning in the hospital.

**Sport or activity:** Beach volleyball, semiprofessional and masters levels (2-person games)

**Greatest athletic achievement:** I have won 39 beach volleyball tournaments in my career so far, spanning three different countries, including championships in the United States, Canada, and Australia. Prior to being diagnosed with diabetes, my greatest achievement was winning two King of the Beach style tournament titles in two different countries in the same year (2004), in Sydney, Australia, and Toronto, Canada. King of the Beach is an individualized tournament format consisting of the top 16 ranked players of the season. Each athlete plays with every other player in their pool, and the two players from each pool with the highest win records move into the next round, and this is repeated until the final four players remain to repeat it one last time. The crowned winner is the player with the highest win record of the final four players. I have competed in two full beach volleyball seasons (2016 and 2017) since my diagnosis and have placed in the top three a total of nine times in 16 tournaments. I plan to get my 40th tournament win this season and my first with type 1 diabetes.

***Current insulin and medication regimen:*** I use the Omnipod pump with Humalog insulin, along with a Dexcom CGM. I wear both on my lower back during tournaments to avoid diving directly on them. I also wear an Apple Watch with the Dexcom mobile app that lets me know where my blood glucose levels are before, during, and after matches. I have learned to use these values and adjust insulin dosing, along with fueling, accordingly.

***Training tips:*** My best advice is to learn all that you can about your body and how it reacts to insulin while competing—fully understand how long insulin is active in your body, how much you need up front and while competing, and how competing and training might bring down your blood glucose naturally without more insulin. Many times, before a match I will see a spike in my glucose, which is usually due to mental anxiety before a match. I rarely take any large doses of insulin before starting, though, to avoid even a chance of crashing low during a match. As I settle into the flow and progression of the match, my levels will steady themselves out, and they usually come down on their own afterward. I wear my Apple Watch during my matches so I have full knowledge of what my CGM glucose levels are doing. I will always test my blood glucose after a match to ensure my CGM is accurate, and it usually is because I always put a new sensor on 2 days before a tournament. If needed, I may take a correction if I have enough time between matches for my insulin to take effect and be gone before the next one. Likewise, if I see a blood glucose crash start to occur during a match, I will use all timeouts allowed, including a medical one if needed, so I can fuel with some quick-acting carbs like a Honey Stinger gel or waffle.

***Typical daily and weekly training and diabetes regimen:*** Time in the sand over time in the gym is my biggest tip for beach volleyball. In a gym setting, it's very hard to duplicate what you do in tournament situations, so I focus on time in the sand to practice and train. I train in the most humid weather, on very windy days, in the pouring rain, and in about any other weather-related situation imaginable. You can't control what the weather will be on any given day, so you have to be prepared for all of it. Also, the only thing that truly makes me ready for a tournament is practicing against other athletes as much as possible, which I can only do down on the beach. I do work out in the gym two to three times a week for around 45 minutes to do volleyball-specific weight training and core muscle work. I have been doing this routine for 30 years, and it has definitely been the key to my success.

▶ ***Monday:*** Always a rest day because I am usually coming off a 2-day tournament weekend and possibly travel. Recovery is just as important as training. I focus on proper nutritional recovery as well and making sure my protein intake is plentiful.

▶ ***Tuesday:*** Every day starts with a couple cups of good strong coffee. I usually do a 4-mile (6.4-kilometer) run sometime around noon. The sun is at its hottest during that time, and I need to train in that heat. I also get a trip to the gym in for a leg and lower body workout, as well as shoulders and a core-specific workout. I head to the beach around 4:00 p.m., set up my net, and start to run some drills with my teammate and other athletes. By 5:30 p.m., we are playing full-on matches for the rest of the night.

continued ➡

*Paul Madau continued*

▶ **Wednesday:** More coffee. I head to the beach around 11:00 a.m. for my own speed interval work in the sand. I like to do sprint/recovery work in the deep sand as I feel this helps me move quicker during tournament play. The sand I play in can get very deep, depending what beach I am playing on, so I need to have my legs ready to move and my endurance at its peak. I will break at about 2:00 to get my work for my job completed and grab some food, then head back to the beach by 4:00. Wednesdays are the most popular training days for other beach volleyball players, so from then until dark my teammate and I will play as many matches as we can against other teams.

▶ **Thursday:** More coffee. I will do another light run around 11:00, usually no more than 3 miles (4.8 kilometers) and also go to the gym for another leg and core workout, as well as some very volleyball-specific upper body work, focusing on shoulder, upper back, and triceps work. I am usually at the beach no later than 3:00 for some more interval cardio training. My teammate and I have a coach who works with us on Thursdays and will run some very intense drills for us to replicate tournament match situations. Defense drills and transitions to offense are key for me because I am primarily the defender in my partnership with my teammate, and my job is to keep the ball from hitting the sand and to transition right into playing offense. Our coach will give his feedback on what we are doing well and what we need to improve. After practice, we compete against other athletes who start showing up at the beach for the rest of the evening. I will always put a new Dexcom sensor on so it has a full 24 hours on my body to become acclimated to my glucose fluctuations and for the adhesive to stick well. Two days before a tournament is sufficient time for my numbers to read extremely accurate while competing.

▶ **Friday:** This is never the same day, week to week. If I am traveling to a tournament out of my city, state, or country, I am usually getting stuff ready to go. I may do a very light run early in the day, but it's usually a day of mental preparation. I go over in my mind what my teammate and I have worked on over the week and make myself mentally prepared for the tournament. I always put a new Omnipod on my body on Friday evenings. Just like for the Dexcom, I like to give the adhesive time to adhere to my body well before the tournament and have plenty of time for the basal program to start working.

▶ **Saturday:** Tournament day 1. My mornings still start with a giant cup of coffee. I always test my blood glucose first thing in the morning and again before my first match to ensure my Dexcom is reading accurately. I hardly ever eat on the morning of a tournament—maybe half a Honey Stinger waffle, and usually am fine for the first hour or two. My glucose tends to be higher than normal before and during a match, so crashing is usually not a problem. It's only afterward and between matches that I have to keep a close eye on them. I fuel with Honey Stinger gels and waffles as needed and snack intermittently on higher protein foods. I also stay hydrated all day because humidity and the sun are a huge factor in exhausting me and jacking up my blood glucose. My teammate and I put all of our work into action as we progress through the day. Our focus is always on the match we are in at that time. If we have done everything right, and I have managed my diabetes correctly, we will usually have a great day of competition.

▶ **Sunday:** Tournament day 2. Coffee. (Do you see a pattern here?) Sundays are usually the second day of the men's tournament if it is a 2-day event. If my teammate and I have advanced to the second day, and we usually do, Sunday is a basic repeat of Saturday except the matches are more intense. We are usually playing teams who have advanced the way we have, and the caliber of competition is much stronger. My diabetes management is very important on Sundays because we have made it to the money rounds. Higher placings of course mean more prize money. I stay on top of my blood glucose numbers and manually test before and after every match and ensure my Dexcom is reading accurately. I fuel as I need to with Honey Stinger and correct any highs with slight doses of insulin to ensure my body cooperates with the rest of the tournament. I take each match as it comes and work through everything, diabetes and opponents (as best I can), draw from the positivity and team dynamic my teammate and I have, and plan for as much success as we can have until we finish the tournament. When I am done, it's then time to just relax and enjoy the evening at the beach.

***Other hobbies and interests:*** I enjoy coaching younger athletes who are starting their beach volleyball careers and climbing through the ranks. I have worked with many Junior Olympic beach volleyball programs in the United States and Canada. It is amazing to see the next generation of athletes starting to formulate their future in sport, and hope I can inspire them in some way. In addition, many years ago I was in three bands in my city. I love to sing, but do not have time for bands anymore. I have a group of friends who also sing, and we hit a couple of karaoke bars when we have time. I also give my time to my sponsors, and I work expos with the companies as my availability allows. My sponsors have been awesome throughout my career going back to 1995, and more importantly, they have been very supportive of me since my type 1 diagnosis. I really like being around other athletes from different sports at the expos and getting to know them. Once in a while, I will meet other athletes with type 1, and we compare stories. It becomes a very small world in that regard.

***Good diabetes and exercise story:*** In 2016, during my first full season postdiagnosis, my Omnipod came off during a tournament. I dove for a ball and landed directly on the pod, ripping it out. I had brought two spare pods with me, so I used both timeouts to fill a new pod with insulin and get it on me. The problem was that I was sweating a lot, and I had sand all over me, so the adhesive wasn't sticking to my body. I had to get some duct tape from the tournament director and use it over the pod and around the adhesive to make it stick. Two plays later, the pod started its "scream of death," which meant it failed. I called a medical timeout, pulled the new (failed) pod off me, and checked my blood with a fingerstick. It was pretty close to my Dexcom readout—a bit high, but not so high as to worry about. This was the final match of the day, and we needed to win it to advance to Sunday. I didn't want to chance my last pod coming off me, so I played the rest of the match with no pump and focused on winning the match as fast as possible. I got the new pod on quickly after we won it, and I hydrated quickly. It was pretty amazing to see how my body adapted to the situation when it absolutely needed to, but also extremely nerve wracking. I don't think I have ever looked at my watch so many times in 30 minutes before.

# 12

# Outdoor Recreation and Sports

**H**ave you ever dreamed of walking or cycling across mountains and deserts, backpacking for weeks, scuba diving in crystal blue waters, or rafting down a dangerous river? Maybe you have watched the Winter Olympics and dreamed about being one of the athletes skiing down mountains at incredible speeds. Or maybe the slower pace and scenery of hiking or kayaking on a lake or simply playing yard games is more to your liking. In any case, people with diabetes have done all these activities and many, many more, all while managing their blood glucose effectively.

This chapter gives recommendations for regimen changes and real-life examples for myriad outdoor physical activities and sports, including hiking and backpacking, rock climbing and bouldering, mountain biking and cyclo-cross, scuba diving and snorkeling, snowboarding, paddleboarding, sailing, skateboarding, and many others—even curling, adventure racing, orienteering, dog mushing, and gardening. These recreational sports and activities vary widely in intensity. Some activities are brief, primarily fueled by adenosine triphosphate (ATP) and creatine phosphate (CP), whereas others involve the lactic acid system and some muscular endurance, such as rock climbing and bouldering. Most of these activities rely on aerobic energy sources, however, especially prolonged activities such as backpacking and mountaineering. (See chapter 2 for a review of how all these energy systems work.)

## GENERAL RECOMMENDATIONS FOR OUTDOOR ADVENTURES

Giving overall general recommendations for regimen changes for all these activities is problematic because they run the gamut from extremely low-level activities to intense ones, and from short to very prolonged in duration. Some activities can vary greatly in how they are performed (e.g., downhill skiing), both in terms of the person doing them and due to environmental factors like cold or windy conditions. For each sport or activity you will find general recommendations based on the type of movement required and real-life examples of athletes' specific regimen changes.

*Making general recommendations on how to handle all outdoor sports and activities is difficult, given their diversity across a spectrum. For each one, consider both the impact of the activity itself on your blood glucose and the environment in which you will be active.*

## General Adjustments for Any Type of Diabetes

For lower-intensity activities like recreational horseback riding with a trail guide, you may not need to reduce your insulin doses or increase your food intake. For more intense activities like mountain biking, you are likely to need to eat more and take less insulin, depending on how long you do it. If you are mountaineering or backpacking, you are likely to need even greater changes to keep your blood glucose stable during and after the activity.

## Other Effects to Consider

As mentioned, this wide array of outdoor and recreational activities will elicit many different blood glucose responses, depending on how long and how hard you are working, and even how hot or cold, or above or below sea level you are. Low-intensity activities like snorkeling may have a minimal effect on your blood glucose unless you do it for several hours, whereas dog mushing will require diligence on your part to prevent lows throughout the activity (especially if you are participating in an extended race like the Iditarod in extreme weather conditions). In fact, the effects of heat, cold, or high altitude can be sizable, causing greater than normal use of your muscle glycogen and blood glucose and occasionally a higher level of insulin resistance, managed only with appropriate regimen changes.

*Outside environmental conditions can impact your blood glucose more than you expect. Learn all you can about how heat, humidity, cold, windchill, altitude, and other extremes can affect blood glucose, and take action to keep yours in check.*

## Dealing With Environmental Extremes

Many people have noticed significant effects on their blood glucose while exercising in extreme environments, which generally increase your metabolic rate along with your reliance on glucose as a fuel. Warm or hot environments may also speed up your insulin absorption by increasing blood flow to your skin (which happens for sweating and cooling purposes). The more prolonged your activity is, the greater the effect may be on your blood glucose and muscle glycogen use. How extreme an environment is affects your responses as well: hot and humid conditions increase your glucose use more than hot ones alone, wind chill exacerbates the effects of a cold environment, and high altitudes can affect you in ways you seldom experience at lower elevations. Refer to the next section, then see the specific activities for athlete examples of regimen changes under environmental extremes.

## Dealing With Meters and Insulin in Extreme Environments

Colorado resident Lisa Seaman has had extensive experience with managing her glucose while mountaineering. "In my experience, all blood glucose meters function poorly at low temperatures. Our (mountaineering group's) solution to this problem was to design a small fleece bag that straps onto your base layer with a chest harness system. This keeps your meter and insulin warm and accessible. I usually have a strip of Velcro on the back of my meter and on the bag so that I don't have to worry about dropping it. Also, the lancet is tied to it with a little piece of cord. I try not to keep my strips all in one container in case I drop it. (I keep some extras in my first aid kit or pack.) Using this system, the meters tend to be within operational temperature range even in the worst of conditions."

She has more advice for hot conditions. "For hot climates, I have a different system altogether. I spent a year in Costa Rica as a guide for Outward Bound. I used a little pelican box designed for cameras to carry my meter. It's completely waterproof, so I could even wear it in my personal flotation device when kayaking or rafting. I still use Velcro on the inside of the box and on the back of my meter, and I keep my strips and lancet in there as well. For insulin, I use the FRIO (insulin cooling) bags, which are really great! They just need to be wet, and they will keep your insulin cool in hot temperatures."

### *How Athletes Deal with Environmental Extremes, Sweating, Insulin, and More*

Active people with diabetes have the added burden of carrying their insulin and supplies with them during athletic endeavors (such as backpacking and mountaineering), keeping insulin from freezing or overheating, making sure their glucose meters work in extreme temperatures, getting their pumps or continuous glucose monitoring (CGM) devices to stay on when they sweat a lot, and using them during water sports. Here are just some of the tips and advice that have come from their personal experiences in handling all these potential issues.

> "Put glucose gels in plastic bags to avoid bursting issues (from freezing). Have multiple pockets (some inside shell layers in extreme cold). Use a bumbag (fanny pack) slung under one shoulder under a shell jacket to keep insulin, gels, and glucose meter warm (the meter is in a waterproof pouch on a lanyard clipped in—very useful when climbing to prevent dropping). Carry a spare blood glucose meter in a rucksack (backpack)."
> —Peter Arrowsmith (Wales)

> "Be aware that extremes of cold or heat can give a false low or high on the CGM."
> —Cindy Ski (Sault Ste. Marie, Canada)

> "Carrying solar chargers and power banks takes away the stress of losing power for a diabetes device when backpacking."
> —Jen Hanson (Toronto, Canada)

"If going in cold weather, make sure to put your pump close to your body, and don't expect to be able to read it in the cold. It will do its job, and you don't need to worry too much."

—Danielle Okuly (Seattle, Washington)

"During extreme weather (i.e., hot and humid), try to remain hydrated as dehydration seems to cause the body to react as if under severe stress and blood glucose levels go way up."

—Mark Robbins (Victor, New York)

"Cold weather makes me go high, and hot weather makes me go low, so I have to change my insulin intake depending on the weather. Altitude also makes me go low."

—Declan Irvine (Raymond Terrace, Australia)

"At 4,500 meters (~ 15,000 feet), the altitude makes me massively insulin resistant. It seems this happens in some people. In such an inhospitable environment, stopping to rest is not an option. I have to do careful monitoring, plenty of corrections (via syringe), 200 percent basal rates, and rehydration to summit the mountain."

—Paul Coker (Cardiff, United Kingdom)

"In very cold weather (Arctic conditions), keep your insulin at body temperature by wearing it in a pouch bag next to your skin and under your clothing. Consider the location of pumps, infusion sets, and CGM carefully. You don't want them to get in the way of rucksack straps or fanny packs."

—Paul Coker (Cardiff, United Kingdom)

"Keep your blood glucose meter close to your body as cold temperatures will give you inaccurate readings on the low end. Try to keep your meter as unexposed to the elements as possible, and check your blood glucose in your coat with the meter sticking in your armpit in cold conditions to get a more accurate reading. Sometimes I pop the batteries out and warm them up if my meter is giving an error message from being too cold."

—Sean Busby (Whitefish, Montana)

"In cold weather, keep your blood glucose meter close to your body heat. Wear gloves to keep your fingers warm so you bleed easier."

—Jim Schuler (United States)

"I always wrap my CGM in a snack ziplock bag and carry it in my SPIbelt or flip belt. For rainy days that has worked, and in extremely cold weather it hasn't been a problem either."

—Emily Tiberio (Beaver, Pennsylvania)

"For weather extremes, wrap everything in plastic. For carrying everything, wear a fanny pack. Wear medical ID, have someone who knows your projected location, have a syringe for a backup system, and carry twice the amount of fast-acting glucose you think you need."

—Courtney Duckworth (Washington, D.C.)

"I love using the FRIO insulin cooling cases to carry my emergency insulin around in hot weather. For all day adventures, I have to be prepared in case my pump fails, so I carry an insulin pen and a couple of needle tips in a small FRIO case. I once sweated off the adhesive to my pump site and was really glad I had backup insulin with me."

—Jeannette Styles (Eugene, Oregon)

"Start two pump sites before an event. If one goes bad or comes off, you can just switch to the second one without having to completely start a new one. I wear my pump site on my butt cheek and my CGM on the outside of my upper thigh. They are under my compression shorts for swimming and biking and stay on. I cut a hole in the top of all my pants pockets and put my pump in my pocket and feed the tubing through the hole so I am less likely to break it or bump into anything."

—John Boyer (Mount Airy, Maryland)

"I use a flip belt to hold my pump or insulin while skiing. I depend on my CGM being in my chest pocket so I can check my blood glucose on the slopes. When I was on a pump, I had a remote so I could bolus or suspend my pump very easily when needed."

—Michael Horgan (Northborough, Massachusetts)

"I use GrifGrips on my CGM for racing ultras due to excessive sweat, ice, and water on my body and time exercising. My previous pump with tubes clipped to the inside of my shorts, which kept it secure. Put on a new site 24 hours (pump) or 48 hours (CGM) before a race. Carry a small meter if you don't use CGM. Stuff a cotton bud inside the test strip container to avoid them shaking around."

—Stephen England (New York City, New York)

"Skin Tac and RockaDex patches have been super helpful to keep my Dexcom CGM attached in sweaty weather. CGM alarms help me to pay attention to my blood glucose occasionally when beautiful surroundings and great company monopolize my attention."

—A.J. Krebs (Medford, Oregon)

"I use benzoin tincture for all adhesive sites. I have tried all the other medically available adhesive boosters, and they haven't worked. I have to have something on my skin in order to make my pump or CGM stay at all."

—Dean McColl (Bremerton, Washington)

"I tape my sensor down with Opsite Flexifit/Flexigrid, a clear waterproof tape. Cut the corners off the square tape (to round them off) because otherwise the corners start peeling off first."

—Bec Johnson (Perth, Australia)

"I use Hypafix medical tape over my CGM to keep it in place while in the pool. This works well with sweating too. I carry a small bag that holds my receiver, meter, and snack."

—Cathy DeVreeze (Ontario, Canada)

"Use spray-on deodorant for infusion sites before placement to prevent excessive sweating. Keep your CGM in a wet/dry bag for water sports and also place it in a ziplock bag. Listen for beeps and alarms through the bag, and check as you're able to."

—Dan Stone (Middletown, Pennsylvania)

"If you have a CGM, find a place to put it where it's easily monitored: on the bookshelf of the treadmill, your life jacket (use a cell phone bag to keep it dry), the handle bars of your bike or motorcycle, etc. Have liquid glucose just as accessible. Also, for swimmers or those like me who sweat a lot, use an adhesive gel or glue to further secure the sensor or transmitter to your skin (like Skin Tac)."

—Greg Cutter (Norfolk, Virginia)

"Have friends carry extra carbs for you on long trips just in case. Choose pants that don't rub the infusion sets and CGM off. Bring tape and spare infusion sets with you at all times."

—Jane (Montpelier, Virginia)

"If your sport is contact sports, put the pump site in a spot that will not come in contact with other people or objects."

—Paul Madau (Rochester, New York)

"Putting CGM sensors and the Omnipod pump on the back of your arm (triceps) keeps it out of the way, and there's less sweat there so it sticks better."

—Rosalind Sutch (Philadelphia, Pennsylvania)

"I always carry antiseptic wipes to keep my hands clean when I am testing my blood glucose during exercise."

—Rachel Rylands (Liverpool, United Kingdom)

"The Omnipod pump works great for swimmers!"

—Sarah McManus (Pittsburgh, Pennsylvania)

## ADVENTURE RACING, TRAIL RUNNING, ORIENTEERING, ROGAINING, AND FELL RACING

All these activities are highly aerobic in nature and have other elements in common. Adventure races vary widely in terms of their duration and difficulty, but take place over more natural terrain and trails (and sometimes without marked paths), making them challenging from that perspective. Trail running is not that different from other running races and training, but it is done in a more natural environment, usually over rougher terrain or on trails in more remote areas, making it more difficult than running on roads or sidewalks. Cross country running is most similar to trail running, but the former uses more cultivated paths.

Other variations of adventure racing and trail running include orienteering and rogaining. Originally a land training exercise for the military, orienteering is a sport that requires the participants to use their navigational skills with a map and compass to get from point to point in diverse and usually unfamiliar terrain as fast as possible. Participants get a specially prepared orienteering (topographical) map that they use to find these points.

With its origins in Australia, rogaining is another type of orienteering sport, one that includes long distance cross country navigation. The participants work on teams of two to five people together on route planning and navigation between checkpoints, using a variety of map types. Rogaine team members choose which checkpoints to reach within a scheduled time limit to maximize their score. These events can be as short as 2 hours or as long as 24 hours or more.

A sport originating on the fells of northern Britain, fell (or hill) running and races involve running off road over upland country where gradient climbs are a significant component of the difficulty. This sport has elements of trail, cross country, and mountain running, but it is distinct from all these. The terrain covered can vary widely, but usually it includes significant ascents and rocky ground, making these races much harder than straight trail running. The participants in fell races must have some mountain navigation skills (like orienteering requires) and must carry adequate survival equipment with them during events.

If you take insulin, you may get by using mostly basal doses without a need for much bolus insulin to cover most of the carbohydrates you eat during any of these events. In any case, you will likely need to consume more carbohydrates to cover for the glycogen and blood glucose that you are using to fuel your activity, along with protein and fat to replace all the calories that your body is expending. Expect that the effects on your insulin action may last for 2 to 3 days beyond finishing your event, especially if it was prolonged or physically grueling.

## Athlete Examples

Due to the intensity and duration of these activities, you will likely have to eat more and lower your insulin to participate effectively. Other activities are similar in some ways, different in others. For regular trail runs lasting 1 to 2 hours, the examples given for running in chapter 9 may apply. For extreme events that involve grueling and unusual environmental conditions and sleep deprivation during the longer events, the most analogous activity is ultradistance events (also covered in chapter 9), but even those do not fully compare to adventure racing and these other outdoor challenges. Also see the athlete examples for mountaineering and backpacking in this chapter.

## Combined Regimen Changes

**Trail Running.** For trail running, Bend, Oregon, resident Jamie Flanagan cuts back his basal rate by 25 to 50 percent. He also checks his blood glucose many times during exercising and always has enough food with him to prevent lows. He tries to keep his glucose around 130 to 150 mg/dL (7.2 to 8.3 mmol/L) while running.

Similarly, Kory Seder of Madison, Wisconsin, views trail running like any other endurance activity. For running on trails, he usually sets a 30 to 50 percent temporary basal reduction 45 minutes before exercise that lasts throughout the run. He adjusts this basal reduction as needed, depending on the intensity of the trail run and his blood glucose responses. If he starts to get low, he treats it with glucose tablets.

For trail running and other activities, Meghan N. from Pennsylvania lowers her basal rates. She also increases her carbohydrate ratio from 1:15 to 1:20, meaning that she takes less insulin for the same amount of carbohydrates before running.

**Adventure Racing.** Tim Godfrey of Seattle, Washington, participates in adventure racing, which typically lasts from 5 to 24 hours per event, although some races take 3 or more days. These events can include a water portion (such as kayaking), mountain biking, and trekking or trail running. All you know when you start is the approximate amount of time it should take to finish, but you do not know the actual length of each leg, the order in which they will occur, or where you will be going (hence the "adventure" part of these races). To compensate, he almost never takes any Humalog during them, and he cuts his basal Lantus dose by a third to a half of usual the night before racing. He finds it easiest to use Hammer gels and Perpetuem drink additive, taking in about 50 grams of carbohydrate per hour, and he checks his blood glucose frequently. With the erratic nature of such racing, he tends to let his glucose climb to as high as 200 mg/dL (11.1 mmol/L) without correcting it to prevent lows, and he stays hydrated with electrolyte drinks with no carbohydrates.

**Rogaining.** Melbourne, Australia, resident Andrew Baker's main sports are orienteering, rogaining, and adventure racing with the occasional ultradistance trail run thrown in. Rogaining is his primary sport, and he participates in events lasting from 6 to 24 hours. For these, he slightly drops his Lantus dose on the morning of the event (down to 25 from its usual level of 28 to 32 units). He tries to eat something every hour during the event without taking any bolus of Humalog unless his blood glucose level is getting high. If the event goes into a second day, he only takes 20 to 22 units of Lantus that morning (down from 25). After events like this, he needs to take a Humalog dose if he eats anything afterward, unlike while he is exercising.

**Orienteering.** For Andrew Baker to compete in 1-hour orienteering events, he typically eats two slices of bread with honey about 30 minutes before the event. He only covers this with a dose of Humalog if his blood glucose is above 180 mg/dL

(10.0 mmol/L), and he only takes a small correction while ignoring the food. He carries a small bag of hard candy with him. If the event is longer than an hour, he brings some food and eats it around the 1-hour mark.

**Fell Racing.**   Edwin Sherstone of the United Kingdom participates in fell racing. For races lasting 3 to 7 hours, he reduces his bolus insulin by 1 to 2 units for any food that he eats in the hour or 2 before starting, and he reduces his morning dose of basal Levemir as well. In addition, he increases his morning carbohydrate intake by 30 to 50 grams.

### Other Effects to Consider

**Effect of Isolation and Environment.**   Andrew Baker from Melbourne, Australia, finds that during long and multiday events, the biggest challenge is making sure he is carrying appropriate diabetes supplies and food, particularly when he is headed a long way from civilization. He recounted that some friends recently did a 7-day adventure race where one of the legs was estimated to take 40 hours but actually required 60 to 70 hours; many of the teams ran out of food. Most people aim to finish with no food left, but with diabetes he is not willing to take that risk, so he overcompensates. On a recent 24-hour rogaining event, he came back with half the food he left with, meaning he had to carry it all the way around the course.

## AIRSOFT, PAINTBALL, AND LASER QUEST

Popular among teenagers and preteens, airsoft, paintball, and laser tag are variable activities, sometimes requiring bursts of running and other times being more sedentary. Airsoft tournaments involve eliminating your opponents (i.e., other participants) by shooting them with plastic ball bearings (BBs) launched from airsoft guns. Organized tournaments may involve using replicas of real guns, tactical gear, and other accessories used by the military and police. Paintball is similar, but it involves marking your opponents by shooting them with paintballs shot from a compressed gas–powered gun. Laser tag takes place in a dark environment (often with ultraviolet lights) with participants carrying laser guns that allow them to "shoot" or mark their opponents on laser targets and earn points during a specified amount of time each game. The duration of play varies widely among these activities, but how much movement you do affects your blood glucose response the most. Almost all airsoft games are held outdoors, paintball can take place indoors or outside, and laser tag is always played indoors.

### Athlete Example

Carter Gillespie of Arizona occasionally participates in organized airsoft and paintball games that are mini-war scenarios lasting up to 8 hours. The games are set up in facilities with buildings, military vehicles, and more. The playing time averages 3 to 4 hours, and may involve 15-minute spurts of running and then short breaks. To compensate for these physically active games, he usually eats snacks with 15 grams of carbohydrates 2 or 3 times during play without taking a bolus to cover them.

He also has to check his blood glucose more often the day after playing because he tends to run low then.

## BOULDERING, OUTDOOR

Bouldering outdoors is analogous to rock climbing, but it varies in the techniques and equipment used. It is usually done on small and low rock formations (or indoors on artificial rock walls) or boulders, without the use of ropes or harnesses. Most climbers wear specialized climbing shoes to help secure footholds, put chalk on their hands for a firmer grip, and (more often when done indoors) use bouldering mats to prevent injuries from falls. Bouldering problems (the path you take to complete the climb) are usually less than 20 feet (6 meters) high and vary widely in difficulty and complexity. It also is possible to do traverses that make you climb horizontally rather than vertically. Bouldering was originally done as training for roped climbs and mountaineering, to practice certain moves closer to the ground and to work on stamina and finger strength. Nowadays, bouldering competitions take place in both indoor and outdoor settings. The diabetes regimen adjustments are similar whether you are bouldering or rock climbing, though.

## Athlete Examples

Given the anaerobic nature and intensity of this activity, you may need no immediate changes in your regimen. Be on the lookout for lows afterward due to the greater use of muscle glycogen. For other athlete examples, see the section on rock and ice climbing later in this chapter and the indoors climbing section in chapter 8.

### No Changes Necessary

Patrick Bowyer of Britain usually expects to see a decline in his blood glucose after about 30 minutes of steady activity, but it declines less when he is bouldering. Instead, he often experiences postexercise high glucose due to the intensity of this activity. He may let this elevation come down on its own, as he often gets low later after bouldering.

### Combined Regimen Changes

A resident of Middletown, Pennsylvania, Dan Stone considers bouldering to be an anaerobic activity. For this activity, he does nothing beforehand, and he usually reduces his basal rate by 30 percent for up to 12 hours afterward or increases his fat and protein intake during a postworkout meal to prevent later-onset lows.

## CANOEING AND KAYAKING

Canoeing and kayaking on relatively calm water (not white water) are prolonged and aerobic in nature, especially when done at lower intensities. (White-water activities, which can be more intense and cause greater use of anaerobic energy sources, are addressed later in this chapter.) For low-level paddling, you will need minimal changes, but the longer you do it (especially if you are working hard), the more regimen adjustments you may need to maintain your blood glucose levels. For example, for longer or more intense paddling (such as against ocean waves instead of on a placid lake or river), you may have to eat more and lower your insulin doses to prevent lows. For multiday trips or outings, you may benefit by lowering your basal insulin because you will have glycogen to replace in your upper-body muscles, making you more insulin sensitive.

## Athlete Examples

These examples illustrate regimen changes that depend on the duration of canoeing or kayaking. For more intense variations on these activities, see the white-water section later in this chapter.

### Diet Changes Alone

For sea kayaking, United Kingdom resident David Hillebrandt aims to keep his glucose level between 126 and 198 mg/dL (7.0 and 11.0 mmol/L) with snacks like muesli bars and chocolate; this is slightly higher than he keeps his glucose during other activities such as downhill skiing. He uses Toujeo as his basal insulin, and he does not adjust it for this activity.

Canadian Vicky Hollingsworth brings glucose or other sugary foods along when she does these activities. She finds that all outdoor activities make her glucose drop more. She uses Lantus and Humalog, and she does not make adjustments to her doses of either one.

For these activities, Rebekah Lindsay of Sevierville, Tennessee, just takes extra snacks, if needed. If she gets low, she treats it with in Hammer gels, Clif Shot Bloks, glucose tablets, or regular jelly beans.

### Combined Regimen Changes

For kayaking, Marin Desbois of Montreal, Canada, reduces his basal to 50 percent. Normally, he kayaks 4 hours a week during the summer months, but he has also participated in 6-day kayak expeditions. During those trips, he often eats additional carbohydrate without boluses. He treats low blood glucose with glucose gels and fruit juices.

Although she does this activity infrequently, when she does go kayaking Scotland resident Janet G. needs to set a lower temporary basal rate during the activity. She also carries juice with her in the kayak as well as glucose.

For kayaking for longer than an hour, AnneLisa Butcher of California reduces her basal rate to 65 percent of her normal. In addition, if her blood glucose is in her target range to start, she eats an extra snack.

## CURLING

Although you may not know much about it, curling has been a medal sport in the Winter Olympics since 1998. It currently includes men's, women's, and mixed doubles tournaments. Akin to shuffleboard on ice, this unique sport involves players sliding stones (heavy, polished granite stones, or rocks) across a sheet of ice toward a target area, known as the "house," composed of four concentric circles. Two teams of four players (with two stones each) take turns sliding a stone across the ice curling sheet toward the house. The curler can attempt to curve the path of the stone by making it turn while it is sliding, and two teammates armed with brooms ("sweepers") can brush and rub the ice in front of the stone as it slides to decrease or increase the ice's surface friction.

A lot of strategy and teamwork go into choosing the ideal path and placement of a stone each time, and the skills of the curlers affect where the stone finally stops. A game usually consists of 8 or 10 ends, and the team with the highest score (determined by the position of their stones relative to the center of the house) wins the game. Whether you need to adjust your insulin or food for curling may depend on your position and how long you play.

## Athlete Example

Sarah McGaugh from Ontario, Canada, finds that she needs to reduce her insulin levels before the game. She has only curled a couple of times this past year, but when she did it was a day-long bonspiel (curling tournament). For that, she sets up a temporary basal rate when she starts that is 20 percent below normal and tries to keep her blood glucose around 126 mg/dL (7.0 mmol/L). She has found that the more games she plays in one day, the more aggressively she needs to lower her basal rate (more like 30 percent) later in the day. How much she lowers it also depends on her position: when she sweeps a lot rather than walking up and down the sheet, her blood glucose may rise a bit instead.

## CYCLO-CROSS

Cyclo-cross is a specialized type of cycle racing involving many laps on a shorter course, usually 1.5 to 2.0 miles per lap (2.5 or 3.5 kilometers), and races typically occur in the autumn and winter. The race courses feature different types of terrain (pavement, wooded trails, grass, and steep hills), along with obstacles that force riders to dismount and carry their bikes to navigate around them. The relative brevity of cyclo-cross races combined with the challenging terrain and mental stress of competition may result in an increase in blood glucose that will require extra insulin. The intensity of the competition may result in a greater use of muscle glycogen and increase your risk of later-onset lows. Cyclo-cross training may be done at a lower intensity for longer and require more regimen changes.

## Athlete Example

Natalie Koch from Syracuse, New York, usually takes 1 unit of bolus insulin about 5 minutes before starting a cyclo-cross race to prevent a glucose high. Sometimes her blood glucose goes up from races anyway, but she has found that taking even that small amount of insulin keeps it a little more in check. Her usual regimen for lower-adrenaline training days is to exercise before taking her daily Lantus injection because she has found that she is more likely to get low if working out after having taken her basal insulin for the day. She also tries to minimize the amount of bolus insulin she takes beforehand to have less on board that could drop her glucose.

## DOG MUSHING

Dog mushing is a sport unto itself. The most famous of the dog sled races, the Iditarod, is run across the state of Alaska, with the goal of being the first to get from Anchorage to Nome with a team of 12 to 16 dogs pulling the musher and gear on a sled. As the official website states, the Iditarod is a "race over 1,150 miles of the most extreme and beautiful terrain known to man: across mountain ranges, frozen rivers, dense forests, desolate tundra, and windswept coastline. Add to that, temperatures far below zero, winds that can cause a complete loss of visibility, the hazards of overflow, long hours of darkness, and treacherous climbs and side hills, and you have the Iditarod."

As you can imagine, this activity includes many elements that potentially affect your blood glucose, including extreme environmental conditions, lack of sleep, higher-intensity exercise, multiple days of prolonged activity in a row (the average competition time is 10 to 17 days), and more. Because of the extreme nature of this sport, dog mushers have to adjust both food and insulin intake during training and races. You may need insulin on board and have to eat frequently to maintain your blood glucose and body temperature.

### Athlete Example

Bruce Linton, a resident of Soldotna, Alaska, takes in more carbohydrates during periods of exercise, which include the Iditarod dog sled race and Ironman triathlons. He takes much less insulin during the Iditarod because he runs the race on little sleep, sometimes needing no insulin at all during the day while sled racing (or during an Ironman race). In addition, racing outdoors across Alaska in March exposes him to extremely cold temperatures, for which he has to eat more just to maintain his body temperature. His first Iditarod took him more than 15 days to complete. His repeated days of activity during the race also heightened his insulin action.

## DOWNHILL SKIING AND SNOWBOARDING

These activities use a mix of anaerobic and aerobic fuels, depending on your skill level. A skilled skier or snowboarder going down difficult slopes may ski more intensely. If you are constantly shifting and moving, you will rely more on your muscle glycogen and blood glucose. Conversely, skiing straight downhill and letting gravity do most of the work may have a minimal impact on your blood glucose. Spending time in chairlift lines, on the chairlift, or in the lodge warming up will also reduce your blood glucose use. Snow conditions (powdery versus icy), outside temperature, and windchill on the slopes can also affect how your body responds, with more extreme conditions causing you to use more blood glucose to stay warm and requiring greater regimen changes.

## Athlete Profile: **Bruce Linton**

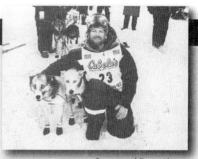

Courtesy of Bruce Linton.

*Hometown:* Soldotna, Alaska

*Diabetes history:* Type 1 diabetes diagnosed in 1993 (at age 30)

*Sport or activity:* Dog mushing, triathlons, running

*Greatest athletic achievement:* Completing the Iditarod dog sled race 6 years in a row, from 2007 through 2012. I have also finished 14 marathons and three full Ironman triathlons with diabetes. I have even qualified for the Boston Marathon, which I have completed three times. Both the Iditarod and the triathlons are extremely challenging, but for different reasons.

*Current insulin and medication regimen:* Insulin pump

*Training tips:* You don't want to be worried about your blood glucose going low during a race, so figure out beforehand how much insulin you need to cut out to keep it stable. It is incredible that your body does not need much insulin and becomes sensitive to it when you are exercising all day long! Also, remember to reduce your basal after you have completed an exercise workout during the night or you will likely go low.

*Typical daily and weekly training and diabetes regimen:* The Iditarod race is a 1,150-mile (1,850-kilometer) dog sled race across Alaska from Anchorage to Nome that occurs day and night and has taken mushers from less than 9 days to more than 32 days to complete. I adjust my insulin intake based on the run and rest schedule of my dogs. When I am out there on the sled, I take less insulin because I am exercising. I also lower it for an all-night run (to avoid going low in the middle of the night while running the sled).

After completing a few marathons, I have found that for this event it is best for me not to take any insulin until the race is over. Most marathons are run in the morning, so I will not take any insulin beforehand, and after 26 miles (42 kilometers) my blood glucose is usually pretty good even though I have not taken any insulin and have consumed a lot of carbohydrate along the way. I learned this the hard way during my first Ironman triathlon when I took about half of the insulin that I normally take. That time, I had too much insulin on board when I got about 15 miles (24 kilometers) into the run, after already completing the 2-mile (3.2-kilometer) swim and 112-mile (180-kilometer) cycling portions, and I could not get my blood glucose up no matter how much carbohydrate I ingested. The next two Ironmans I did were the only 2 full days in my life with diabetes that I did not take any insulin, and I completed them with blood glucoses of 135 and 140.

*Sample training day:* I use a basal of 0.95 units of Humalog per hour and then bolus with a ratio of 1 unit of insulin for every 10 grams of carbohydrate. In an endurance event or training, I reduce my bolus intake when ingesting food to compensate for the exercising that I am doing. I also reduce my basal dose as well if the endurance event occurs over a long period (like the Iditarod or Ironmans).

*Other hobbies and interests:* Raising my 9- and 10-year-old children with my wife while both of us have full-time jobs takes up most of my time. I like to go fishing here on the Kenai Peninsula

continued ➡

*Bruce Linton continued*

in Alaska, and the entire family gets annual downhill ski passes in the winter at Alyeska Resort in Girdwood, Alaska.

**Good diabetes and exercise story:** As I mentioned, 15 miles (24 kilometers) into my 26.2-mile (42-kilometer) run in my first Ironman triathlon, my blood glucose was below 70 mg/dL (3.9 mmol/L). My body was so tired that after every aid station I would check my blood glucose again and ingest more food and liquid. For a long while, no matter how much I ate, my blood glucose would not rise. Finally, after gorging myself with more than 200 grams of carbohydrate, I was able to get it to rise a little bit. It was scary that I was not responding to my food intake. When I finished that race, I was probably the only person in the field to have gained weight after exercising for 13 hours! I learned that day that you really have to lower your insulin a lot when you exercise over a long time.

## Athlete Examples

Regimen changes vary widely with the intensity and duration of skiing or snowboarding as well as the environmental conditions. For regimen changes for cross-country skiing, refer to chapter 9.

### No Changes Necessary

Nina Horvath (Vancouver, Canada) does not adjust anything for downhill skiing. She does not find it sufficient enough exertion to impact her blood glucose.

Scotland resident Becs Badger does not make any immediate changes to her regimen for skiing. She just checks her blood glucose more frequently and treats lows as required with glucose tablets if her glucose drops to less than 72 mg/dL (4.0 mmol/L).

### Insulin Changes Alone

A reduction in insulin needs during these activities is fairly common. For example, Canadian Dessi Zaharieva sets an 80 percent temporary basal rate on her pump for 6 to 8 hours while snowboarding. Similarly, for downhill skiing, Jeff Mazer of Bozeman, Montana, reduces his basal rates on his pump by 20 percent during the activity.

Likewise, Martin Berkeley of Wales sets his pump on a temporary 40 percent of normal basal rate while downhill skiing, whereas Annie Auerback of Madison, Connecticut, reduces hers by 50 percent and checks her blood glucose often. Belgium resident Aline Verbeke simply lowers her bolus for breakfast by 25 to 50 percent before doing these activities, depending on how difficult the day will be, without adjusting her basal insulin.

For skiing, Michael Horgan of Northborough, Massachusetts, also lowers his basal insulin. He watches his CGM and keeps his pump strapped to his chest with a flip belt. He has had problems with his insulin freezing while he is skiing, so he tries to keep it close to his body.

Conversely, Daniel Schneider, a resident of Denver, Colorado, finds that downhill skiing is significantly different than other sports and that during chairlift-accessed skiing he needs to take insulin boluses with snacks and cannot rely on the intermittent skiing activity to lower his blood glucose enough to compensate. He has found that the stress of the cold as well as the high intensity of skiing followed by the low intensity of sitting on a chairlift between runs ultimately leads to hyperglycemia for him.

Canadian Scott Lahrs from West Kelowna, British Columbia, finds snowboarding similarly frustrating. Going from the chairlift to a hard run then repeating that cycle all day keeps his blood glucose level elevated. When he snowboards, he eats very little throughout the day, but then he must consume a lot later when he is back home to prevent overnight lows.

## Diet Changes Alone

Naomi from Spokane, Washington, find that skiing requires her to take in extra carbohydrates. She checks her CGM often, and when she is trending low she eats glucose because it does not freeze. Although Claire T. of Alexandria, Virginia, rarely skis, when she does she merely checks her CGM reading and snacks as needed.

For downhill skiing, Steven Rausch of Navarre, Florida, has to remember to check the pump screen (where his CGM displays) to monitor his blood glucose level often. With all the clothing he wears skiing, he has to keep his pump under the outer layer, usually in a jacket front pocket. He eats about 50 grams of carbohydrates (Clif Bars and dried apricots) if it gets below 90 mg/dL (5.0 mmol/L).

## Combined Regimen Changes

Medford, Oregon, resident A.J. Krebs finds downhill skiing to be tricky to manage. The cold can make fingerstick blood glucose readings hard to obtain and CGM unreliable, and every ski day is different. She always carries glucose and hopes for the best. Some days, a 75 percent reduction in her basal rate works great, but other days it does not. In either case, she finds that cutting her bolus doses for the food she eats during the day is critical to not ending up low on the slopes.

D. Jones from Illinois turns his pump down to 30 percent of his normal basal rate for the entire day he is on the mountain doing downhill skiing. He also checks his glucose every hour. If he is going below 120 mg/dL (6.7 mmol/L), he eats up to three Clif Shot Bloks and slows his pace for a while.

A professional snowboarder, Sean Busby (who is profiled in chapter 5) reduces his basal insulin for this activity. The amount depends on the altitude and temperature, but generally he makes a 30 to 40 percent reduction. He also carries extra prefilled syringes in his coat during competitions and training in case he cannot access his pump quickly under his clothing. To treat lows, he consumes honey (especially if he is on a chairlift). He generally eats a granola or energy bar every 45 to 60 minutes, depending on how hard he has been working. During competitions, he usually lowers his basal rate by only 10 to 20 percent because adrenaline keeps his blood glucose higher.

Karen Stark of Minnesota has found that downhill skiing has a profound effect on her blood glucose. To compensate, she often takes her basal insulin but no bolus (NovoLog) while skiing. She grazes on food throughout the day, and her blood glucose levels stay fairly constant.

When Matt Green of Massachusetts goes skiing or snowboarding, his blood glucose tends to rise even though he keeps his pump on. If he starts out with a blood glucose level of 150 mg/dL (8.3 mmol/L), he does not make any adjustments initially. He checks his glucose frequently, however, to pick up trends and adjust accordingly.

Alex Oppen of Wisconsin finds that snowboarding drops his blood glucose faster than many of his other activities. Sometimes he reduces his basal rate by 10 percent, but more often he simply eats extra carbohydrate to compensate. He treats lows with soda.

### Other Effects to Consider

**Effect of Environmental Conditions and Multiple Days of Activity.** To compete in snowboarding professionally, Sean Busby often trains extremely hard over several days, and he reduces his basal rate further (down to 70 to 80 percent total). He usually makes large reductions during cold spells (−20 to 10 degrees Fahrenheit, or −29 to −12 Celsius) because he finds that his blood glucose drops faster in colder temperatures.

Massachusetts resident Matt Green's biggest problem during downhill skiing or snowboarding is using his glucose meter in the cold. If he takes it out of his jacket pocket, condensation often forms inside its plastic housing. As for his insulin pump, he keeps it close to his body underneath at least one base layer of clothing to protect it from the cold weather.

## HIKING AND BACKPACKING

Both hiking and backpacking are aerobic in nature, requiring the endurance to cover long distances at a relatively slow pace. Backpackers in particular often carry extra weight. While hiking at slower speeds, your body may be able to use quite a bit of fat as fuel, but increasing your speed, going uphill, or climbing will increase your use of blood glucose and muscle glycogen. For hiking, you can simply eat more or lower your insulin; for backpacking, you may need to make changes in your intake of both insulin and food. Of course, the duration of these activities (hours or days), the amount of extra weight that you carry, the temperature, and the altitude can all affect your blood glucose responses and the adjustments you will need to prevent lows (or highs).

Higher altitudes and colder temperatures can increase your blood glucose use, but they may make you insulin resistant at the same time. Hot and humid conditions can predispose you to dehydration (due to increased sweating), as can high altitudes (due to faster breathing rates), so you should be especially careful to drink plenty of fluids because being dehydrated can make your blood glucose appear higher. The terrain can also affect you, as uphill climbing requires more energy

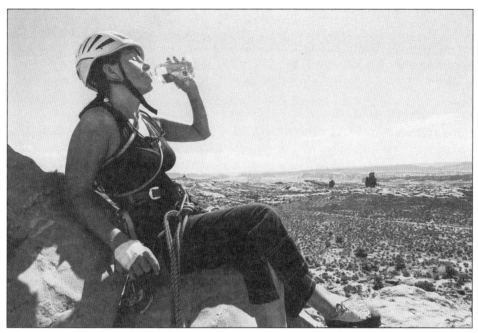

Many outdoor activities pose extra concerns for athletes with diabetes. Along with the activities' intensity and duration, higher altitudes can increase your blood glucose use, making it a good idea to check your level often.

than downhill portions. Your risk for later-onset lows, especially overnight, after such strenuous activities means that you may need to lower your insulin levels and possibly eat a bedtime snack, particularly during several days of hiking or while on multiday backpacking trips.

## Athlete Examples

These examples show the changes that you may need to make for hiking and backpacking to compensate for harsher environmental conditions. Backpackers who use insulin cannot get by with making diet changes alone (without insulin adjustments), although hikers often can. For additional backpacking examples in more extreme environments, see the section on mountaineering later in this chapter.

### Insulin Changes Alone

Jeff Mazer of Bozeman, Montana, usually reduces his basal rates on his pump by 40 to 50 percent for hiking and may lower his boluses as well. If everything goes as planned with his pump settings, he makes minimal adjustments to his carbohydrate intake.

Andrea Limbourg of France reduces her basal rate by about 15 percent during hiking. She checks her glucose occasionally and makes adjustments as needed.

Illinois resident Janet Switzer lowers her basal rate down to 30 percent of normal and starts her hike with a blood glucose reading of at least 150 mg/dL (8.3 mmol/L).

Likewise, Susan Shaw of California lowers her basal to 60 percent of normal if she is going to hike for over an hour.

For hiking, Adelaide Lindahl of Minnesota reduces her basal rate by 0.5 units per hour. But she also has to take a bolus for small meals or snacks (e.g., granola bars) at least every 4 hours to prevent her blood glucose from rising over time.

## Diet Changes Alone

Virginia resident Greg Cutter usually takes day hikes. On these days, he typically has a protein-rich breakfast with moderate carbohydrates and fruit juice. On the trail, he monitors his CGM and eats snacks or sports bars instead of meals. He finds it easy to monitor and make adjustments as needed during his hikes.

For hiking or walking, Linda Frischmeyer of Vancouver, Washington, eats extra carbohydrates without adjusting her insulin doses. Similarly, Pat Shermer of South Dakota exercises regularly and already has her insulin adjusted for it, so when she is hiking she just takes in extra carbohydrates to compensate.

Japan resident Renée McNulty finds that high-altitude hiking above 2,000 meters (6,560 feet) makes her feel nauseated. She drinks a watered-down sports drink to keep her blood glucose up.

## Combined Regimen Changes

For hikes of 10 miles (16 kilometers) or more, Sarah Bancroft from the United Kingdom reduces her basal rates by 50 percent during the walk and for an hour afterward. She also eats about three jelly babies each hour of the walk.

During hikes, Dean McColl of Washington State makes at least a 50 percent reduction in her basal rate, depending on the grade and difficulty of the trail. On difficult and steep trails, she may go without any basal insulin delivery for the duration of the hike. She also eats gluten-free snack bars with 20 grams of carbohydrates every hour and hydrates well because her hydration status also affects her blood glucose levels.

Toronto resident Michael Riddell usually reduces his basal insulin delivery on his pump by about 80 percent 1 hour before he starts his long hikes. When he eats a snack along the way, he only boluses for about half the carbohydrate content in the snack. Using CGM, he can fine-tune the insulin delivery on his pump and/or eat an extra high-GI (glycemic index) snack if needed.

When hiking, Debbie Lewin of Toronto lowers her basal rate starting 2 to 3 hours beforehand. She wears a small backpack with snacks and her treatment for lows in it, along with her favorite activity snacks (protein bars and homemade granola) and her glucagon kit.

When she is backpacking, A.J. Krebs from Oregon finds that having some protein on board helps keep her glucose stable over the longer term. She eats a few more carbohydrates on heavy activity days, but still typically has fewer than 50 grams of carbohydrates total (unless she is treating lows). If her blood glucose is on the low side, she cuts her basal doses. If it is running higher, she leaves the basal rate alone. If her glucose is really high, she increases her basal (which she often has to do after a site change) until she starts trending down. If she has been running reduced basal rates all day and eating low-carbohydrate, high-protein snacks without boluses, she often boluses a little when stopping to set up camp to cover the protein that has not hit her system yet.

Florida resident Mike Joyce enjoys both hiking and trail running, and he intends to hike the Appalachian Trail in the eastern United States soon. He finds that protein and fat intake works best for long-distance hiking, keeping his blood glucose stable without a spike. He also finds that keeping his bolus insulin minimal prevents lows, although on longer backpacking trips he also ends up reducing his doses of Tresiba (long-acting basal insulin).

Jared Sibbitt of Arizona, who is a backpacking instructor, often takes 30-day backpacking trips during the summer. During these trips, he reduces his bedtime Lantus dose by 10 percent and takes smaller Humalog doses (10 to 40 percent lower) with breakfast and dinner. While actively backpacking, he eats small snacks all day long without bolusing for them; these snacks include trail mix, gorp, sesame sticks, nuts, and some low-GI carbohydrates.

For backpacking about a week every year, Garrick Neal of Canada makes adjustments based on the number of hours he is hiking each day and the elevation gain. Usually he makes about a 40 percent reduction in Lantus basal doses and Humalog for meals and snacks.

For hiking or backpacking, Jude Restis of Washington State lowers his basal rates by 40 to 60 percent. In addition, he increases his carbohydrate intake to 20 to 40 grams per hour. To treat lows, he uses glucose tablets, Clif Shot Bloks, and Hammer gels.

Canadian Jen Hanson (who is profiled in chapter 4) often leads groups doing 6- to 8-day trips of remote backpacking, which cover 10 to 25 kilometers (6.2 to 15.5 miles) per day over very rugged terrain with significant elevation changes. She typically sets a 40 percent reduced basal rate for the entire duration of these trips, and she does not return her basal to normal until 2 days after the whole trip ends. On top of the initial 40 percent reduction in her basal rate, she reduces it another 40 percent (down to 80 percent lower than nontrip days) 1 hour before leaving a camp. She resets her basal to the early morning value about 30 minutes before arriving at a camp in view of setting up the campsite, collecting firewood, preparing meals, and so on. On the trail, she boluses 50 percent of normal for lunch, although she takes full boluses for breakfast and dinner. She does not typically bolus for trail snacks, which she consumes every 1 to 1.5 hours. She stays as hydrated as possible, recognizing that water can be scarce. For the scarcer water days, she drinks at least a liter before leaving camp, and she packs another 2 liters for the trail.

## Other Effects to Consider

**Effect of Training.** Jamie Flanagan of Oregon has backpacked across the entire state of Oregon on the Pacific Crest Trail (about 550 miles, or 900 kilometers) in 30 days. He struggled with some lows during the first week, but after that his body adjusted to the daily hiking, even though he was covering 15 to 18 miles (24 to 30 kilometers) a day wearing a 30- to 40-pound pack (14 to 18 kilograms).

**Effect of Dehydration.** At the ages of 58 and 60 Dwain Chapman of Highland, Illinois, hiked the Grand Canyon rim down to the river; after an overnight stay at Phantom Ranch, he hiked back up to the rim. For endurance activities like this he compensates by reducing his basal rate by 50 percent, checking his blood glucose at least once every hour, and eating more carbohydrates along the hike (like small Rice Krispies treats with 20 grams of carbohydrate). He also eats a lunch of crackers, peanut butter, and fruit while giving himself an appropriate bolus. On his first trip to the Grand Canyon, the stress of the climb in the heat resulted in some blood glucose changes that likely reflected dehydration. A physician who was hiking with him thought Dwain was low (even though his meter did not indicate it) and suggested he drink some Gatorade. This turned out to be a major mistake: his blood glucose soared up to 500 mg/dL (27.8 mmol/L), and he had to take a big bolus and rest for about an hour before continuing. When he repeated his hike 2 years later, he had no problems because he worked harder to stay hydrated, checked his blood glucose even more frequently, and nibbled consistently throughout each day.

## HORSEBACK RIDING, RECREATIONAL

Recreational horseback riding is usually a low-intensity activity that mainly requires using your postural muscles to stay on your horse. The faster the horse goes, the more energy you will have to expend to remain in the saddle. Recreational riding generally does not affect your blood glucose much, but going on all-day trail rides or riding while your horse is cantering or galloping can have a greater impact. You may need to increase your carbohydrate intake to keep your blood glucose stable or slightly lower your basal insulin. By way of example, Janet G. from Scotland just monitors her blood glucose carefully and takes glucose when necessary while riding, although she rides infrequently. For athlete examples of similar but more intense riding, see the section on competitive horseback riding in chapter 10.

## HUNTING, FISHING, AND SHOOTING

These activities largely involve endurance, but they usually involve periods of inactivity interspersed with movement. Because they are outdoors activities, environmental extremes (e.g., heat, humidity, coldness, and altitude) can affect blood glucose responses. Fly fishing may be done standing in a cold stream or river and is more active, so it may cause your blood glucose levels to decrease more than hunting or other types of fishing that are stationary.

## Athlete Examples

Given the lower intensity of most of these activities, any regimen changes you need may reflect how much movement you do and possibly the impact of environmental conditions.

### *No Changes Necessary*

For fishing, D. Jones of LaGrange, Illinois, does not usually need to make any changes to his regimen. If he were to start going low, he would either suspend the basal insulin delivery on his pump, eat Clif Shot Bloks, or do a combination of both.

For duck hunting, Thomas Pintar of Indiana does not make any changes because the activity is low intensity compared with his training for triathlons. However, he always carries glucose tablets to treat lows to be on the safe side.

### Insulin Changes Alone

For duck hunting, Kansas City, Missouri, resident N. Hanway suspends his insulin pump during the activity to keep his glucose above 200 mg/dL (11.1 mmol/L). He has a MiniMed 670G hybrid pump that he uses on auto mode most of the time, but it does not do the best job of keeping his blood glucose from crashing, especially when he is active.

### Diet Changes Alone

Scott Dunton enjoys hunting and fishing when he is not surfing. To compensate for these activities, he usually just snacks more, particularly if he is walking a lot while hunting.

Missouri resident Brandon Hunter both hunts and fishes. Because he may be outside for extended periods by himself during these activities, he takes extra food and drinks along with him, but he does not adjust his insulin.

### Combined Regimen Changes

Mike McMahon of Alaska works on commercial fishing boats during the summers, an activity that involves a lot of manual labor. A morning Lantus user, he decreases his dose by about half to avoid lows while he is working, and he eats extra snacks throughout the day as well.

## JET SKIING

For larger jet skis, this activity mainly involves holding on to the handlebars. On certain smaller models, you may have to stand up during this activity. The greatest potential effect on your blood glucose with jet skiing comes from intensity. Short, intense bouts on your jet ski will maintain your blood glucose, but if you ride for long periods you may experience a decrease. For comparable activities, see the athlete examples listed under water skiing and snowmobiling later in this chapter.

## Athlete Example

Cara Gabriel of Green Bay, Wisconsin, says that her family spends a great deal of time on the water at their lake house in the summer (but on ice in the winter). Before she goes jet skiing, she checks her blood glucose and corrects with an insulin bolus or eats something. Out on the water, she has a hard time telling whether she is high or low, but her glucose usually runs on the high side because of the adrenaline. She takes fruit snacks along in case she has a low because sometimes she gets far out on the lake.

## KITEBOARDING AND KITESURFING

A newer fad, these activities involve holding onto a kite while standing on a specialized board (kiteboarding) or a surfboard (kitesurfing) while on the water. The kiteboard is similar in size to a wakeboard, and you are strapped to it with bindings. Kiteboarding combines aspects of wakeboarding, snowboarding, windsurfing, surfing, paragliding, skateboarding, sailing, and gymnastics into one extreme sport. Kitesurfing differs only in that it uses a standard surfboard, usually with no bindings. Kitesurfing focuses more on riding the waves (in an ocean location where waves break) than on hitting the big air and doing tricks like in freestyle kiteboarding.

The intensity of these activities has the greatest potential effect on your blood glucose. Short, intense sessions may maintain your blood glucose. But if you kiteboard or kitesurf for long periods, your blood glucose may decline over time, especially when the winds are strong. See other comparable examples listed under surfing or water skiing in this chapter.

### Athlete Examples

While kiteboarding, Jen Hanson (who is profiled in chapter 4) attempts to keep her blood glucose in the range of 117 to 171 mg/dL (6.5 to 9.5 mmol/L). For her, doing this activity often involves remote locations where it is not safe to leave an insulin pump on shore. Because ocean water, dirt, and adhesives for her insulin pump and CGM have posed problems, she often switches to injections during these outings, despite preferring to use a pump the rest of the time.

Rhet Hulbert from Boise, Idaho, considers this an activity for which he needs very little insulin on board. He occasionally eats some carbohydrates to keep him going.

## MOTORCYCLE RIDING AND RACING (OFF-ROAD)

This activity mainly involves holding on to the handlebars of your motorcycle and navigating across frequently rough terrain, which can involve prolonged contractions in your arms and legs. The biggest effect on your blood glucose during this activity likely comes from the release of adrenaline because of the thrill and danger involved. In the short run, the release of this hormone and others will keep your blood glucose stable or higher, but if you ride for long enough your blood glucose may drop over time. Because of the nature of this activity, adjusting your insulin doses to compensate may be easiest. If you do not use insulin, you may or may not need to eat anything.

### Athlete Examples

Greg Cutter of Norfolk, Virginia, enjoys the adrenaline rush associated with doing off-road motorcycle racing. He always checks his blood glucose before doing this activity, but because getting low during the activity could be fatal, he errs on the high side with his blood glucose (staying greater than 150 mg/dL [8.3 mmol/L]) when he is riding. To accomplish this, he takes a minimal amount of Humalog at breakfast before riding with a higher-protein meal but does not adjust his Lantus dose. He keeps his CGM on the tank bag for easy viewing, so unless his glucose numbers on his CGM suggest that he stop and adjust his blood glucose, he keeps going and going until it is time for a meal. Also, he finds that the adrenaline release tends to keep his blood glucose higher while racing.

United Kingdom resident Kathryn Latham also enjoys off-road motorcycle riding. She has noticed that she has higher blood glucose while riding when she becomes excited, and she finds it difficult to control her stress hormone release during the activity.

Alex Oppen of Wisconsin does a related sport—junior drag racing (which can involve motorcycles or cars). He finds that he needs to check his blood glucose often during this activity because adrenaline release raises his level, but he also avoids going too low, which would affect his ability to focus and race well. For the latter reason, he is cautious about making too many adjustments that may lower his blood glucose while racing.

## MOUNTAIN BIKING

This activity is mostly a prolonged endurance sport, but it requires occasional bursts of anaerobic energy to climb hills and inclines. The adjustments that you will need to make depend mainly on how long and hard you bike and the terrain that you cover. More intense biking, such as what you do during climbs or over difficult terrain, may maintain your blood glucose better from the greater release of glucose-raising hormones, but you will have to watch out for lows after you stop. Mountain biking for long periods will use more of your glycogen stores and blood glucose, increasing your risk for hypoglycemia both during and after the activity. You will need to consume more food and reduce your insulin doses to compensate.

## Athlete Examples

These examples show that mountain biking usually requires changes in both insulin and diet to compensate. For additional cycling examples, refer to the cycling section in chapter 9 and to cyclo-cross earlier in this chapter.

### *Insulin Changes Alone*

New Jersey resident Joe LoCurcio finds that he can usually prevent hypoglycemia with basal rate alterations alone. The changes that he makes depend on how much insulin he has on board. If he boluses for a meal within an hour of riding, he may suspend his pump during a 45-minute to 2-hour ride. The longer and more intense his workouts are, the more likely he is to get low. After an intense 2-hour workout, he keeps his basal rate reduced for more than 4 hours, and his carbohydrate ratio may stay at 50 percent of normal for up to 8 hours.

When mountain biking, D. Jones reduces his basal rate to 30 percent of normal. He checks his blood glucose every hour while doing this activity.

## Diet Changes Alone

Steve Clement from Lewis Center, Ohio, does a lot of mountain bike training for races that last 1 to 6 hours. For that activity, he has been doing low-carbohydrate eating and then slowly running out of steam during the ride. He eats a glucose gel when he feels his energy decrease, but he has not had any issues with low blood glucose. He just avoids taking any insulin boluses close to when he rides.

## Combined Regimen Changes

For Australia native Bec Johnson, her blood glucose generally stays stable or possibly drops a little bit if training longer than an hour. She manages this activity with a low-carbohydrate, protein-rich snack (like nuts, cheese, or a boiled egg) eaten at least 1 to 2 hours beforehand; she finds the slow spike from protein keeps her glucose steady. She also uses caffeine if anticipating a drop during training and has some coffee beforehand (which also keeps her levels higher). If it is too late for her to follow either of these strategies, she consumes small, controlled amounts of glucose to manage a blood glucose level that is trending down.

Canadian Scott Lahrs has a similar regimen for ultradistance mountain biking (as well as cross-country skate skiing). For mountain biking events lasting 3 hours or less, he does not reduce his basal insulin, but for 3 to 6 hours, he reduces it by 25 percent. For 6- to 12-hour events, his reduction is 40 percent; for 12 to 18 hours he lowers it 60 percent; and for over 18 hours, he uses an 80 percent reduction. During the event, he averages taking in 80 to 100 grams of carbohydrates per hour, usually in the form of Tailwind Nutrition, jelly beans, gels, and Clif Shot Bloks. (He never eats sports bars because he finds them too heavy in his stomach and hard to chew.) His carbohydrate intake is moderated by his starting blood glucose: if above 180 mg/dL (10 mmol/L), he does not consume any carbohydrates until it drops below that. His correction carbohydrate amounts depend on how fast his blood glucose is dropping and how hard he is riding. He typically still has 30 to 60 grams per hour, along with backing off his pace a little, and waits to see what happens. If he starts out too high (above 234 mg/dL [13 mmol/L]), he takes a correction bolus dose of 0.5 to 1 unit of insulin. If it becomes that high during a ride, he also takes half a unit and watches it carefully. Once he finishes a ride of 3 hours or less, he eats normally. After longer rides, he goes to bed with his blood glucose over 180 mg/dL (10 mmol/L) to prevent overnight lows. If he rides longer than 6 hours, he usually needs to eat more than double his usual carbohydrates for a normal dinner bolus. After 24-hour solo rides, he just constantly eats carbohydrates after the event. (He says his mind is pretty fried in those cases, and he is just in survival mode.)

North Carolina resident Jimmy Dodson participates in long-distance mountain biking. To maintain his blood glucose, he generally eats 30 to 45 grams of carbohydrates beforehand and supplements at least every 30 to 60 minutes with another 30 to 60 grams. He starts a lower, temporary basal rate (50 to 70 percent of normal) on his pump 20 to 45 minutes before starting, depending on the activity that he will be doing, the expected intensity, the weather, and other factors.

Troy Willard of Georgia challenges himself with mountain biking endurance races, including 12- and 24-hour, 100-mile (160-kilometer), and off-road events. He typically eats a breakfast higher in fat and protein at least 3 hours before starting to balance out his blood glucose early in a race. During it, he sets his basal rate at 50 percent, and he consumes Hammer gels and Clif Bars throughout, taking in about 30 to 45 grams of carbohydrates per hour, but he avoids glucose gels. For training rides, he mixes a recovery drink containing four times more carbohydrates than protein (usually 100 grams of carbohydrates and 25 grams of whey protein), for which he boluses with 8 to 10 units of NovoLog, depending on his blood glucose after a ride. He feels that drinking these protein/carbohydrate shakes helps his legs feel fresher during cycling the next day.

Elise Rayner of Colorado rides daily, doing either road cycling or mountain biking. For her daily workouts lasting 45 to 90 minutes, she reduces her NovoLog by 50 percent for any meal that she eats within 2 hours of riding, but if she rides after that she makes no changes in bolus insulin. For rides longer than 2.5 hours, she reduces her boluses by 80 percent but does not adjust her basal Lantus. Every 45 minutes, she takes in 15 to 20 grams of carbohydrates (typically gels); if her rides last more than 2 hours, she consumes that much every 30 minutes instead and alternates sips of water and electrolyte drinks every 15 minutes. She often needs a postmeal bolus of 1 to 3 units to cover glucose spikes when eating after strenuous rides.

For Renée McNulty of Japan, mountain biking for long periods requires adjustments in both her insulin and food intake. She decreases the basal rates on her pump by almost 60 percent, 60 to 90 minutes before biking more than 2 hours; if she bikes for 3 or more hours, she keeps it reduced for another 12 hours or so. She eats a banana before she begins as well as a 25-gram glucose gel every hour, switching to a 40-gram bar every third hour. Her glucose highs after rides frequently resolve themselves, so she does not always treat them immediately after stopping.

For mountain or road biking, Carrie Czerwonka of Blanchardville, Wisconsin, reduces her basal rate by 50 percent a half-hour before starting and then takes her pump off during 2-hour rides. Afterward she keeps her basal at 50 percent. She mainly eats when disconnecting from and reconnecting to her pump. For longer rides, she leaves her pump on at a basal rate that is 30 to 50 percent below normal, and she eats during the ride. After these workouts, she may have heightened insulin sensitivity for 2 or 3 days afterward.

## *Other Effects to Consider*

Chad Lawrence, a resident of Kingston, New York, enjoys all sorts of bicycling, including road cycling and racing, downhill mountain bike racing, dual slalom racing, and cross-country mountain biking. Dual slalom is a head-to-head competition down a man-made course, usually with gated turns (much like ski racing) and with obstacles such as berms, jumps, bumps, and occasional drops or rock piles. Many of these activities are short and intense (about 30 seconds per dual slalom run), and he finds that the adrenaline rush from these competitions often raises his blood glucose, which he offsets with an increase in his basal rates. He loads with carbohydrates before endurance events and usually lowers his basal rates, depending on how intense and long the ride will be.

# MOUNTAINEERING

Mountaineering is similar to backpacking but generally includes more intense elements. Also known as alpinism in Europe, this activity involves walking, hiking, trekking, and climbing mountains. Originally people just tried to reach the highest points of unclimbed, unconquered mountains, but today the sport has specialized into rock craft, snow craft, and skiing, depending on whether you are ascending rock, snow, or ice. On ice you can wear crampons, spiked footwear that you attach to your boots to give better traction, and on snow you can wear snowshoes or skis. The trips can last for days, during which you carry all your own gear. You may have to contend with freezing temperatures, sudden snowstorms or thunderstorms, and other hazards. The goal of many participants in this sport is summiting peaks that are at least 14,000 feet (4,267 meters) above mean sea level ("the 14ers"), of which there are 54 in Colorado alone.

Mountaineering requires you to deal with high altitudes and cold temperatures, both of which can affect your blood glucose responses. In general, physical stressors like these can increase insulin resistance, keeping your glucose higher overall. If being at altitude gives you mountain sickness, you may not feel like eating, will become dehydrated more easily, and may experience high blood glucose levels. Being really cold also may increase your risk of hypoglycemia, particularly if you are shivering (which counts as activity). Any type of mountaineering requires significant food intake during the activity, along with altered insulin levels to prevent hypoglycemia or hyperglycemia, depending on the conditions. See other (less extreme) athlete examples under hiking and backpacking, found earlier in this chapter.

## Athlete Examples

These examples show the extreme changes in food and medications that you will likely need to make for mountaineering. They also point out how other factors such as cold environments and high altitudes affect blood glucose as well.

### Combined Regimen Changes

Ginny Barndollar of Bethel Park, Pennsylvania, loves the outdoors. She says, "Just put me on a trail, and I am one happy person." On mountaineering and backpacking trips, she typically covers 15 to 20 miles (24.1 to 32.1 kilometers) a day. As a low-carbohydrate athlete, she mainly eats protein and fats on the trail (and a few carbohydrates) and stays hydrated. She prepares all her backpacking meals, so she knows the carbohydrate counts and ingredients. However, even for her, extreme weather has been a concern during her mountaineering treks, especially when her pump is buried under two heavy jackets and is hard to access. Also, she has found her CGM to be finicky in cold weather. She uses the MiniMed 670G hybrid closed-loop system, which has helped some with these issues, and she sets a temporary glucose target. Before she had the 670G, she used to disconnect her pump and use pens to inject insulin on many expeditions. So far, she has not had any issues with her hybrid system malfunctioning in extreme weather conditions.

For mountain climbing in winter, Dan Stone from Middletown, Pennsylvania, puts his insulin and blood glucose testing equipment in an insulated pouch next to his skin to prevent it from freezing, and he keeps a backup vial of insulin with a hiking partner. He manages his blood glucose using a lower temporary basal rate on his pump and carbohydrate intake based on his CGM readings and how long he is active. He finds that mountain climbing and hiking require changes similar to marathon running. He sets his basal rate at 0.2 to 0.4 units per hour and ingests carbohydrates as needed (when his CGM reading is less than 100 mg/dL [5.6 mmol/L]) because he aims to keep his blood glucose between 100 and 140 mg/dL (7.8 mmol/L) throughout.

A participant in various aspects of mountaineering, including hiking, rock and ice climbing, and high-altitude climbing, David Panofsky of Wisconsin enjoys summiting mountains and helping other athletes do the same, starting with IDEA 2000—the International Diabetic Expedition to Aconcagua, in Argentina. From personal experience, he knows that this activity involves juggling many factors along with diabetes, including high altitude, cold weather, lack of sleep, emotional stress, and malfunctioning diabetes equipment in harsh environments, just to name a few. In general, he finds that the trekking approach to a mountain (backpacking to the base camp) requires a 75 percent decrease in his basal insulin rates, followed by some boluses or a slight increase over 8 hours. For the high-altitude mountaineering portion, he may need either to decrease or to increase his basal rates by 25 percent. During certain aspects of mountaineering (e.g., leading, soloing, or scrambling), he believes that letting his blood glucose stay slightly higher may be safer than risking a low. Although eating extra is important throughout the activity, he treats lows with licorice, Clif Bars and gels, Clif Shot Bloks, soda, and sports drinks.

## Other Effects to Consider

A resident of North Carolina, Jimmy Dodson finds that his biggest challenge with mountaineering has been adjusting to the altitude. Until he acclimatizes to a new altitude, his blood glucose runs higher, as though he were sick—he does experience acute mountain sickness. For elevations above about 8,000 feet (2,400 meters), he has to increase his basal rates by 20 to 40 percent of normal for 1 to 3 days. He monitors his body's acclimatization by checking his resting heart rate (when he wakes up) and his basal insulin needs, both of which go back down to normal once his body adapts to a certain altitude.

For winter mountaineering, Maggie Crawford of San Diego, California, keeps her insulin and electronics on her body to keep them warm. She considers the remoteness of her location and may run her glucose a little high or bring extra food if she finds herself in a remote location with any risk of going low. Her blood glucose runs on the high side when she is at higher altitudes, so she ends up working hard to keep it in an appropriate range while spending lots of time pushing herself in the mountains.

Monica Tusch of Brighton, United Kingdom, has found that when she reaches a certain altitude during high-altitude mountaineering, it is difficult for her to measure her blood glucose levels accurately due to the effect of the altitude on her meter.

She also becomes insulin resistant. She has found that it is a fine line between reducing her basal rates while trekking but then increasing them once she reaches that threshold altitude.

Although his primary activity is mountaineering, David Hillebrandt of Holsworthy, Devon in the United Kingdom also does a lot of hill walking, skiing, rock and ice climbing, and kayaking. His diabetes management depends on weather, ascent, descent, length of planned activity, and the potential risk if a low occurs.

Paul Coker of Cardiff, Wales, found that being at high altitude (4,500 meters, or ~15,000 feet) on Mount Kilimanjaro made him massively insulin resistant. To compensate, he switched to fasting and taking correction boluses every hour to keep his blood glucose below 600 mg/dL (33.3 mmol/L). The effects of altitude can mimic the symptoms of diabetic ketoacidosis (DKA), and being insulin resistant in such an inhospitable environment often means that stopping to rest is not an option; he had to do careful monitoring, make plenty of corrections (via syringe) for 200 percent basal rates, and maintain his hydration to reach the summit.

## PADDLEBOARDING, STAND-UP

Paddleboarding used to be an activity that involved lying prone or kneeling on a surfboard and paddling with both arms in an overhead swimming motion. However, the modern offshoot involves standing balanced on a long paddleboard (or occasionally kneeling) and propelling yourself forward using a long paddle (rather than your arms) on one side of the board or the other, either on the ocean or in a lake. This type of paddleboarding is called either stand-up paddleboarding or stand-up paddlesurfing. (See other similar athlete examples under windsurfing later in this chapter.)

## Athlete Examples

Sara Pomish of Michigan normally does not change her regimen for paddleboarding. She keeps her blood glucose between 80 and 130 mg/dL (4.4 and 7.2 mmol/L) for all activities. If she is around 70 mg/dL (3.9 mmol/L) before she starts, she may eat a few jelly beans to start to bring her glucose up a little.

Idaho resident Rhet Hulbert considers paddleboarding to be an activity where he is moving at a slower endurance pace. He finds he needs very little insulin on board and occasionally some carbohydrates to keep him going. His target during this activity is a blood glucose of 120 to 150 mm/dL (6.7 and 8.3 mmol/L).

## POWERBOAT RACING

Powerboat racing is an extreme activity that involves racing point to point on ocean-going, inflatable powerboats. This sport is a very physically demanding, full-body workout, especially for the back and arms. The boats can reach up to 100 kilometers (62 miles) per hour on the open ocean waters. Adrenaline release is also a factor and can raise blood glucose, although the duration of the races can lead blood glucose to drop over time without adjustments.

## Athlete Example

South Africa resident Lyndon Collins worked with his diabetes specialist to come up with a plan that would allow him to do powerboat racing with type 1 diabetes (which he did regularly for 15 years, only stopping for about 6 years due to work commitments and having kids). His two-man team won a circuit racing world title in 2009 in the P750 class with a record time that still stands with the Union Internationale Motonautique (UIM).

Although Lyndon uses basal–bolus injections, his diabetes management plan only included raising his blood glucose above 216 mg/dL (12.0 mmol/L) with glucose and then checking it after every circuit race (each lasting about 20 minutes) when doing three races per day over 2 days. By the end of each race day, his glucose would normally come down on its own to a reasonable level. He usually did surf circuit racing, consisting of 12 laps on a course set out in the waves. He also participated in long-haul racing out at sea, which was 120 to 180 kilometers (75 to 112 miles) per race. This involved constant racing with only seconds-long pit stops for fuel—not long enough to easily check his glucose. Leaving a pit stop required navigating and holding on while punching back waves and heading back out to sea. He always carried water to counter the dehydration caused by having higher blood glucose for the first couple of hours, or he used a camel pack to stay hydrated during long races. Although he managed to never get too low in all his years of racing, he ended up with other physical issues, such as dislocated shoulders and broken ribs, fingers, and toes. The adrenaline release and his competitive nature also assisted in racing and keeping his blood glucose up.

## ROCK AND ICE CLIMBING

Outdoor rock climbing, bouldering, and ice climbing all have some aerobic aspects, but many of the movements that these activities require are quick, powerful, and intense (e.g., grabbing and pulling) with rest periods in between moves. Bouldering requires less equipment, but for climbing you need proper gear and safety equipment while you ascend difficult rock faces, particularly when they are covered in ice. Carrying your gear can weigh you down and increase the intensity of your workout. More difficult climbing may initially maintain your blood glucose better (because of the greater hormone release), but you will use more muscle glycogen and have a greater risk of later-onset lows. Prolonged climbing also increases your muscle glycogen use and requires you to make greater regimen changes. The more intense your activity is and the longer it lasts, the greater your risk is for lows during the later stages and afterward. Harsher environmental conditions (like cold) can also impact your blood glucose responses and the necessary adjustments.

## Athlete Examples

You can use changes in insulin, diet, or usually both to compensate for this activity. The regimen adjustments differ when you climb for longer periods or more intensely. For other relevant athlete examples, see bouldering earlier in this chapter and climbing indoors in chapter 8.

## No Changes Necessary

Washington State resident Dean McColl finds that outdoor climbing—unlike climbing in a gym—may not require her to make many adjustments. Depending on the intensity of her climbing route, her blood glucose may not drop at all, with no insulin changes due to the adrenaline release she gets while climbing.

For free climbing, Mauro Sormani of Italy leaves his basal rates the same as normal. The physical and emotional stresses associated with this activity keep his blood glucose from dropping while he is doing it.

When rock climbing, Jared Sibbitt of Arizona does not make many adjustments because this is more of an anaerobic activity for him. When climbing at high altitude, however, he experiences some insulin resistance; this keeps his blood glucose from dropping as much, so he keeps his insulin about the same as usual.

## Insulin Changes Alone

Dan Stone of Pennsylvania considers rock climbing and bouldering anaerobic activities and adjusts his regimen accordingly. For such activities, he does not make any adjustments beforehand and sometimes reduces his basal rate for 12 hours afterward.

## Combined Regimen Changes

A.J. Krebs from Medford, Oregon, finds that her blood glucose response while climbing depends on her starting blood glucose. Climbing sometimes makes her glucose spike, so if she is starting out above 150 mg/dL (8.3 mmol/L), she sets a temporary basal rate on her pump that is 150 percent of normal. If she is in the range of 100 to 150 mg/dL (5.6 to 8.3 mmol/L), she makes no change to her basal rate. If she is under 100 mg/dL (5.6 mmol/L), she has carbohydrates available and keeps an eye on her CGM readings.

Wisconsin resident David Panofsky finds it important to eat more during both ice and rock climbing to prevent lows, and he even keeps his blood glucose slightly higher during certain portions of climbing. In addition, he initially lowers his basal rates by 25 percent, but if the activity is prolonged, he lowers them by 50 percent total, along with bolusing 50 percent less for meals and giving it slowly over a few hours (with an extended bolus on a pump) instead of all at once.

For Jimmy Dodson of North Carolina, ice climbing requires him to cut his basal rates to 30 percent of normal. On many days while he is climbing he can eat up to 30 grams of carbohydrates per hour without taking any bolus insulin. The cold temperatures he experiences during this activity increase his body's use of blood glucose to try to stay warm.

While walking the approach to where he will be ice climbing, Edwin Sherstone of Southport in the United Kingdom has to increase his carbohydrate intake by 30 to 50 grams and reduce his fast-acting insulin by a unit or two. During the actual climbing portion, he does not need to supplement at all due to the intensity of the climb.

## SAILING

Sailing is mainly an anaerobic activity, requiring short, powerful movements, such as pulling a rope to adjust a sail. You may not move that much between pulls other than to maintain your balance while standing (or sitting) on the deck. The intensity of your activities may also vary with the size of the boat, the number of crew members, and the strength of the wind. Strong winds may not affect larger boats, which usually carry more crew members and thus require less work from each person. Particularly on smaller boats, strong winds will require more effort and more directional changes to control your course. For most recreational sailing, you may need no changes in your insulin or food intake. For intensive sailing, involving more physical labor, you may need to reduce your insulin doses and eat more.

## Athlete Example

For sailboat races lasting all day and sometimes overnight, Greg Cutter of Virginia checks his blood glucose on his CGM frequently and errs on the high side (greater than 150 mg/dL [8.3 mmol/L]) because getting low during this activity can be dangerous. The level of his nutrition intake depends on the size of the boat: for small racing dinghies, he keeps sports bars in his pockets, and for larger racing boats, he tends to eat real sandwiches instead of just snacking.

## SCUBA DIVING

Scuba (self-contained underwater breathing apparatus) diving is a low-intensity aerobic activity that involves slow kicking and some arm movement. The main concern, as far as diabetes goes, is the high environmental pressure experienced underwater. This pressure can increase your absorption of insulin from your skin (where you injected or pumped it) and may cause low blood glucose while you are underwater, which can go unrecognized or be difficult to treat. Historically, insulin users have not been allowed to obtain certification from the National Association of Underwater Instructors (NAUI) to allow them to scuba dive legally, although you can be certified through the Professional Association of Diving Instructors (PADI), which has allowed many athletes taking insulin to dive safely.

*Since 1997, the Diver Alert Network (DAN) has recognized that insulin users with diabetes can engage in scuba diving. They created a set of guidelines on how to dive safely, which is accessible at www.diversalertnetwork.org /files/DiabetesSummaryGuidelines.pdf.*

There are many contraindications to scuba diving (including bad sinus infections), but the guidelines for safe diving for people with diabetes focus primarily on managing blood glucose levels. If you use insulin, you should determine whether your predive blood glucose level is stable, rising, or falling by checking it at 60 minutes, 30 minutes, and immediately beforehand. Aim to be slightly higher than normal, such as 150 to 180 mg/dL (8.3 to 10.0 mmol/L), and stable. If your glucose is lower but rising, do not dive until it reaches at least 145 mg/dL (8.1 mmol/L). Under no circumstances should you start your dive if your blood glucose is dropping. Consume carbohydrates until your blood glucose is stable or rising and carry some with you in a waterproof container (e.g., gels or cake frosting) to eat when you surface, if you need to. Avoid injecting bolus doses of insulin within 2 hours of dives to lower your risk of having to deal with a low underwater.

To dive safely, you should be able to recognize and treat your own lows, have no advanced diabetes complications (such as unstable proliferative retinopathy, because increases in your intraocular pressures may cause hemorrhages), and dive with a buddy who is educated about your diabetes care. If you develop a low while underwater, signal your buddy with an "L" sign using your thumb and forefinger (meaning "low" in this case, not "loser"), and begin to surface. A dive depth limit of 90 feet (27.4 meters) is recommended to keep you from confusing the symptoms of nitrogen narcosis with low blood glucose and to avoid needing decompression therapy. Keep in mind that colder water will increase your metabolic rate while you are diving, even if you wear a wet suit, and may require you to make greater changes in insulin or carbohydrate intake before diving than needed in warmer water.

## Athlete Examples

The following examples show that most people try to reduce their insulin level and raise their blood glucose for dives by taking less insulin and eating more beforehand.

### Diet Changes Alone

For scuba diving, Arizona resident Jared Sibbitt runs his blood glucose slightly higher than normal to avoid any chance of becoming hypoglycemic underwater. He checks his glucose frequently before diving to get an idea of his trends, and he eats additional snacks if he needs to before diving.

### Combined Regimen Changes

Steve Prosterman (profiled later in this chapter) teaches scuba diving and is in charge of groups of diving researchers and college students on a regular basis, so it is very important for him to maintain his awareness and not go low while diving. He has figured out very good protocols for himself that can help others avoid lows as well. He uses serial checks of his blood glucose to find out which way it is heading. (Using a CGM can help, but its values need to be checked with a meter, and it cannot be worn during a dive.) He checks his glucose a few times within an hour before diving to make sure it is not dropping, and he eats some snacks with carbohydrates (apples, fruit snacks, or bars) if it is lower than 140 to 150 mg/dL (7.8 to 8.3 mmol/L) before starting a dive.

Troy Sandy from Indiana makes sure he has very little insulin on board before scuba diving. He checks his blood glucose at 1 hour, half an hour, and just before diving to make sure he is not trending down. He keeps a glucose gel in his pocket during the dive. (He admits that he has needed a gel underwater before, but found it is not as tasty with some saltwater mixed in.) He checks his glucose again as soon as he comes up from a dive and gets out of the water. He wears a CGM before and after diving (not during), but always verifies its readings with a blood glucose meter before starting a dive.

Canadian Dessi Zaharieva has a set of rules she follows to scuba dive safely. First, she takes her pump off completely. She tries to start with blood glucose levels that are higher than normal, in the range of 180 to 216 mg/dL (10 to 12 mmol/L) because going low underwater is not an option. She checks her blood glucose during breaks and eats snacks if she needs them to raise her blood glucose. She finds that wet suit diving is not as challenging as dry suit diving due to the greater impact of the cold water temperature on her glucose when diving without her wet suit to warm her up.

To scuba dive safely, Greg Cutter of Virginia checks his blood glucose before diving and eats enough snacks to raise his glucose to over 150 mg/dL (8.3 mmol/L) to avoid dangerous lows while underwater, especially because he cannot use his CGM while diving or snorkeling. Before diving, he takes a bolus for breakfast that is only 50 percent of his usual as he prefers to err on the high side rather than be too low during submersion. Because this activity only lasts for an hour or two, he makes other insulin adjustments later to lower his glucose if it is on the high side afterward.

Massachusetts teenager Jackson Burke plans ahead for scuba diving because he cannot easily eat if he goes low underwater. He and his doctor decided that he should start a dive with his blood glucose at 180 mg/dL (10.0 mmol/L), have no active insulin on board, disconnect his pump and CGM, eat a snack before going down, and check his glucose again whenever he surfaces at intervals and make adjustments then as needed. He typically comes up from a dive with the same blood glucose level as when he goes down. He reconnects to his pump after diving and runs an increased temporary basal to cover for going without any insulin for about 3 hours.

Oregon resident Jeannette Styles has found scuba diving to be a learning experience. When she goes on dive trips with her husband, which involve diving three to four times a day, she changes her insulin usage completely. She switches from just using a pump to combining pump use with injections of basal insulin. She takes about 50 percent of her normal daily basal as Lantus (split between morning and evening doses) on the night before she starts her dives, and she reduces the basal rate on her pump by 50 percent to avoid having too much basal on board after the Lantus starts working. Because she dives with her pump off, she eats small snacks with protein if her starting glucose is below 150 mg/dL (8.3 mmol/L). About an hour after finishing diving each day, she reconnects her pump and checks her blood glucose. She then corrects any elevations and boluses for her next meal. Although she does not find scuba diving to be very strenuous, she has found in the past that if she disconnects without using Lantus to cover the missed basal, her blood glucose creeps up all day long, and she wants to avoid having to give a short-acting bolus before diving because that increases her risk of going low underwater. She says that going low would ruin a good dive (not to mention be potentially dangerous).

Emily Marrama from Lynn, Massachusetts, switches from using her pump (which she cannot take underwater) to a basal–bolus injection regimen for scuba diving. In addition to checking her glucose before and after each dive, she tends not to correct it unless it is over 200 mg/dL (11.1 mmol/L), just to be on the safe side underwater. She did notice an increase in her A1C after a 6-week dive vacation after using this regimen because she let it run higher most of that time.

# Prevailing Over a Diabetes-Related Obstacle to Scuba Diving

In this book, you can see that diabetes does not keep people from participating in every conceivable sport and recreational physical activity! Before you read the last athlete profile, I want to tell you a story about how this athlete helped me overcome the only seemingly insurmountable obstacle that I have encountered while having diabetes for most of my life.

When I was working on my master's degree back in 1987, I happily enrolled in a scuba diving certification course through my university. A friend of mine was one of the instructors, and I was so excited about finally learning how to dive because I love the ocean—although we were supposed to be diving at Lake Tahoe. I had already bought all the gear I needed to get started—only to be unceremoniously booted from the class after I had uttered the words "I have diabetes" during my required predive physical. It was a NAUI certification course, and that organization does not certify anyone with diabetes "on insulin therapy or oral anti-hyperglycemia medication" (their exact wording).

NAUI to this day contends that "even if diabetes is well controlled, exercise lowers the need for insulin; for such a person, any unexpected exertion needed for self or buddy rescue would make the normal insulin dose excessive, thus favoring a reaction." Not only are their statements obsolete, but so are their policies. I know this now, but I did not at the time, and

I was devastated by this setback. Diabetes had never before kept me from doing anything I wanted to, even though I had only gotten my first blood glucose meter the year before. (In high school, without a way to measure my blood glucose, I was the jack of all team sports, master of none.) I also did not know back then that PADI, the other primary scuba diving organization, does certify people with type 1 diabetes to dive, and thousands of individuals with diabetes have dived safely over the years. The Diver Alert Network has also advised people with diabetes about how to stay safe while diving, and many of their recommendations are based on the input and extensive diving experience of a person I was soon to meet, who has type 1 diabetes.

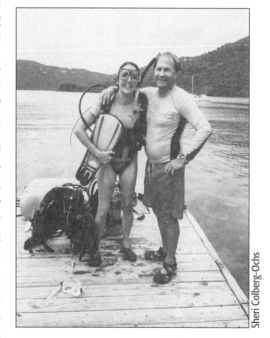

Sheri Colberg-Ochs

In 1990 while I was working on my PhD in exercise physiology at the University of California, Berkeley, I attended a meeting of the now-defunct International Diabetic Athletes Association (IDAA) in Phoenix, Arizona, where I attended a presentation about scuba diving by scuba instructor Steve Prosterman of the University of the Virgin Islands, who had already been living with type 1 diabetes for a year longer than my own two plus decades with it. When I spoke to him afterward, he invited me to come down to St. Thomas anytime to learn how to dive. At that time, he was running weeklong summer camps for adults with type 1 diabetes to learn scuba diving and other water sports. I did not have the money or the time while I was in graduate school to consider going there, but his offer always stayed in the back of my mind.

A few years ago, as I contemplated reaching the half-century milestone of my life, I decided that I really wanted to go somewhere tropical to celebrate. I contacted Steve Prosterman, and he said the offer for him to teach me how to dive was still good, although more than 20 years had passed. Putting aside my few remaining reservations, I ditched the kids for a few days, grabbed my husband, and took Steve up on it. Finally, I fulfilled my almost lifelong dream of going scuba diving—on my 50th birthday! It was the best way I could have ever celebrated a half-century of life and almost 46 years with type 1 diabetes. I will always be indebted to Steve for helping me make my dream finally come true. Final score: Sheri (and Steve), 1, type 1 diabetes and NAUI, 0. Take that!

## SKATEBOARDING

This activity is mainly anaerobic, involving short bursts of intense activity such as jumping, and more prolonged and aerobic use of postural muscles to maintain balance. Usually, you will need minimal changes in your insulin or food intake for recreational skateboarding (depending on how long you skate), but if you use it as a form of transportation, the activity is more aerobic in nature and may require greater adjustments to compensate. See inline skating in chapter 8 for comparable athlete examples.

## Athlete Example

For New Jersey resident Michael Luzzi, skateboarding usually makes his blood glucose go low. Because he usually skateboards after breakfast when his insulin levels are higher, he can do this activity for only 45 minutes or so without becoming low. If it is hot, he has to check his level more frequently because he may not detect the symptoms of his lows as easily.

## SKI TOURING

Ski touring is skiing in the backcountry on unmarked or unpatrolled areas, similar to backcountry skiing. Typically, ski touring is done off piste (off trail) and outside of ski resorts and may last more than 1 day. A defining characteristic of this type of skiing is that your heels are free of bindings, which allows you to have a more natural gliding motion while traversing and ascending terrain that ranges from perfectly flat to extremely steep. Touring gives you potential access to areas of new snow, and may involve your having some independent navigational skills. Some routes may lead to less stable areas (that is, potential avalanche terrain). Given that ski touring is similar to hiking and wilderness backpacking (but with snow), how much you alter your insulin or food intake likely depends on the duration of the activity, how hard your terrain is to traverse, the altitude, and cold temperatures. You also have to worry about carrying all your supplies and keeping them from freezing during long tours.

## Athlete Examples

For ski touring, special preparations and precautions are likely to be necessary for managing diabetes and making changes in diet and insulin.

### *Insulin Changes Alone*

For all-day ski touring, Nina Horvath (Vancouver, British Columbia) checks her blood glucose every hour and snacks then as well. She usually likes higher fat and protein snacks like nuts and eating half an energy bar to keep from dropping too low.

### *Combined Regimen Changes*

For Wales resident Peter Arrowsmith, ski touring off piste is probably the most endurance-based activity he does. For long ski-touring routes, he lowers his insulin doses and takes in constant small amounts of carbohydrates. (He says a couple of beers in mountain huts help.) For basal insulin, he uses Humulin I (isophane, or NPH, an intermediate-acting insulin), and for meals he uses Humalog. For minor lows, he takes jelly beans or jelly babies, but he uses energy gels for more severe drops. He once skied a world cup run fine as low as 27 mg/dL (1.5 mmol/L) because it was too stormy to wait at the top of the mountain.

For backcountry ski touring, Sean Busby, a resident of Montana and Alaska (profiled in chapter 5), can be stricter with his diabetes management than he used to be when traveling to remote areas. Although climbing and hiking in the cold on touring skis lowers his blood glucose quickly, his management is now tighter based on trends he can see using CGM. If he is in avalanche terrain, he will treat with carbohydrates at readings of 90 to 100 mg/dL (5.0 to 5.6 mmol/L), depending on how long he will be exposed when it is imperative that he keep moving to stay safe. Sometimes he is in avalanche terrain for hours, which requires that he read the terrain and know what he is doing before going into lengthy climbs; having CGM for his diabetes management has helped immensely. He makes basal rate changes frequently, depending on the climate and how many days of strenuous exercise he does in a row.

During ski touring, Hans Timmermans of the Netherlands consumes mostly glucose, fruit, or bread. He must also cut back on his insulin doses to prevent lows. He only takes Lantus at bedtime, but he covers his insulin needs for meals during the day with bolus insulin doses.

## SKYDIVING, PARASAILING, AND HANG GLIDING

These activities mainly involve the muscular contractions required to hold on to your parachute lines, parasail, or hang glider and have little or no immediate impact on your blood glucose. But these activities may cause an increase in your anxiety level and a release of adrenaline, which can raise your glucose. Skydivers in particular should monitor their blood glucose before and after diving. If your blood glucose increases, you may need some insulin to lower it afterward. Neither decreases in insulin beforehand nor food intake during these activities is usually necessary. The only exception is if you have to carry your hang glider, parasail, or parachute a long distance after landing, in which case you may need to eat some extra food to compensate for that aerobic activity.

## SNORKELING

Snorkeling is a low-intensity aerobic exercise. This activity is slower and less intense than regular swimming because you do not use your upper body as much to snorkel. Even though kicking with swim fins is a harder workout for your legs, you often kick more slowly with fins on, so the intensity of snorkeling can vary somewhat with your kicking speed and whether you spend time floating or minimally kicking. Because of its low intensity, you will need few, if any, regimen changes to maintain your blood glucose. The most important variable is how long you snorkel. For short durations you may not need to make any changes, but if you snorkel for an hour or longer, you may have to increase your food intake and decrease your insulin somewhat. Also, if you are kicking harder for a long time, expect a drop in your blood glucose and make adjustments to prevent lows.

## Athlete Example

Washington State resident Naomi only finds snorkeling to be a challenge due to dealing with her diabetes technology in the ocean water. She makes sure that her blood glucose is a little higher to start, disconnects her pump during snorkeling, and then gets out of the water to check her CGM monitor every half-hour or so.

When snorkeling in warm water in Hawaii or the Caribbean, California resident Sheri Ochs finds she needs to make minimal changes to her food intake and no insulin adjustments for this activity. She gives her usual Lantus in both the morning and the evening on a snorkeling trip day, and she checks her blood glucose before and after doing an hour of snorkeling. If her blood glucose is on the low side before snorkeling, she may eat a small snack first, but she does not expect it to drop much with only basal insulin on board.

## SNOWMOBILING

Snowmobiling is primarily an anaerobic activity that involves holding on while you are riding, but it also involves more aerobic use of your postural (core) muscles. How hard you are working due to the terrain and how long you ride will affect your blood glucose responses, especially if the activity becomes more aerobic as its duration increases. You may need to eat more and possibly reduce your insulin doses for this activity when it lasts for longer than an hour. Your responses may also be affected by how cold it is. Generally, colder temperatures and lower windchill will increase your glucose use and require greater regimen changes.

## Athlete Examples

Sean Busby of Whitefish, Montana, tries to be well prepared when going snowmobiling in the backcountry. He takes extra precautions, such as bringing extra insulin, food, and water with him, and he checks his blood glucose frequently to see how the elements (along with the exercise) are affecting him. Bringing extra batteries for his insulin pump is also important because he has found that cold weather drains them more quickly.

For snowmobiling, D. Jones of LaGrange, Illinois, reduces his basal rate on his pump down to only 10 percent of normal. In addition, he checks his blood glucose every hour and eats Clif Shot Bloks if his glucose goes under 120 mg/dL (6.7 mmol/L). When doing cold weather exercise, he keeps his glucose meter in an inside pocket to keep it close to body temperature or it will not work.

## SNOWSHOEING

Snowshoeing is usually a slower movement than regular walking, but it can be more intense because of the resistance of pulling your snowshoe up and out of the snow with each step, especially in powdery snow conditions. The terrain covered is similar to what you might encounter when hiking, backpacking, or cross-country skiing. How much you alter your insulin or carbohydrate intake will depend on the duration of the activity and other environmental factors such as high altitude and low temperatures.

## Athlete Examples

For most people engaging in moderate snowshoeing, a combination of diet and insulin changes appears to work best to maintain blood glucose.

### Diet Changes Alone

For snowshoeing, Mark Robbins of Victor, New York, makes sure that his blood glucose is at least 140 mg/dL (7.8 mmol/L) when he starts. To stay balanced, he eats snacks as needed during this activity.

Oregon resident A.J. Krebs eats more protein to keep her glucose more stable while snowshoeing. She eats a few more carbohydrates on heavy activity days but still typically has fewer than 50 grams of carbohydrates total a day (unless she is treating lows) because she follows a low-carbohydrate regimen.

### Combined Regimen Changes

While he is snowshoeing, Illinois resident D. Jones suspends his pump. He also checks his blood glucose every 20 to 30 minutes.

Alisa Krakel of Colorado goes on long snowshoeing outings during which she tries to eat some additional carbohydrates every hour. She also reduces the basal rate on her pump to 30 to 40 percent of normal because this activity is strenuous and prolonged when she does it.

Although Bob Paxson of California generally does not make adjustments in his basal rate for snowshoeing, he eats more carbohydrates during the activity. He lowers his basal somewhat when he experiences low blood glucose that he cannot bring up easily, even with food and glucose. He says this happens to him more frequently during extremely cold weather.

## SURFING AND BOOGIEBOARDING

Surfing and boogieboarding both require you to use your postural muscles more aerobically to maintain your balance while riding a wave. A more anaerobic component arises when you paddle hard with your arms to get out to the waves or quickly recruit additional muscles to help you adjust to changes in the waves while surfing. The duration of a ride can be rather short, making these activities more intermittent than continuous. You may need to make regimen changes depending on how long you are active and how large and how rough the waves are. Riding on or paddling against stronger waves for a longer period will use more of your blood glucose than riding or paddling in calmer conditions. The water and outside temperatures can also affect your glucose responses.

## Athlete Examples

These examples show that you can manage these activities with a variety of regimen changes. Duration and wave conditions can affect the changes you will need to make.

### Insulin Changes Alone

While surfing, Jamie Flanagan of Oregon takes his pump off. He generally checks his blood glucose every 20 to 30 minutes during the activity.

Likewise, Benny Privratsky of California removes his pump for surfing. He adjusts after checking his glucose and before disconnecting. If he starts with his blood glucose at a good level, he can usually surf or bodysurf for 30 to 40 minutes without needing many changes. He always takes some snacks with him to the beach.

### Diet Changes Alone

For California resident Alexis Pollak, surfing requires her to monitor her blood glucose more closely because she is less aware of lows while she is in the water. She generally likes to start with a higher level (around 200 mg/dL [11.1 mmol/L]) because the water and waves make lows more dangerous. To raise it beforehand, she usually eats some glucose tablets and keeps GU energy gel on hand to treat lows.

### Combined Regimen Changes

Southern California resident Peter Nerothin applies his situational approach to managing his blood glucose to surfing as well. He avoids surfing with any fast-acting bolus insulin on board whenever possible, preferring to only have basal Levemir in his system whenever he is active. He also carries supplies with him to treat lows. Knowing that he cannot use his CGM while surfing, he tends to play it safe and let his glucose run a little higher during this activity (but never over 200 mg/dL [11.1 mmol/L]).

A former professional surfer, Scott Dunton takes his pump off before surfing, and he tries to have his blood glucose at 140 mg/dL (7.8 mmol/L) or higher. His glucose is usually relatively stable during this activity, although how long he surfs varies depending on what the waves are like. He does not adjust his basal rates before or after this activity. When he first started surfing, his blood glucose dropped a lot during the activity, and he used to keep his pockets full of candy bars to eat during the first 15 minutes of surfing. Once his body had adjusted to doing up to 3 hours of surfing at a time, his blood glucose dropped much less.

## WATER SKIING AND WAKEBOARDING

Water skiing mainly involves prolonged muscular contractions while you hold onto the rope and stabilize your body on the skis, but it includes a more intense component when you push with your legs to stand up on your skis or when you have to deal with crossing a wave while skiing. Unless you ski for an extended period, you will usually need only minimal changes to regulate your blood glucose because of the brief, intense nature of this activity. If you take insulin, you may reduce your insulin or eat a snack. If you are a pump user, you may choose to remove your pump during this activity. Regimen changes for water skiing or wakeboarding vary depending on how long you do them and how accustomed to the activity you are.

### Athlete Examples

Sarah McGaugh from Canada finds she does not need to make any regimen changes for water skiing or wakeboarding. Neither does Kory Seder of Madison, Wisconsin, who considers these low-level activities.

For water skiing for 45 to 60 minutes or longer, Anne Butcher from California usually lowers her basal rate by 35 percent. If her blood glucose is in a normal range when she starts this activity, she eats a snack.

## WHITE-WATER SPORTS (CANOEING, KAYAKING, AND RAFTING)

White-water sports usually have both aerobic and anaerobic aspects and may be quite prolonged. For low-level paddling (i.e., going downstream without much effort), you will need to make only minimal changes to manage your blood glucose. For longer or more intense paddling, however, you may need more food or lower insulin levels to prevent lows, even if a greater release of adrenaline in the short run keeps your glucose higher during the activity. For multiday trips, you may need to reduce basal insulin doses and be on the lookout for later-onset lows.

### Athlete Examples

These examples show that the required changes depend on the intensity and duration of your white-water paddling activity. The environmental conditions (such as water temperature) may also play a role.

#### Insulin Changes Alone

Lisa Seaman from Colorado finds that the stress of white-water kayaking causes enough adrenaline release for her blood glucose to rise during the activity. To compensate, she either increases her basal rate or keeps it the same, whereas she would normally lower it during other physical activities.

## Diet Changes Alone

For white-water paddling in cold water, Jennifer Roche of Melbourne, Australia, usually eats jelly beans throughout the day when she is doing this activity. She needs fewer of them during the trickier parts of the paddling due to the greater release of adrenaline that keeps her glucose higher.

## Combined Regimen Changes

Before 2 to 4 hours of white-water kayaking, Steven Long from Wakefield in the United Kingdom typically reduces his dose of Toujeo basal insulin the night before by 20 percent. The morning of the activity, he gives a smaller bolus for the carbohydrate-based breakfast he eats (muesli, porridge, and toast, about 116 grams of carbohydrates). After kayaking, he eats more carbohydrates (sandwiches with 77 grams), covered with a reduced bolus dose of insulin. He keeps using a smaller insulin-to-carbohydrate ratio for the next couple of days as well.

Oregon resident Jamie Flanagan cuts his basal rate by about 20 percent when white-water kayaking. He finds that his blood glucose does not drop as rapidly as it does during more aerobic sports. He likes to be around 180 mg/dL (10.0 mmol/L) when kayaking because going low would be life-threatening and he has few opportunities to get out of his kayak and dry off his hands to test his glucose. In addition, he supplements with snacks throughout this activity to prevent lows.

For Alisa Krakel, a resident of Colorado, white-water rafting trips lasting several days can be challenging to her blood glucose management. The heat, constant exercise, and adrenaline highs all affect her responses in varying ways. To compensate, she usually has to adjust both her insulin and her food intake.

## WINDSURFING

This activity usually involves prolonged muscular work to hold onto the sail and stand upright on the board without losing your balance, along with muscle strength and endurance in your upper body to hold the sail up and control it with the wind. The intensity of this activity will depend on wind conditions and your skill level, while necessary diabetes management adjustments result from how long you do the activity and how hard it is. Stronger winds will increase the intensity of your workout and the amount of blood glucose and muscle glycogen that you use. You may need less insulin and more food under more challenging conditions if you windsurf for longer. Lighter winds or shorter bouts of windsurfing reduce your blood glucose use and may require minimal changes.

## Athlete Example

St. Thomas (U.S. Virgin Islands) resident Steve Prosterman (profiled at the end of this chapter) always carries a glucose source with him when windsurfing or paddleboarding. Because he does not use an insulin pump, he eats extra carbohydrates to bump his glucose up to the high 100s mg/dL (at least 10 mmol/L) before starting because he will be in an isolated environment out on the ocean while active. If his

346 The Athlete's Guide to Diabetes

glucose is too high at the start (over 250 mg/dL [13.9 mmol/L]), he takes a very small bolus to cover it. After exercise, he checks and corrects his blood glucose, if needed.

## YARD GAMES (BOCCE, CORNHOLE, CROQUET, HORSESHOES, ETC.)

People participate in a number of outdoor and yard games, especially during recreational time spent with family and friends. Among these are bocce, cornhole, croquet, horseshoes, lawn bowling, lawn darts, nerf football, shuffleboard, and many others. For instance, spikeball is a trendy beach or park activity that is a bit like volleyball except you bounce the ball off a horizontal round net on the ground. Most of these are low-level activities that are likely to have minimal impact on your blood glucose levels. If you participate long enough over time, it is possible that your blood glucose may start trending down.

### Athlete Examples

For Kerri Sparling from Rhode Island, neither yard games nor yard work requires her to do much except for monitoring her CGM. Having access to CGM makes all the difference for her because it lets her to know about low or high glucose as it approaches, not after it has arrived.

Likewise, Jorden Rieke of Cleveland, Ohio, does not treat these activities as real exercise. She treats a low if she gets one or if her CGM tells her she is trending that way.

## YARD WORK AND GARDENING

The effect of these outdoor activities on your blood glucose can vary. In general, working out in your yard requires you to use postural muscles to maintain your balance (an aerobic activity) and use other muscles to perform repetitive motions, such as raking, mowing with a push mower, weeding, and watering. If you are just weeding or watering, your blood glucose will probably remain more stable, but doing harder work can have a greater impact on your blood glucose. When you perform more forceful activities such as carrying or chopping wood, digging a hole, hoeing, mowing high grass, or even shoveling snow, your blood glucose is likely to decrease if you do it for long, and you will likely have to take in some food or lower your insulin levels to compensate.

### Athlete Examples

The following examples show that yard work and gardening can be compensated for in various ways, depending on how long and how hard you work. For instance, Elizabeth Drabble from Canada admits that when she gardens, her blood glucose will often drop low. It certainly can vary with circumstances, though.

## Insulin Changes Alone

Jeff Foot of Scotland reduces his basal insulin by half starting about 1 hour before he starts gardening and until about 1 hour before he stops. Doing so prevents all lows for him.

While doing yard work (especially mowing the lawn), Illinois resident D. Jones reduces his basal rate to 30 percent of his normal. He occasionally checks his blood glucose.

Rebekah Lindsay (of Sevierville, Tennessee) adjusts for gardening or yard work like she does for many other activities. She lowers her basal rate 1 hour before by 50 percent and then sets her basal to zero during the activity itself.

## Diet Changes Alone

Emily Tiberio of Beaver, Pennsylvania, finds that she has more trouble than normal managing her blood glucose while gardening. Because she forgets to think of it as physical activity, she is always having lows while she is working in the yard—and yet she finds she can run for 15 miles with no issues.

Likewise, Daniel Schneider of Denver, Colorado, says that doing gardening or yard work does lead to lower blood glucose if he does it more than an hour. To compensate, he snacks frequently when working in the yard.

San Diego, California, resident Peter Nerothin finds that he needs no basal adjustments when working in the yard or cleaning around the house. He simply fuels when trending down. It also works best if he has not had an insulin bolus within 4 to 6 hours.

James Ruggiero from East Aurora, New York, finds that doing repetitive movements with his upper body and arms, such as chopping wood, is most likely to make his blood glucose drop. To prevent this from happening, he consumes more carbohydrates in advance of doing these activities.

For doing lawn care (e.g., using a weed eater), snow blowing, or shoveling snow, Minnesota resident Gary Taylor simply eats some extra carbohydrates before and during these activities. He does not do any of them regularly, so it is easier just to snack extra for them.

## Combined Regimen Changes

Australia native Betty Murdock reports that lawn mowing in particular sends her blood glucose low. She has learned to pre-emptively drink juice (15 grams of carbohydrates) before she starts, and she suspends her insulin for the duration.

Minnesota resident Bren Gauvin-Chadwick deals with gardening the same as walking: by making sure that she is not trending down on her blood glucose. She then treats it with a Clif Shot Blok (8 carbohydrates each) or a snack. On occasion, she needs to decrease her basal rate on her pump.

Australian Ron C. monitors his blood glucose more during activities he does not do on a regular basis, including gardening. His regimen for this activity is generally the same as for others: reduce or suspend his basal insulin and consume plenty of food in the form of bars, fruit, or gels (~20 to 25 grams of carbohydrates every 30 minutes or so, depending on his blood glucose level). Gardening often throws him for a loop—at 324 mg/dL (18.0 mmol/L) one minute and low the next (or so it feels like to him). He is still working out the best way to prevent this from occurring.

D. Hollander of New York finds that doing any outdoor work like chopping wood, planting, or doing physical labor around his property drops his blood glucose quickly. To prevent lows, he drinks orange juice or milk to start with blood glucose in the range of 175 to 200 mg/dL (9.7 to 11.1 mmol/L) because he anticipates a decrease of 50 to 100 mg/dL (2.8 to 5.6 mmol/L) in the first 30 minutes of activity. He prefers to eat only when he is hungry, so he reduces his basal rate or disconnects from his pump if his blood glucose starts to decrease too much.

Gary Scheiner of Philadelphia, Pennsylvania, finds that yard work lowers his blood glucose more than just about anything. He has to compensate by reducing his pre–yard work bolus by 50 percent and consuming 20 to 30 grams of carbohydrates every hour (usually in the form of juice or regular soda).

In this book, you have found out everything you need to know to be active with diabetes. You even learned what to do if you take up some of the newer sports like kiteboarding and the latest fitness fads. So go ahead—learn how to scuba dive, climb a mountain, ski the Alps, play pickleball, take up CrossFit, participate in an adventure race, or just do some gardening—whatever makes you happy. The important point is to stay physically active for the rest of your (long and healthy) life with diabetes. Your mind and your body will thank you.

## Athlete Profile: **Steve Prosterman**

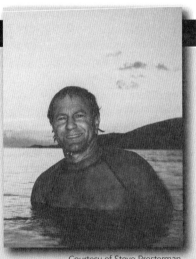

*Courtesy of Steve Prosterman.*

**Hometown:** St. Thomas, U.S. Virgin Islands

**Diabetes history:** Type 1 diabetes diagnosed in 1967 (at age 9)

**Sport or activity:** Scuba diving, windsurfing, ocean swimming, and free diving

**Greatest athletic achievement:** I wrote the scuba diving protocols for people with type 1 diabetes that are still used around the world. I was the first diving instructor to really come out of the closet for diving with diabetes and prove we can do this and do it safely. Since then I have been a tech diving instructor, mixed gas operator and diving safety officer for the University of the Virgin Islands, and a member of the American Academy of Underwater Sciences. In these positions, I have been able to help decision makers understand that we—people with type 1 diabetes—need to be looked at as individuals who have the power to care for ourselves and be safe, with good understanding of our diabetes and how it relates to exercise along with precautions we can take to ensure no hypoglycemia occurs underwater while diving. I also run the hyperbaric chamber in St. Thomas for the region, which is sometimes used to speed up the healing of foot ulcers related to diabetes.

*Current insulin and medication regimen:* Two shots of Levemir (a.m./p.m.), one shot per meal of NovoLog, and six to seven blood glucose checks daily or use Dexcom plus check two to three times per day.

*Training tips:* Find the direction of your blood glucose before activity, and stop the drop! Then go for it.

*Typical daily and weekly training and diabetes regimen:*

▶ *Monday:* Gym workout on a stationary bike and weights in the morning, teaching swimming/snorkeling in the afternoon, and going for an ocean swim if I have time.

▶ *Tuesday:* Stationary bike workout and weights in the morning, and teaching diving in the afternoon.

▶ *Wednesday:* Stationary bike workout and weights in the morning, and teaching diving, swimming, or windsurfing in the afternoon.

▶ *Thursday:* Stationary bike workout and weights in the morning, and teaching diving in the afternoon.

▶ *Friday:* Stationary bike workout and weights in the morning, and teaching diving, swimming, or windsurfing in the afternoon.

▶ *Saturday:* Stationary bike workout and weights in the morning, windsurfing or boating with adventure ocean swim/free diving in the afternoon (or currently, repairing hurricane-damaged house).

▶ *Sunday:* Stationary bike workout and weights in the morning, windsurfing or boating with adventure ocean swim/free diving in afternoon (or, again, repairing hurricane-damaged house).

*Other hobbies and interests:* Biking, climbing, travel—mostly limited to family trips now, and small sail boating.

*Good diabetes and exercise story:* I tried to work for NOAA (the National Oceanic and Atmospheric Administration) in the late 1980s at the underwater habitat in St. Croix, but I was told that they didn't allow insulin users with diabetes to do scuba diving, and I couldn't be hired for that reason. Luckily, the University of the Virgin Islands (UVI) had not caught on to that line of thinking yet and hired me on a merit and individual case basis. I have been at UVI for 30 years now, and wrote protocols for diving and diabetes at my adventure camp held throughout the 1990s (along with Diver Alert Network) that are now used around the world.

As a person who has diabetes who dives, I feel that we all have an obligation to be safe and avoid problems while diving or doing any adventure sport. This obligation is not only to ourselves, but to those who accompany us (dive buddies, adventure partners, etc.) and to others with diabetes who wish to do these sports in the future to ensure they are not shut out of that sport because of the mistakes of a few.

APPENDIX

# A

—— Diabetes, Sport, and Related ——
## Organizations

**Academy of Nutrition and Dietetics (AND)**
120 South Riverside Plaza, Suite 2190, Chicago, IL 60606
(800) 877-1600 or (312) 899-0040
www.eatright.org

**American Association of Diabetes Educators (AADE)**
200 W. Madison Street, Suite 800, Chicago, IL 60606
(800) 338-3633
www.diabeteseducator.org

**American College of Sports Medicine (ACSM)**
401 W. Michigan Street, Indianapolis, IN 46202
(317) 637-9200
www.acsm.org

**American Council on Exercise (ACE)**
4851 Paramount Drive, San Diego, CA 92123
(888) 825-3636, Ext. 782 or (858) 576-6500
www.acefitness.org

**American Diabetes Association (ADA)**
2451 Crystal Drive, Suite 900, Arlington, VA 22202
(800) DIABETES (800-342-2383)
www.diabetes.org

**Cecelia Health**
205 East 42nd Street, New York, NY 10017
(866) 411-0254
www.ceceliahealth.com

### Children With Diabetes
8216 Princeton-Glendale Road, PMB 200, West Chester, OH 45069
www.childrenwithdiabetes.com

### College Diabetes Network
50 Milk Street, 16th Floor, Boston, MA 02109
www.collegediabetesnetwork.org

### Diabetes Education & Camping Association (DECA)
16681 McGregor Blvd, Suite 205, Fort Myers, FL 33908
(239) 984-3554
info@diabetescamps.org
www.diabetescamps.org

### Diabetes Training Camp Foundation
109 North Mansfield Avenue, Margate City, NJ 08402
www.diabetestrainingcamp.com

### Integrated Diabetes Services
333 E. Lancaster Avenue, Suite 204, Wynnewood, PA 19096
(877) SELF-MGT (877-735-3648) or (610) 642-6055
gary@integrateddiabetes.com
www.integrateddiabetes.com

### JDRF
120 Wall Street, New York, NY 10005-4001
(800) 533-CURE (2873)
info@jdrf.org
www.jdrf.org

# B

## —— Diabetes, Sport, and Nutrition —— Websites

### acefitness.org

American Council on Exercise

The American Council on Exercise (ACE) is an organization that provides certification and education for fitness professionals and fitness information for everyone.

### ars.usda.gov/ba/bhnrc/ndl

Nutrient Data Laboratory: Beltsville, MD

This government site provides access to the U.S. Department of Agriculture (USDA) food nutrient data laboratory, where you can access data about the nutritional content of any food or drink.

### beyondtype1.org

Beyond Type 1

Founded in 2015 by Juliet de Baubigny, Nick Jonas, Sarah Lucas, and Sam Talbot, this organization educates people about diabetes using the power of social media and technology.

### calorieking.com

CalorieKing

The CalorieKing website provides products and services designed to educate, motivate, and inspire lifelong weight control.

### ceceliahealth.com

Cecelia Health

This site gives access to personalized fitness and nutritional coaching by certified diabetes educators to help people with fitness goals, diabetes management, and weight loss.

### childrenwithdiabetes.com

Children With Diabetes

Children With Diabetes offers a variety of conferences and events as well as an online community for kids with type 1 diabetes and their parents and siblings.

**choosemyplate.gov**

Choose My Plate

This U.S. Department of Agriculture (USDA) website provides guidance on the latest nutritional guidelines and physical fitness recommendations for everyone.

**collegediabetesnetwork.org**

College Diabetes Network

This group provides young adults with diabetes the peer connections and resources to successfully manage the challenging transition to independence at college and beyond.

**connect1d.org**

ConnecT1D

ConnecT1D runs a family diabetes camp and retreats for adults and middle-school students in Washington State, along with hosting meetups and providing expertise to the community.

**connectedinmotion.ca**

Connected In Motion

Founded as a way of breathing new life into diabetes education for adults living with type 1 diabetes, this group fosters participation in sports and outdoor adventures in both Canada and the United States.

**diabetesdestiny.org**

Diabetes DESTINY

Diabetes "Diabetes Exercise and Strategies—Together in Network with You" (DESTINY) offers camps and programs involving sports and activities for youth and people of all ages.

**diabetesincontrol.com**

Diabetes In Control

This site reviews all the latest diabetes, fitness, and nutrition news on a weekly basis, posts articles about these research findings, and sends out weekly e-newsletters.

**diabetesmotion.com**

Diabetes Motion

Founded by Dr. Sheri Colberg, this website offers free educational information about being active with any type of diabetes, along with troubleshooting tips and advice.

**diabetesstrong.com**

Diabetes Strong: Healthy Life With Diabetes

The Diabetes Strong (formerly TheFitBlog) website features an educational blog run by Christel Oerum, who shares expert advice about living well and being fit and active with any type of diabetes.

**diabetestrainingcamp.com**

Diabetes Training Camp

Founded by Dr. Matt Corcoran, Diabetes Training Camp offers a variety of sports training camps around the United States for adults with diabetes.

**dLife.com**

dLife

One of the first sites started to enhance diabetes education, dLife offers educational information, expert columns, and recipes, among other features.

**dmacademy.com**

Diabetes Motion Academy

Founded by Dr. Sheri Colberg, this site offers approved continuing education courses for fitness and other allied health professionals.

**eparmedx.com**

Official Website: The New PAR-Q+ and ePARmed-X+

On this site, you can access the Physical Activity Readiness Questionnaire for Everyone (PAR-Q+) and the related Physical Activity Readiness Medical Examination.

**excarbs.com**

ExCarbs

This site is focused on providing education to help people with diabetes using insulin feel comfortable with taking up exercise and avoiding activity-related hypoglycemia.

**glucoseadvisors.com**

Glucose Advisors

This site, founded by Ironman triathlete Cliff Scherb, gives you access to coaches, educators, and physicians, along with decision-making support tools.

**glucosezone.com**

GlucoseZone

Founded by Charlie O'Connell, a fitness professional with type 1 diabetes, GlucoseZone is available to help others living with diabetes reach their fitness goals.

**grifgrips.com**

GrifGrips

This site carries a wide array of "Grif Grips," which attach to your skin over your pump or CGM to promote better adhesion, as well as other portability gear.

**health.gov**

Office of Disease Prevention and Health Promotion

This U.S. federal government website lists the latest physical activity and dietary guidelines for Americans.

**hypoactive.org**

HypoActive

Based in Australia, HypoActive promotes an active lifestyle for people with type 1 diabetes and who enjoy outdoor activities.

**integrateddiabetes.com**

Integrated Diabetes Services

Founded by certified diabetes educator Gary Scheiner, this company provides remote coaching to help people navigate the complexities of living with type 1 diabetes.

**myfitnesspal.com**

My Fitness Pal

A popular website and downloadable app, My Fitness Pal gives you free access to calorie counters and fitness trackers to help you reach your fitness and weight goals.

**ridingoninsulin.org**

Riding on Insulin (ROI)

The stated mission of this organization is to empower, activate, and connect the global diabetes community through shared experience and action sports (and outdoor adventures).

**rockadex.net**

RockaDex Diabetes Supplies

This site sells patches to hold pumps and CGM in place on your skin, along with a variety of other diabetes supplies (like insulin cooling cases).

**shericolberg.com**

Dr. Sheri Colberg: Diabetes Motion Expert

Dr. Sheri Colberg's website contains articles about exercise, diabetes, fitness and more, an exercise blog, information about her books, and contact information.

**tcoyd.org**

Taking Control of Your Diabetes (TCOYD)

This organization offers informational conferences around the United States, as well as newsletters, books, and additional educational materials and programs.

**teamnovonordisk.com**

Team Novo Nordisk

Team Novo Nordisk is a global all-diabetes sports team of cyclists, triathletes, and runners, spearheaded by the world's first all-diabetes professional cycling team.

**teamusa.org**

Team USA

This official website of the United States Olympic team contains information about all Olympic sports and Team USA athletes.

# Suggested Reading

Brand-Miller, Jennie, Thomas M.S. Wolever, Kaye Foster-Powell, and Stephen Colagiuri. *The Low GI Handbook: The New Glucose Revolution Guide to the Long-Term Health Benefits of Low GI Eating*. New York: Da Capo Lifelong Books, 2010.

Colberg, Sheri. *Diabetes and Keeping Fit for Dummies*. New York, NY: Wiley, 2018.

Colberg, Sheri, and Steven V. Edelman. *50 Secrets of the Longest Living People With Diabetes*. New York, NY: Marlowe & Company, 2007.

Edelman, Steven V. *Taking Control of Your Diabetes*. 5th ed. Caddo, OK: Professional Communications, 2018.

Hayes, Charlotte. *The "I Hate to Exercise" Book for People With Diabetes*. 3rd ed. Alexandria, VA: American Diabetes Association, 2013.

Riddell, Michael C. *Getting Pumped: An Insulin Pump Guide for Active Individuals With Type 1 Diabetes*. Brampton, ON: Medtronic of Canada, 2016.

Scheiner, Gary. *Practical CGM: Improving Patient Outcomes Through Continuous Glucose Monitoring*. Alexandria, VA: American Diabetes Association, 2015.

Scheiner, Gary. *Think Like a Pancreas: A Practical Guide to Managing Diabetes With Insulin*. New York, NY: Da Capo Lifelong Books, 2012.

Shafer, Sherri. *Diabetes and Carb Counting for Dummies*. New York, NY: Wiley, 2017.

Volek, Jeff S., and Stephen D. Phinney. *The Art and Science of Low Carbohydrate Performance*. Lexington, KY: Beyond Obesity, 2012.

Walsh, John, and Ruth Roberts. *Pumping Insulin: Everything for Success on a Pump and CGM*. 6th ed. San Diego, CA: Torrey Pines Press, 2016.

# ——— Selected Bibliography ———

## Chapter 1

Ahlqvist, E., P. Storm, A. Käräjämäki, M. Martinell, M. Dorkhan, A. Carlsson, P. Vikman, R.B. Prasad, D.M. Aly, P. Almgren, Y. Wessman, N. Shaat, P. Spégel, H. Mulder, E. Lindholm, O. Melander, O. Hansson, U. Malmqvist, Å. Lernmark, K. Lahti, T. Forsén, T. Tuomi, A.H. Rosengren, and L. Groop. 2018. Novel subgroups of adult-onset diabetes and their association with outcomes: a data-driven cluster analysis of six variables. *Lancet: Diabetes and Endocrinology* 6:361-369.

Amati, F., J.J. Dubé, P.M. Coen, M. Stefanovic-Racic, F.G. Toledo, and B.H. Goodpaster. 2009. Physical inactivity and obesity underlie the insulin resistance of aging. *Diabetes Care* 32:1547-1549.

American College of Sports Medicine. 2017. *ACSM's Guidelines for Exercise Testing and Prescription.* 10th ed. Baltimore: Lippincott, Williams & Wilkins.

American Diabetes Association. 2018. 2. Classification and diagnosis of diabetes mellitus: Standards of medical care in diabetes—2018. *Diabetes Care* 41:S13-S27.

Armstrong, M.J., S.R. Colberg, and R.J. Sigal. 2015. Moving beyond cardio: The value of resistance training, balance training and other forms of exercise in the management of diabetes. *Diabetes Spectrum* 28:14-23.

Behm, D.G., A.J. Blazevich, A.D. Kay, and M. McHugh. 2016. Acute effects of muscle stretching on physical performance, range of motion, and injury incidence in healthy active individuals: A systematic review. *Applied Physiology, Nutrition, and Metabolism* 41:1-11.

Colberg, S.R., R.J. Sigal, J.E. Yardley, M.C. Riddell, D.W. Dunstan, P.C. Dempsey, E.S. Horton, K. Castorino, and D.F. Tate. 2016. Physical activity/exercise and diabetes: A position statement of the American Diabetes Association. *Diabetes Care* 39:2065-2079.

Dubé, J.J., N.T. Broskey, A.A. Despines, M. Stefanovic-Racic, F.G. Toledo, B.H. Goodpaster, and F. Amati. 2016. Muscle characteristics and substrate energetics in lifelong endurance athletes. *Medicine and Science in Sports and Exercise* 4:472-480.

Fuchsjager-Mayrl, G., J. Pleiner, G.F. Wiesinger, A.E. Sieder, M. Quittan, M.J. Nuhr, C. Francesconi, H.P. Seit, M. Francesconi, L. Schmetterer, and M. Woltz. 2002. Exercise training improves vascular endothelial function in patients with type 1 diabetes. *Diabetes Care* 25:1795-1801.

Garber, C.E., B. Blissmer, M.R. Deschenes, B.A. Franklin, M.J. Lamonte, I.M. Lee, D.C. Nieman, and D.P. Swain. 2011. American College of Sports Medicine position stand. Quantity and quality of exercise for developing and maintaining cardiorespiratory, musculoskeletal, and neuromotor fitness in apparently healthy adults: guidance for prescribing exercise. *Medicine and Science in Sports and Exercise* 43:1334-1359.

Haskell, W.L., I.-M. Lee, R.R. Pate, K.E. Powell, S.N. Blair, B.A. Franklin, C.A. Macera, G.W. Heath, P.D. Thompson, and A. Bauman. 2007. Physical activity and public health: Updated recommendation for adults from the American College of Sports Medicine and the American Heart Association. *Medicine and Science in Sports and Exercise* 39:1423-1434.

Johnson, S.T., L.J. McCargar, G.J. Bell, C. Tudor-Locke, V.J. Harber, and R.C. Bell. 2006. Walking faster: Distilling a complex prescription for type 2 diabetes management through pedometry. *Diabetes Care* 29:1654-1655.

Tielemans, S.M., S.S. Soedamah-Muthu, M. De Neve, M. Toeller, N. Chaturvedi, J.H. Fuller, and E. Stamatakis. 2013. Association of physical activity with all-cause mortality and incident and prevalent cardiovascular disease among patients with type 1 diabetes: the EURODIAB Prospective Complications Study. *Diabetologia* 56:82-91.

Tinsley, L.J., V. Kupelian, S.A. D'Eon, D. Pober, J.K. Sun, G.L. King, and H.A. Keenan. 2017. Association of glycemic control with reduced risk for large-vessel disease after more than 50 years of type 1 diabetes. *Journal of Clinical Endocrinology and Metabolism* 102:3704–3711.

U.S. Department of Health and Human Services. 2018. *Physical Activity Guidelines for Americans*, 2nd edition. Accessed at https://health.gov/paguidelines/second-edition, November 12, 2018.

# Chapter 2

Adolfsson, P., S. Mattsson, and J. Jendle. 2015. Evaluation of glucose control when a new strategy of increased carbohydrate supply is implemented during prolonged physical exercise in type 1 diabetes. *European Journal of Applied Physiology* 115:2599–2607.

Bak, J., U. Jacobsen, F. Jorgensen, and O. Pedersen. 1989. Insulin receptor function and glycogen synthase activity in skeletal muscle biopsies from patients with insulin-dependent diabetes mellitus: Effects of physical training. *Journal of Clinical Endocrinology and Metabolism* 69:158–164.

Bergman, B.C., G.E. Butterfield, E.E. Wolfel, G.D. Lopaschuk, G.A. Casazza, M.A. Horning, and G.A. Brooks. 1999. Muscle net glucose uptake and glucose kinetics after endurance training in men. *American Journal of Physiology* 277:E81–E92.

Brazeau, A.S., R. Rabasa-Lhoret, I. Strychar, and H. Mircescu. 2008. Barriers to physical activity among patients with type 1 diabetes. *Diabetes Care* 31:2108–2109.

Briscoe, V.J., D.B. Tate, and S.N. Davis. 2007. Type 1 diabetes: Exercise and hypoglycemia. *Applied Physiology, Nutrition, and Metabolism* 32:576–582.

Bruce, C., and J. Hawley. 2004. Improvements in insulin resistance with aerobic exercise training: A lipocentric approach. *Medicine and Science in Sports and Exercise* 36:1196–1201.

Bussau, V.A., L.D. Ferreira, T.W. Jones, and P.A. Fournier. 2006. The 10-s maximal sprint: A novel approach to counter an exercise-mediated fall in glycemia in individuals with type 1 diabetes. *Diabetes Care* 29:601–606.

Bussau, V.A., L.D. Ferreira, T.W. Jones, and P.A. Fournier. 2007. A 10-s sprint performed prior to moderate-intensity exercise prevents early postexercise fall in glycaemia in individuals with type 1 diabetes. *Diabetologia* 50:1815–1818.

Caduff, A., H.U. Lutz, L. Heinemann, G. Di Benedetto, M.S. Talary, and S. Theander. 2011. Dynamics of blood electrolytes in repeated hyper- and/or hypoglycaemic events in patients with type 1 diabetes. *Diabetologia* 54:2678–2689.

Campbell, M.D., M. Walker, R. M. Bracken, D. Turner, E.J. Stevenson, J.T. Gonzalez, J.A. Shaw, and D.J. West. 2015. Insulin therapy and dietary adjustments to normalize glycemia and prevent nocturnal hypoglycemia after evening exercise in type 1 diabetes: a randomized controlled trial. *BMJ Open Diabetes Research and Care* 3:e000085.

Campbell, M.D., D. J. West, S.C. Bain, M.I. Kingsley, P. Foley, L. Kilduff, D. Turner, B. Gray, J.W. Stephens, and R.M. Bracken. 2015. Simulated games activity vs continuous running exercise: a novel comparison of the glycemic and metabolic responses in T1DM patients. *Scandinavian Journal of Medicine and Science in Sports* 25:216–222.

Carlson, J.N., S. Schunder-Tatzber, C.J. Neilson, and N. Hood. 2017. Dietary sugars versus glucose tablets for first-aid treatment of symptomatic hypoglycaemia in awake patients with diabetes: a systematic review and meta-analysis. *Emergency Medicine Journal* 34:100–106.

Colberg, S.R., J.M. Hagberg, S.D. McCole, J.M. Zmuda, P.D. Thompson, and D.E. Kelley. 1996. Utilization of glycogen but not plasma glucose is reduced in individuals with NIDDM during mild-intensity exercise. *Journal of Applied Physiology* 81:2027–2033.

Colberg, S.R., R.J. Sigal, J.E. Yardley, M.C. Riddell, D.W. Dunstan, P.C. Dempsey, E.S. Horton, K. Castorino, and D.F. Tate. 2016. Physical activity/exercise and diabetes: A position statement of the American Diabetes Association. *Diabetes Care* 39:2065–2079.

Coyle, E., A. Coggan, M. Hemmert, and J. Ivy. 1986. Muscle glycogen utilization during prolonged strenuous exercise when fed carbohydrates. *Journal of Applied Physiology* 61:165–172.

De Feo, P., C. Di Loreto, A. Ranchelli, C. Fatone, G. Gambelunghe, P. Lucidi, and F. Santeusanio. 2006. Exercise and diabetes. *Acta Biomedica* 77:14–17.

Dubé, M.-C., S.J. Weisnagel, D. Prud'homme, and C. Lavoie. 2006. Is early and late post-meal exercise so different in type 1 diabetic lispro users? *Diabetes Research and Clinical Practice* 72:128–134.

Fahey, A.J., N. Paramalingam, R.J. Davey, E.A. Davis, T.W. Jones, and P.A. Fournier. 2012. The effect of a short sprint on postexercise whole-body glucose production and utilization rates in individuals with type 1 diabetes mellitus. *Journal of Clinical Endocrinology and Metabolism* 97:4193–4200.

Frier, B.M. 2014. Hypoglycaemia in diabetes mellitus: epidemiology and clinical implications. *Nature Reviews Endocrinology* 10:711–722.

Galassetti, P., D. Tate, R.A. Neill, S. Morrey, D.H. Wasserman, and S.N. Davis. 2003. Effect of antecedent hypoglycemia on counterregulatory responses to subsequent euglycemic exercise in type 1 diabetes. *Diabetes* 52:1761–1769.

Galassetti, P., D. Tate, R.A. Neill, S. Morrey, D.H. Wasserman, and S.N. Davis. 2004. Effect of sex on counterregulatory responses to exercise after antecedent hypoglycemia in type 1 diabetes. *American Journal of Physiology* 287:E16–E24.

Galassetti, P., D. Tate, R.A. Neill, A. Richardson, S.Y. Leu, and S.N. Davis. 2006. Effect of differing antecedent hypoglycemia on counterregulatory responses to exercise in type 1 diabetes. *American Journal of Physiology* 290:E1109–E1117.

Guelfi, K.J., T.W. Jones, and P.A. Fournier. 2005. The decline in blood glucose levels is less with intermittent high-intensity compared with moderate exercise in individuals with type 1 diabetes. *Diabetes Care* 28:1289–1294.

Guelfi, K.J., T.W. Jones, and P.A. Fournier. 2005. Intermittent high-intensity exercise does not increase the risk of early postexercise hypoglycemia in individuals with type 1 diabetes. *Diabetes Care* 28:416–418.

Guelfi, K.J., N. Ratnam, G.A. Smythe, T.W. Jones, and P.A. Fournier. 2007. Effect of intermittent high-intensity compared with continuous moderate exercise on glucose production and utilization in individuals with type 1 diabetes. *American Journal of Physiology* 292:E865–E8670.

Hernandez, J.M., T. Moccia, J.D. Fluckey, J.S. Ulbrecht, and P.A. Farrell. 2000. Fluid snacks to help persons with type 1 diabetes avoid late onset postexercise hypoglycemia. *Medicine and Science in Sports and Exercise* 32:904–910.

Houmard, J.A., C.J. Tanner, C.A. Slentz, B.D. Duscha, J.S. McCartney, and W.E. Kraus. 2004. Effect of the volume and intensity of exercise training on insulin sensitivity. *Journal of Applied Physiology* 96:101–106.

Koivisto, V.A., T. Sane, F. Fyhrquist, and R. Pelkonen. 1992. Fuel and fluid homeostasis during long-term exercise in healthy subjects and type I diabetic patients. *Diabetes Care* 15:1736–1741.

Kreisman, S.H., J.B. Halter, M. Vranic, and E.B. Marliss. 2003. Combined infusion of epinephrine and norepinephrine during moderate exercise reproduces the glucoregulatory response of intense exercise. *Diabetes* 52:1347–1354.

MacDonald, M.J. 1987. Postexercise late-onset hypoglycemia in insulin-dependent diabetic patients. *Diabetes Care* 10:584–588.

McMahon, S.K., L.D. Ferreira, N. Ratnam, R.J. Davey, L.M. Youngs, E.A. Davis, P.A. Fournier, and T.W. Jones. 2007. Glucose requirements to maintain euglycemia after moderate-intensity afternoon exercise in adolescents with type 1 diabetes are increased in a biphasic manner. *Journal of Clinical Endocrinology and Metabolism* 92:963–968.

Mallad, A., L. Hinshaw, M. Schiavon, C. Dalla Man, V. Dadlani, R. Basu, C. Lingineni, C. Cobelli, M.L. Johnson, R. Carter, Y.C. Kudva, and A. Basu. 2015. Exercise effects on postprandial glucose metabolism in type 1 diabetes: a triple-tracer approach. *American Journal of Physiology Endocrinology and Metabolism* 308:E1106–E1115.

Manohar, C., J.A. Levine, D.K. Nandy, A. Saad, C. Dalla Man, S.K. McCrady-Spitzer, R. Basu, C. Cobelli, R.E. Carter, A. Basu, and Y.C. Kudva. 2012. The effect of walking on postprandial glycemic excursion in patients with type 1 diabetes and healthy people. *Diabetes Care* 35:2493–2499.

Maran, A., P. Pavan, B. Bonsembiante, E. Brugin, A. Ermolao, A. Avogaro, and M. Zaccaria. 2010. Continuous glucose monitoring reveals delayed nocturnal hypoglycemia after intermittent high-intensity exercise in nontrained patients with type 1 diabetes. *Diabetes Technology and Therapeutics* 12:763Y8.

Mitchell, T.H., G. Abraham, A. Schiffrin, L.A. Leiter, and E.B. Marliss. 1988. Hyperglycemia after intense exercise in IDDM subjects during continuous subcutaneous insulin infusion. *Diabetes Care* 11:311–317.

Mitranun, W., C. Deerochanawong, H. Tanaka, and D. Suksom. 2014. Continuous vs interval training on glycemic control and macro- and microvascular reactivity in type 2 diabetic patients. *Scandinavian Journal of Medicine and Science in Sports* 24:e69–e76.

Poirier, P., S. Mawhinney, L. Grondin, A. Tremblay, T. Broderick, J. Cleroux, C. Catellier, G. Tancrede, and A. Nadeau. 2001. Prior meal enhances the plasma glucose lowering effect of exercise in type 2 diabetes. *Medicine and Science in Sports and Exercise* 33:1259–1264.

Price, T.B., D.L. Rothman, R. Taylor, M.J. Avison, G.I. Shulman, and R.G. Shulman. 1994. Human muscle glycogen resynthesis after exercise: Insulin-dependent and -independent phases. *Journal of Applied Physiology* 76:104–111.

Rabasa-Lhoret, R., J. Bourque, F. Ducros, and J.L. Chiasson. 2001. Guidelines for premeal insulin dose reduction for postprandial exercise of different intensities and durations in type 1 diabetic subjects treated intensively with a basal-bolus insulin regimen (ultralente-lispro). *Diabetes Care* 24:625–630.

Richter, E., L. Turcotte, P. Hespel, and B. Kiens. 1992. Metabolic responses to exercise: Effects of endurance training and implications for diabetes. *Diabetes Care* 15:1767–1776.

Rickels, M.R., S.N. DuBose, E. Toschi, R.W. Beck, A.S. Verdejo, H. Wolpert, M.J. Cummins, B. Newswanger, M.C. Riddell, and T1D Exchange Mini-Dose Glucagon Exercise Study Group. 2018. Mini-dose glucagon as a novel approach to prevent exercise-induced hypoglycemia in type 1 diabetes. *Diabetes Care* 41:1909–1916.

Riddell, M.C., I.W. Gallen, C.E. Smart, C.E. Taplin, P. Adolfsson, A.N. Lumb, A. Kowalski, R. Rabasa-Lhoret, R.J. McCrimmon, C. Hume, F. Annan, P.A. Fournier, C. Graham, B. Bode, P. Galassetti, T.W. Jones, I.S. Millán, T. Heise, A.L. Peters, A. Petz, and L.M. Laffel. 2017. Exercise management in type 1 diabetes: a consensus statement. *Lancet Diabetes Endocrinology* 5:377–390.

Sandoval, D.A., D.L. Guy, M.A. Richardson, A.C. Ertl, and S.N. Davis. 2004. Effects of low and moderate antecedent exercise on counterregulatory responses to subsequent hypoglycemia in type 1 diabetes. *Diabetes* 53:1798–1806.

Sandoval, D.A., D.L. Guy, M.A. Richardson, A.C. Ertl, and S.N. Davis. 2006. Acute, same-day effects of antecedent exercise on counterregulatory responses to subsequent hypoglycemia in type 1 diabetes mellitus. *American Journal of Physiology* 290:E1331–E1338.

Shetty, V.B., P.A. Fournier, R.J. Davey, A.J. Retterath, N. Paramalingam, H.C. Roby, M.N. Cooper, E.A. Davis, and T.W. Jones. 2016. Effect of exercise intensity on glucose requirements to maintain euglycemia during exercise in type 1 diabetes. *Journal of Clinical Endocrinology and Metabolism* 101:972–980.

Sigal, R.J., C. Purdon, S.J. Fisher, J.B. Halter, M. Vranic, and E.B. Marliss. 1994. Hyperinsulinemia prevents prolonged hyperglycemia after intense exercise in insulin-dependent diabetic subjects. *Journal of Clinical Endocrinology and Metabolism* 79:1049–1057.

Tansey, M.J., E. Tsalikian, R.W. Beck, N. Mauras, B.A. Buckingham, S.A. Weinzimer, K.F. Janz, C. Kollman, D. Xing, K.J. Ruedy, M.W. Steffes, T.M. Borland, R.J. Singh, and W.V. Tamborlane. 2006. The effects of aerobic exercise on glucose and counterregulatory hormone concentrations in children with type 1 diabetes. *Diabetes Care* 29:20–25.

Trout, K.K., M.R. Rickels, M.H. Schutta, M. Petrova, E.W. Freeman, N.C. Tkacs, and K.L. Teff. 2007. Menstrual cycle effects on insulin sensitivity in women with type 1 diabetes: A pilot study. *Diabetes Technology and Therapeutics* 9:176-182.

Tuominen, J., P. Ebeling, H. Vuorinen-Markkola, and V. Koivisto. 1997. Postmarathon paradox in IDDM: Unchanged insulin sensitivity in spite of glycogen depletion. *Diabetic Medicine* 14:301-308.

Turner, D., S. Luzio, B.J. Gray, G. Dunseath, E.D. Rees, L.P. Kilduff, M.D. Campbell, D.J. West, S.C. Bain, and R.M. Bracken. 2015. Impact of single and multiple sets of resistance exercise in type 1 diabetes. *Scandinavian Journal of Medicine and Science in Sports* 25:e99-e109.

West, D.J., R.D. Morton, S.C. Bain, J.W. Stephens, and R.M. Bracken. 2010. Blood glucose responses to reductions in pre-exercise rapid-acting insulin for 24 h after running in individuals with type 1 diabetes. *Journal of Sports Sciences* 28:781-788.

West D.J., J.W. Stephens, S.C. Bain, L.P. Kilduff, S. Luzio, R. Still, and R.M. Bracken. 2011. A combined insulin reduction and carbohydrate feeding strategy 30 min before running best preserves blood glucose concentration after exercise through improved fuel oxidation in type 1 diabetes mellitus. *Journal of Sports Sciences* 29:279-289.

Yardley, J.E., and S.R. Colberg. 2017. Update on management of type 1 diabetes and type 2 diabetes in athletes. *Current Sports Medicine Reports* 16:38-44.

Yardley, J.E., G.P. Kenny, B.A. Perkins, M.C. Riddell, N. Balaa, J. Malcolm, P. Boulay, F. Khandwala, and R.J. Sigal. 2013. Resistance versus aerobic exercise: acute effects on glycemia in type 1 diabetes. *Diabetes Care* 36:537-542.

Yardley, J.E., G.P. Kenny, B.A. Perkins, M.C. Riddell, J. Malcolm, P. Boulay, F. Khandwala, and R.J. Sigal. 2012. Effects of performing resistance exercise before versus after aerobic exercise on glycemia in type 1 diabetes. *Diabetes Care* 35:669-675.

Yardley, J.E., and R.J. Sigal. 2015. Exercise strategies for hypoglycemia prevention in individuals with type 1 diabetes. *Diabetes Spectrum* 28:32-38.

Yardley, J.E., R.J. Sigal, M.C. Riddell, B.A. Perkins, and G.P. Kenny. 2014. Performing resistance exercise before versus after aerobic exercise influences growth hormone secretion in type 1 diabetes. *Applied Physiology Nutrition Metabolism* 39:262-265.

# Chapter 3

Admon, G., Y. Weinstein, B. Falk, N. Weintrob, H. Benzaquen, R. Ofan, G. Fayman, L. Zigel, N. Constantini, and M. Phillip. 2005. Exercise with and without an insulin pump among children and adolescents with type 1 diabetes mellitus. *Pediatrics* 116:e348-e355.

Ahmed, M., M.J. McKenna, and R.K. Crowley. 2017. Diabetic ketoacidosis in patients with type 2 diabetes recently commenced on SGLT-2 inhibitors: An ongoing concern. *Endocrine Practice* 23:506-508.

Ashwell, S.G., J. Gebbie, and P.D. Home. 2006. Optimal timing of injection of once-daily insulin glargine in people with type 1 diabetes using insulin lispro at meal-times. *Diabetic Medicine* 23:46-52.

Bischof, M.G., E. Bernroider, C. Ludwig, S. Kurzemann, K. Kletter, W. Waldhäusl, and M. Roden. 2001. Effect of near physiologic insulin therapy on hypoglycemia counterregulation in type-1 diabetes. *Hormone Research* 56:151-158.

Campbell, M.D., M. Walker, R.M. Bracken, D. Turner, E.J. Stevenson, J.T. Gonzalez, J.A. Shaw, and D.J. West. 2015. Insulin therapy and dietary adjustments to normalize glycemia and prevent nocturnal hypoglycemia after evening exercise in type 1 diabetes: a randomized controlled trial. *BMJ Open Diabetes Research and Care* 3:e000085.

Chokkalingam, K., K. Tsintzas, L. Norton, K. Jewell, I.A. Macdonald, and P.I. Mansell. 2007. Exercise under hyperinsulinaemic conditions increases whole-body glucose disposal without affecting muscle glycogen utilisation in type 1 diabetes. *Diabetologia* 50:414-421.

Cryer, P.E. 2006. Hypoglycemia in diabetes: Pathophysiological mechanisms and diurnal variation. *Progress in Brain Research* 153:361–365.

De Oliveira, L.P., C.P. Vieira, F.D. Guerra, M.S. Almeida, and E.R. Pimentel. 2015. Structural and biomechanical changes in the Achilles tendon after chronic treatment with statins. *Food and Chemical Toxicology* 77:50–57.

DeVries, J.H., I.M. Wentholt, N. Masurel, I. Mantel, A. Poscia, A. Maran, and R.J. Heine. 2004. Nocturnal hypoglycaemia in type 1 diabetes: Consequences and assessment. *Diabetes/Metabolism Research and Reviews* 20:S43–S46.

Ebrahim, S, F.C. Taylor, and P. Brindle. 2014. Statins for the primary prevention of cardiovascular disease. *British Medical Journal* 348:g280.

Everett, J. 2004. The role of insulin pumps in the management of diabetes. *Nursing Times* 100:48–49.

Franc, S., A., Daoudi, A. Pochat, M.H. Petit, C. Randazzo, C. Petit, M. Duclos, A. Penfornis, E. Pussard, D. Not, E. Heyman, F. Koukoui, C. Simon, and G. Charpentier. 2015. Insulin-based strategies to prevent hypoglycaemia during and after exercise in adult patients with type 1 diabetes on pump therapy: the DIABRASPORT randomized study. *Diabetes, Obesity and Metabolism* 17:1150–1157.

Galasso, S., A. Facchinetti, B.M. Bonora, V. Mariano, F. Boscari, E. Cipponeri, A. Maran, A. Avogaro, G.P. Fadini, and D. Bruttomesso. 2016. Switching from twice-daily glargine or detemir to once-daily degludec improves glucose control in type 1 diabetes. An observational study. *Nutrition Metabolism and Cardiovascular Diseases* 26:1112–1119.

Garg, S., R.L. Brazg, T.S. Bailey, B.A. Buckingham, R.H. Slover, D.C. Klonoff, J. Shin, J.B. Welsh, and F.R. Kaufman. 2012. Reduction in duration of hypoglycemia by automatic suspension of insulin delivery: The in-clinic ASPIRE study. *Diabetes Technology and Therapeutics* 14:205–209.

Gomez, A.M., C. Gomez, P. Aschner, A. Veloza, O. Muñoz, C. Rubio, and S. Vallejo. 2015. Effects of performing morning versus afternoon exercise on glycemic control and hypoglycemia frequency in type 1 diabetes patients on sensor-augmented insulin pump therapy. *Journal of Diabetes Science and Technology* 9:619–624.

Gomis, R., and E. Esmatjes. 2004. Asymptomatic hypoglycaemia: Identification and impact. *Diabetes/Metabolism Research and Reviews* 20:S47–S49.

Green, B.D., P.R. Flatt, and C.J. Bailey. 2006. Dipeptidyl peptidase IV (DPP IV) inhibitors: A newly emerging drug class for the treatment of type 2 diabetes. *Diabetes and Vascular Disease Research* 3:159–165.

Handelsman Y., R.R. Henry, Z.T. Bloomgarden, S. Dagogo-Jack, R.A. DeFronzo, D. Einhorn, E. Ferrannini, V.A. Fonseca, A.J. Garber, G. Grunberger, D. LeRoith, G.E. Umpierrez, and M.R. Weir. 2016. American Association of Clinical Endocrinologists and American College of Endocrinology position statement on the association of SGLT-2 inhibitors and diabetic ketoacidosis. *Endocrine Practice* 22:753–762.

Heinemann, L., L. Nosek, C. Kapitza, M.A. Schweitzer, and L. Krinelke. 2009. Changes in basal insulin infusion rates with subcutaneous insulin infusion: time until a change in metabolic effect is induced in patients with type 1 diabetes. *Diabetes Care* 32:1437–1439.

Henderson J.N., K.V. Allen, I.J. Deary, and B.M. Frier. 2003. Hypoglycaemia in insulin-treated type 2 diabetes: Frequency, symptoms and impaired awareness. *Diabetic Medicine* 20:1016–1021.

Herman, W.H., L.L. Ilag, S.L. Johnson, C.L. Martin, J. Sinding, A. Al Harthi, C.D. Plunkett, F.B. LaPorte, R. Burke, M.B. Brown, J.B. Halter, and P. Raskin. 2005. A clinical trial of continuous subcutaneous insulin infusion versus multiple daily injections in older adults with type 2 diabetes. *Diabetes Care* 28:1568–1573.

Joy, S.V., P.T. Rodgers, and A.C. Scates. 2005. Incretin mimetics as emerging treatment for type 2 diabetes. *Annals of Pharmacotherapy* 39:110–118.

Klonoff, D.C. 2014. Afrezza inhaled insulin: the fastest-acting FDA-approved insulin on the market has favorable properties. *Journal of Diabetes Science and Technology* 8:1071–1073.

Kwon, S., and K.L. Hermayer. 2013. Glucocorticoid-induced hyperglycemia. *American Journal of Medicine and Science* 345:274–277.

Linkeschova, R., M. Raoul, U. Bott, M. Berger, and M. Spraul. 2002. Less severe hypoglycaemia, better metabolic control, and improved quality of life in type 1 diabetes mellitus with continuous subcutaneous insulin infusion (CSII) therapy: an observational study of 100 consecutive patients followed for a mean of 2 years. *Diabetic Medicine* 19:746–751.

Ma, Z., J.S. Christiansen, T. Laursen, T. Lauritzen, and J. Frystyk. 2014. Short-term effects of NPH insulin, insulin detemir, and insulin glargine on the GH-IGF1-IGFBP axis in patients with type 1 diabetes. *European Journal of Endocrinology* 171:471–479.

Moon, R.J., L.A. Bascombe, and R.I. Holt. 2007. The addition of metformin in type 1 diabetes improves insulin sensitivity, diabetic control, body composition and patient well-being. *Diabetes, Obesity and Metabolism* 9:143–145.

Moser, O., G. Tschakert, A. Mueller, W. Groeschl, T.R. Pieber, B. Obermayer-Pietsch, G. Koehler, and P. Hofmann. 2015. Effects of high-intensity interval exercise versus moderate continuous exercise on glucose homeostasis and hormone response in patients with type 1 diabetes mellitus using novel ultra-long-acting insulin. *PLoS One* 10:e0136489.

Perkins, B.A., D.Z. Cherney, H. Partridge, N. Soleymanlou, H. Tschirhart, B. Zinman, N.M. Fagan, S. Kaspers, H.J. Woerle, U.C. Broedl, and O.E. Johansen. 2014. Sodium-glucose cotransporter 2 inhibition and glycemic control in type 1 diabetes: results of an 8-week open label proof-of-concept trial. *Diabetes Care* 37:1480–1483.

Peter, R., S.D. Luzio, G. Dunseath, A. Miles, B. Hare, K. Backs, V. Pauvaday, and D.R. Owens. 2005. Effects of exercise on the absorption of insulin glargine in patients with type 1 diabetes. *Diabetes Care* 28:560–565.

Peterson, G.E. 2006. Intermediate and long-acting insulins: A review of NPH insulin, insulin glargine and insulin detemir. *Current Medical Research and Opinion* 22:2613–2619.

Ratner, R.E., I.B. Hirsch, J.L. Neifing, S.K. Garg, T.E. Mecca, and C.A. Wilson. 2000. Less hypoglycemia with insulin Glargine in intensive insulin therapy for type 1 diabetes. *Diabetes Care* 23:639–643.

Rave, K., S. Bott, L. Heinemann, S. Sha, R.H. Becker, S.A. Willavize, and T. Heise. 2005. Time-action profile of inhaled insulin in comparison with subcutaneously injected insulin lispro and regular human insulin. *Diabetes Care* 28:1077–1082.

Smart, C.E., M. Evans, S.M. O'Connell, P. McElduff, P.E. Lopez, T.W. Jones, E.A. Davis, and B.R. King. 2013. Both dietary protein and fat increase postprandial glucose excursions in children with type 1 diabetes, and the effect is additive. *Diabetes Care* 36:3897–3902.

Yamakita, T., T. Ishii, K. Yamagami, T. Yamamoto, M. Miyamoto, M. Hosoi, K. Yoshioka, T. Sato, S. Onishi, S. Tanaka, and S. Fjuii. 2002. Glycemic response during exercise after administration of insulin lispro compared with that after administration of regular human insulin. *Diabetes Research and Clinical Practice* 57:17–22.

Zaharieva, D., L. Yavelberg, V. Jamnik, A. Cinar, K. Turksoy, and M.C. Riddell. 2017. The effects of basal insulin suspension at the start of exercise on blood glucose levels during continuous versus circuit-based exercise in individuals with type 1 diabetes on continuous subcutaneous insulin infusion. *Diabetes Technology and Therapeutics* 19:370–378.

# Chapter 4

Adolfsson, P., S. Mattsson, and J. Jendle. 2015. Evaluation of glucose control when a new strategy of increased carbohydrate supply is implemented during prolonged physical exercise in type 1 diabetes. *European Journal of Applied Physiology* 115:2599–2607.

Albarracin, C., B. Fuqua, J. Geohas, V. Juturu, M.R. Finch, and J.R. Komorowski. 2007. Combination of chromium and biotin improves coronary risk factors in hypercholesterolemic type

2 diabetes mellitus: A placebo-controlled, double-blind randomized clinical trial. *Journal of the Cardiometabolic Syndrome* 2:91–97.

Baker, L.B., I. Rollo, K.W. Stein, and A.E. Jeukendrup. 2015. Acute effects of carbohydrate supplementation on intermittent sports performance. *Nutrients* 7:5733–5763.

Bell, K.J., C.E. Smart, G.M. Steil, J.C. Brand-Miller, B. King, and H.A. Wolpert. 2015. Impact of fat, protein, and glycemic index on postprandial glucose control in type 1 diabetes: implications for intensive diabetes management in the continuous glucose monitoring era. *Diabetes Care* 38:1008–1015.

Bischof, M.G., E. Bernroider, M. Krssak, H. Krebs, H. Stingl, P. Nowotny, C. Yu, G.L. Shulman, W. Waldhausl, and M. Roden. 2002. Hepatic glycogen metabolism in type 1 diabetes after long-term near normoglycemia. *Diabetes* 51:49–54.

Brand-Miller, J., S. Hayne, P. Petocz, and S. Colagiuri. 2003. Low-glycemic index diets in the management of diabetes: A meta-analysis of randomized control trials. *Diabetes Care* 26:2261–2267.

Burani, J., and P.J. Longo. 2006. Low-glycemic index carbohydrates: An effective behavioral change for glycemic control and weight management in patients with type 1 and 2 diabetes. *Diabetes Educator* 32:78–88.

Burke, L.M. 2015. Re-examining high-fat diets for sports performance: did we call the "nail in the coffin" too soon? *Sports Medicine Auckland New Zealand* 45:33–49.

Bursell, S.-E., A.C. Clermont, L.P. Aiello, L.M. Aiello, D.K. Schlossman, E.P. Feener, L. Laffel, and G.L. King. 1999. High-dose vitamin E supplementation normalizes retinal blood flow and creatinine clearance in patients with type 1 diabetes. *Diabetes Care* 22:1245–1251.

Bussau, V.A., T.J. Fairchild, A. Rao, P. Steele, and P.A. Fournier. 2002. Carbohydrate loading in human muscle: An improved 1 day protocol. *European Journal of Applied Physiology* 87:290–295.

Campbell, M.D., M. Walker, R.A. Ajjan, K.M. Birch, J.T. Gonzalez, and D.J. West. 2017. An additional bolus of rapid-acting insulin to normalise postprandial cardiovascular risk factors following a high-carbohydrate high-fat meal in patients with type 1 diabetes: A randomised controlled trial. *Diabetes Vascular Disease Research* 14:336–344.

Campbell, M.D., M. Walker, R.M. Bracken, D. Turner, E.J. Stevenson, J.T. Gonzalez, J.A. Shaw, and D.J. West. 2015. Insulin therapy and dietary adjustments to normalize glycemia and prevent nocturnal hypoglycemia after evening exercise in type 1 diabetes: a randomized controlled trial. *BMJ Open Diabetes Research and Care* 3:e000085.

Cantorna, M.T., Y. Zhu, M. Froicu, and A. Wittke. 2004. Vitamin D status, 1,25-dihydroxyvitamin D3, and the immune system. *American Journal of Clinical Nutrition* 80:1717S–1720S.

Chang, C.K., K. Borer, and P.J. Lin. 2017. Low-carbohydrate-high-fat diet: Can it help exercise performance? *Journal of Human Kinetics* 56:81–92.

Clapp, J.F., III, and B. Lopez. 2007. Low- versus high-glycemic index diets in women: Effects on caloric requirement, substrate utilization, and insulin sensitivity. *Metabolic Syndrome and Related Disorders* 5:231–242.

Coyle, E.F. 1994. Fluid and carbohydrate replacement during exercise: How much and why? *Sports Science Exchange* 7:1–6.

Desbrow, B., and M. Leveritt. 2007. Well-trained endurance athletes' knowledge, insight, and experience of caffeine use. *International Journal of Sports Nutrition and Exercise Metabolism* 17:328–339.

Faure, P., A. Roussel, C. Coudray, M.J. Richard, S. Halimi, and A. Favier. 1992. Zinc and insulin sensitivity. *Biological Trace Element Research* 32:305–310.

Foster, T.S. 2007. Efficacy and safety of alpha-lipoic acid supplementation in the treatment of symptomatic diabetic neuropathy. *Diabetes Educator* 33:111–117.

Foster-Powell, K., S. Holt, and J. Brand-Miller. 2002. International table of glycemic index and glycemic load values: 2002. *American Journal of Clinical Nutrition* 76:5–56.

Francescato, M.P., M. Geat, S. Fusi, G. Stupar, C. Noacco, and L. Cattin. 2004. Carbohydrate requirement and insulin concentration during moderate exercise in type 1 diabetic patients. *Metabolism* 53:1126–1130.

Hernandez, J.M., T. Moccia, J.D. Fluckey, J.S. Ulbrecht, and P.A. Farrell. 2000. Fluid snacks to help persons with type 1 diabetes avoid late onset postexercise hypoglycemia. *Medicine and Science in Sports and Exercise* 32:904–910.

Ivy, J.L., S.L. Katz, C.L. Cutler, W.M. Sherman, and E.F. Coyle. 1988. Muscle glycogen synthesis after exercise: Effect of time of carbohydrate ingestion. *Journal of Applied Physiology* 64:1480–1485.

Jensen, T.E., and E.A. Richter. 2012. Regulation of glucose and glycogen metabolism during and after exercise. *Journal of Physiology* 590:1069–1076.

Kanter, M.M. 1994. Free radicals, exercise, and antioxidant supplementation. *International Journal of Sport Nutrition* 4:205–220.

Lane, J.D., M.N. Feinglos, and R.S. Surwit. 2008. Caffeine increases ambulatory glucose and postprandial responses in coffee drinkers with type 2 diabetes. *Diabetes Care* 31:221–222.

Larsson, S.C., and A. Wolk. 2007. Magnesium intake and risk of type 2 diabetes: A meta-analysis. *Journal of Internal Medicine* 262:208–214.

Laxminarayan, S., J. Reifman, S.S. Edwards, H. Wolpert, and G.M. Steil. 2015. Bolus estimation—rethinking the effect of meal fat content. *Diabetes Technology and Therapeutics* 17:860–866.

Lefavi, R.G., R.A. Anderson, R.E. Keith, G.D. Wilson, J.L. McMillan, and M.H. Stone. 1992. Efficacy of chromium supplementation in athletes: Emphasis on anabolism. *International Journal of Sport Nutrition* 2:111–112.

Lennerz, B.S., A. Barton, R.K. Bernstein, R.D. Dikeman, C. Diulus, S. Hallberg, E.T. Rhodes, C.B. Ebbeling, E.C. Westman, W.S. Yancy Jr, and D.S. Ludwig. 2018. Management of type 1 diabetes with a very low-carbohydrate diet. *Pediatrics* 141:e20173349.

Maughan, R.J. 1995. Creatine supplementation and exercise performance. *International Journal of Sport Nutrition* 5:94–101.

McKewen, M.W., N.J. Rehrer, C. Cox, and J. Mann. 1999. Glycaemic control, muscle glycogen and exercise performance in IDDM athletes on diets of varying carbohydrate content. *International Journal of Sports Medicine* 20:349–353.

Mettler, S., N. Mitchell, and K.D. Tipton. 2010. Increased protein intake reduces lean body mass loss during weight loss in athletes. *Medicine and Science in Sports and Exercise* 42:326–337.

Nielsen, F.H. 2014. Effects of magnesium depletion on inflammation in chronic disease. *Currents Opinions in Clinical Nutrition and Metabolic Care* 17:525–530.

Nielsen, F.H., and H.C. Lukaski. 2006. Update on the relationship between magnesium and exercise. *Magnesium Research* 19:180–189.

Norris, J.M., X. Yin, M.M. Lamb, K. Barriga, J. Seifert, M. Hoffman, H.D. Orton, A.E. Barón, M. Clare-Salzler, H.P. Chase, N.J. Szabo, H. Erlich, G.S. Eisenbarth, and M. Rewers. 2007. Omega-3 polyunsaturated fatty acid intake and islet autoimmunity in children at increased risk for type 1 diabetes. *Journal of the American Medical Association* 298:1420–1428.

Phillips, S.M., S. Chevalier, and H.J. Leidy. 2016. Protein "requirements" beyond the RDA: Implications for optimizing health. *Applied Physiology Nutrition and Metabolism* 41:565–572.

Pittas, A.G., J. Lau, F.B. Hu, and B. Dawson-Hughes. 2007. The role of vitamin D and calcium in type 2 diabetes. A systematic review and meta-analysis. *Journal of Clinical Endocrinology and Metabolism* 92:2017–2029.

Rosenfalck, A.M., T. Almdal, L. Viggers, S. Madsbad, and J. Hilsted. 2006. A low-fat diet improves peripheral insulin sensitivity in patients with Type 1 diabetes. *Diabetic Medicine* 23:384–392.

Rosenthal, M.J., D. Smith, L. Yaguez, V. Giampietro, D. Kerr, E. Bullmore, M. Brammer, S.C. Williams, and S.A. Amiel. 2007. Caffeine restores regional brain activation in acute hypoglycaemia in healthy volunteers. *Diabetic Medicine* 24:720–727.

Sawka, M.N., L.M. Burke, E.R. Eichner, R.J. Maughan, S.J. Montain, and N.S. Stachenfeld. 2007. Exercise and fluid replacement. *Medicine and Science in Sports and Exercise* 39:377-390.

Thomas, D.T., K.A., Erdman, and L.M. Burke. 2016. Position of the Academy of Nutrition and Dietetics, Dietitians of Canada, and the American College of Sports Medicine: Nutrition and athletic performance. *Journal of Academy of Nutrition and Dietetics* 116:501-528.

Thornalley, P.J., R. Babaei-Jadidi, H. Al Ali, N. Rabbani, A. Antonysunil, J. Larkin, A. Ahmed, G. Rayman, and C.W. Bodmer. 2007. High prevalence of low plasma thiamine concentration in diabetes linked to a marker of vascular disease. *Diabetologia* 50:2164-2170.

Volek, J.S., D.J. Freidenreich, C. Saenz, L.J. Kunces, B.C. Creighton, J.M. Bartley, P.M. Davitt, C.X. Munoz, J.M. Anderson, C.M. Maresh, E.C. Lee, M.D. Schuenke, G. Aerni, W.J. Kraemer, and S.D. Phinney. 2016. Metabolic characteristics of keto-adapted ultra-endurance runners. *Metabolism* 65:100-110.

Volek, J.S., T. Noakes, and S.D. Phinney. 2015. Rethinking fat as a fuel for endurance exercise. *European Journal of Sport Science* 15:13-20.

West D.J., J.W. Stephens, S.C. Bain, L.P. Kilduff, S. Luzio, R. Still, and R.M. Bracken. 2011. A combined insulin reduction and carbohydrate feeding strategy 30 min before running best preserves blood glucose concentration after exercise through improved fuel oxidation in type 1 diabetes mellitus. *Journal of Sports Sciences* 29:279-289.

Wolever, T.M., S. Hamad, J.L. Chiasson, R.G. Josse, L.A. Leiter, N.W. Rodger, S.A. Ross, and E.A. Ryan. 1999. Day-to-day consistency in amount and source of carbohydrate associated with improved blood glucose control in type 1 diabetes. *Journal of the American College of Nutrition* 18:242-247.

Yardley, J.E., and S.R. Colberg. 2017. Update on management of type 1 diabetes and type 2 diabetes in athletes. *Current Sports Medicine Reports* 16:38-44.

Zaharieva, D.P., L.A. Miadovnik, C.P. Rowan, R.J. Gumieniak, V.K. Jamnik, and M.C. Riddell. 2016. Effects of acute caffeine supplementation on reducing exercise-associated hypoglycaemia in individuals with type 1 diabetes mellitus. *Diabetic Medicine* 33:488-496.

Zajac, A., S. Poprzecki, A. Maszczyk, M. Czuba, M. Michalczyk, and G. Zydek. 2014. The effects of a ketogenic diet on exercise metabolism and physical performance in off-road cyclists. *Nutrients* 6:2493-2508.

Zunino, S.J., D.H. Storms, and C.B. Stephensen. 2007. Diets rich in polyphenols and vitamin A inhibit the development of type I autoimmune diabetes in nonobese diabetic mice. *Journal of Nutrition* 137:1216-1221.

# Chapter 5

Adolfsson, P., S. Mattsson, and J. Jendle. 2015. Evaluation of glucose control when a new strategy of increased carbohydrate supply is implemented during prolonged physical exercise in type 1 diabetes. *European Journal of Applied Physiology* 115:2599-2607.

Bally, L., T. Zueger, N. Pasi, C. Carlos, D. Paganini, and C. Stettler. 2016. Accuracy of continuous glucose monitoring during differing exercise conditions. *Diabetes Research and Clinical Practice* 112:1-5.

Breton, M.D., S.A. Brown, C.H. Karvetski, L. Kolla, K.A. Topchyan, S.M. Anderson, and B.P. Kovatchev. 2014. Adding heart rate signal to a control-to-range artificial pancreas system improves the protection against hypoglycemia during exercise in type 1 diabetes. *Diabetes Technology and Therapeutics* 16:506-511.

Colberg, S.R., R. Laan, E. Dassau, and D. Kerr. 2015. Physical activity and type 1 diabetes: Time for a rewire? *Journal of Diabetes Science and Technology* 9:609-618.

Colberg, S.R., R.J. Sigal, J.E. Yardley, M.C. Riddell, D.W. Dunstan, P.C. Dempsey, E.S. Horton, K. Castorino, and D.F. Tate. 2016. Physical activity/exercise and diabetes: A position statement of the American Diabetes Association. *Diabetes Care* 39:2065-2079.

Davidson, J. 2005. Strategies for improving glycemic control: Effective use of glucose monitoring. *American Journal of Medicine* 118:27S–32S.

Englert, K., K. Ruedy, J. Coffey, K. Caswell, A. Steffen, L. Levandoski, and Diabetes Research in Children (DirecNet) Study Group. 2014. Skin and adhesive issues with continuous glucose monitors: A sticky situation. *Journal of Diabetes Science and Technology* 8:745–751.

Francescato, M.P., G. Stel, E. Stenner, and M. Geat. 2015. Prolonged exercise in type 1 diabetes: Performance of a customizable algorithm to estimate the carbohydrate supplements to minimize glycemic imbalances. *PLoS One* 10:e0125220.

Heinemann, L., L. Nosek, C. Kapitza, M.A. Schweitzer, and L. Krinelke. 2009. Changes in basal insulin infusion rates with subcutaneous insulin infusion: Time until a change in metabolic effect is induced in patients with type 1 diabetes. *Diabetes Care* 32:1437–1439.

Herrington, S.J., D.L. Gee, S.D. Dow, K.A. Monosky, E. Davis, and K.L. Pritchett. 2012. Comparison of glucose monitoring methods during steady-state exercise in women. *Nutrients* 4:1282–1292.

Garg, S., and L. Jovanovic. 2006. Relationship of fasting and hourly blood glucose levels to HbA1c values: Safety, accuracy, and improvements in glucose profiles obtained using a 7-day continuous glucose sensor. *Diabetes Care* 29:2644–2649.

Jayawardene, D.C., S.A. McAuley, J.C. Horsburgh, A. Gerche, A.J. Jenkins, G.M. Ward, R.J. MacIsaac, T.J. Roberts, B. Grosman, N. Kurtz, A. Roy, and D.N. O'Neal. 2017. Closed-loop insulin delivery for adults with type 1 diabetes undertaking high-intensity interval exercise versus moderate-intensity exercise: a randomized, crossover study. *Diabetes Technology and Therapeutics* 19:340–348.

Kelly, D., J.K., Hamilton, and M.C. Riddell. 2010. Blood glucose levels and performance in a sports camp for adolescents with type 1 diabetes mellitus: a field study. *International Journal of Pediatrics* 2010:216167.

Kominiarek, M.A., and P. Rajan. 2016. Nutrition recommendations in pregnancy and lactation. *Medical Clinics of North America* 100:1199–1215.

Matuleviciene, V., J.I. Joseph, M. Andelin, I.B. Hirsch, S. Attvall, A. Pivodic, S. Dahlqvist, D. Klonoff, B. Haraldsson, and M. Lind. 2014. A clinical trial of the accuracy and treatment experience of the Dexcom G4 sensor (Dexcom G4 system) and Enlite sensor (Guardian REAL-time system) tested simultaneously in ambulatory patients with type 1 diabetes. *Diabetes Technology and Therapeutics* 16:759–767.

Radermecker, R.P., C. Fayolle, J.F. Brun, J. Bringer, and E. Renard. 2013. Accuracy assessment of online glucose monitoring by a subcutaneous enzymatic glucose sensor during exercise in patients with type 1 diabetes treated by continuous subcutaneous insulin infusion. *Diabetes and Metabolism* 39:258–262.

Riddell M.C., and J. Milliken. 2011. Preventing exercise-induced hypoglycemia in type 1 diabetes using real-time continuous glucose monitoring and a new carbohydrate intake algorithm: An observational field study. *Diabetes Technology and Therapeutics* 13:819–825.

Sherr, J.L., E. Cengiz, C.C. Palerm, B. Clark, N. Kurtz, A. Roy, L. Carria, M. Cantwell, W.V. Tamborlane, and S.A. Weinzimer. 2013. Reduced hypoglycemia and increased time in target using closed-loop insulin delivery during nights with or without antecedent afternoon exercise in type 1 diabetes. *Diabetes Care* 36:2909–2914.

T1D Exchange. 2016. Why do some people with T1D stop using a pump and CGM? April 20, https://t1dexchange.org/pages/why-do-some-people-with-t1d-stop-using-a-pump-and-cgm.

Yardley, J.E., R.J. Sigal, G.P. Kenny, M.C. Riddell, L.E. Lovblom, and B.A. Perkins. 2013. Point accuracy of interstitial continuous glucose monitoring during exercise in type 1 diabetes. *Diabetes Technology and Therapeutics* 15:46–49.

# Chapter 6

Allami, N., Y. Paulignan, A. Brovelli, and D. Boussaoud. 2008. Visuo-motor learning with combination of different rates of motor imagery and physical practice. *Experimental Brain Research* 184:105–113.

Arvinen-Barrow, M., D. Clement, J.J. Hamson-Utley, R.A. Zakrajsek, S.M. Lee, C. Kamphoff, T. Lintunen, B. Hemmings, and S.B. Martin. 2015. Athletes' use of mental skills during sport injury rehabilitation. *Journal of Sport Rehabilitation* 24:189–197.

Covassin, T., E. Beidler, J. Ostrowski, and J. Wallace. 2015. Psychosocial aspects of rehabilitation in sports. *Clinics in Sports Medicine* 34:199–212.

Dolenc, P. 2015. Anxiety, self-esteem and coping with stress in secondary school students in relation to involvement in organized sports. *Zdravstveno Varstvo* 54:222–229.

Eaves, D.L., M. Riach, P.S. Holmes, and D.J. Wright. 2016. Motor imagery during action observation: A brief review of evidence, theory and future research opportunities. *Frontiers in Neuroscience* 10:514.

Hardy, J., C.R. Hall, and L. Hardy. 2005. Quantifying athlete self-talk. *Journal of Sports Science* 23:905–917.

Ma, Z., J.S. Christiansen, T. Laursen, T. Lauritzen, and J. Frystyk. 2014. Short-term effects of NPH insulin, insulin detemir, and insulin glargine on the GH-IGF1-IGFBP axis in patients with type 1 diabetes. *European Journal of Endocrinology* 171:471–479.

Marsh, H.W., J.P. Chanal, and P.G. Sarrazin. 2006. Self-belief does make a difference: A reciprocal effects model of the causal ordering of physical self-concept and gymnastics performance. *Journal of Sports Science* 24:101–111.

Newmark, T.S., and D.F. Bogacki. 2005. The use of relaxation, hypnosis, and imagery in sport psychiatry. *Clinical Sports Medicine* 24:973–977.

Oishi, K., and T. Maeshima. 2004. Autonomic nervous system activities during motor imagery in elite athletes. *Journal of Clinical Neurophysiology* 21:170–179.

Papaioannou, A., E. Bebetsos, Y. Theodorakis, T. Christodoulidis, and O. Kouli. 2006. Causal relationships of sport and exercise involvement with goal orientations, perceived competence and intrinsic motivation in physical education: A longitudinal study. *Journal of Sports Science* 24:367–382.

Ridderinkhof, K.R., and M. Brass. 2015. How kinesthetic motor imagery works: a predictive-processing theory of visualization in sports and motor expertise. *Journal of Physiology, Paris* 109:53–63.

Wang, J., D. Marchant, T. Morris, and P. Gibbs. 2004. Self-consciousness and trait anxiety as predictors of choking in sport. *Journal of Science and Medicine in Sport* 7:174–185.

# Chapter 7

Amati, F., J.J. Dubé, P.M. Coen, M. Stefanovic-Racic, F.G. Toledo, and B.H. Goodpaster. 2009. Physical inactivity and obesity underlie the insulin resistance of aging. *Diabetes Care* 32:1547–1549.

Arroll, B., and F. Goodyear-Smith. 2005. Corticosteroid injections for painful shoulder: A meta-analysis. *British Journal of General Practice* 55:224–228.

Cheuy, V.A., M.K. Hastings, P.K. Commean, and M.J. Mueller. 2016. Muscle and joint factors associated with forefoot deformity in the diabetic neuropathic foot. *Foot and Ankle International* 37:514–521.

Cosca, D.D., and F. Navazio. 2007. Common problems in endurance athletes. *American Family Physician* 76:237–244.

Cymet, T.C., and V. Sinkov. 2006. Does long-distance running cause osteoarthritis? *Journal of the American Osteopathic Association* 106:342–345.

De Jonge, S., R. Rozenberg, B. Vieyra, H.J. Stam, H.J. Aanstoot, H. Weinans, H.T. van Schie, and S.F. Praet. 2015. Achilles tendons in people with type 2 diabetes show mildly compromised structure: an ultrasound tissue characterisation study. *British Journal of Sports Medicine* 49:995-999.

De Oliveira, L.P., C.P. Vieira, F.D. Guerra, M.S. Almeida, and E.R. Pimentel. 2015. Structural and biomechanical changes in the Achilles tendon after chronic treatment with statins. *Food and Chemical Toxicology* 77:50-57.

Flann, K.L., P.C. LaStayo, D.A. McClain, M. Hazel, and S.L. Lindstedt. 2011. Muscle damage and muscle remodeling: No pain, no gain? *Journal of Experimental Biology* 214:674-679.

Fredericson, M., and A.K. Misra. 2007. Epidemiology and aetiology of marathon running injuries. *Sports Medicine* 37:437-439.

Fullem, B.W. 2015. Overuse lower extremity injuries in sports. *Clinics in Podiatric Medicine and Surgery* 32:239-251.

Janghorbani, M., D. Feskanich, W.C. Willett, and F. Hu. 2006. Prospective study of diabetes and risk of hip fracture: The Nurses' Health Study. *Diabetes Care* 29:1573-1578.

Khan, T.S., and L.A. Fraser. 2015. Type 1 diabetes and osteoporosis: From molecular pathways to bone phenotype. *Journal of Osteoporosis* 2015:174186.

Kimmerle, R., and E. Chantelau. 2007. Weight-bearing intensity produces Charcot deformity in injured neuropathic feet in diabetes. *Experimental and Clinical Endocrinology and Diabetes* 115:360-364.

Kwon, S., and K.L. Hermayer. 2013. Glucocorticoid-induced hyperglycemia. *American Journal of Medicine and Science* 345:274Y7.

Mota, M., C. Panus, E. Mota, V. Sfredel, A. Patrascu, L. Vanghelie, and E. Toma. 2000-2001. Hand abnormalities of the patients with diabetes mellitus. *Romanian Journal of Internal Medicine* 38-39:89-95.

Napoli, N., M. Chandran, D.D. Pierroz, B. Abrahamsen, A.V. Schwartz, S.L. Ferrari, and IOF Bone and Diabetes Working Group. 2017. Mechanisms of diabetes mellitus-induced bone fragility. *Nature Reviews. Endocrinology* 13:208-219.

Nelson, N.L., and J.R. Churilla. 2016. A narrative review of exercise-associated muscle cramps: Factors that contribute to neuromuscular fatigue and management implications. *Muscle and Nerve* 54:177-185.

Pujalte, G.G., and M.L. Silvis. 2014. The injured runner. *Medical Clinics of North America* 98:851-868.

Vignon, E., J.P. Valat, M. Rossignol, B. Avouac, S. Rozenberg, P. Thoumie, J. Avouac, M. Nordin, and P. Hilliquin. 2006. Osteoarthritis of the knee and hip and activity: A systematic international review and synthesis (OASIS). *Joint Bone Spine* 73:442-455.

Wilder, R.P., and S. Sethi. 2004. Overuse injuries: Tendinopathies, stress fractures, compartment syndrome, and shin splints. *Clinical Sports Medicine* 23:55-81.

Zreik, N.H., R.A. Malik, and C.P. Charalambous. 2016. Adhesive capsulitis of the shoulder and diabetes: A meta-analysis of prevalence. *Muscles, Ligaments, and Tendons Journal* 6:26-34.

# Chapters 8-12

Armstrong, M.J., S.R. Colberg, and R.J. Sigal. 2015. Moving beyond cardio: The value of resistance training, balance training and other forms of exercise in the management of diabetes. *Diabetes Spectrum* 28:14-23.

Brubaker, P.L. 2005. Adventure travel and type 1 diabetes: The complicating effects of high altitude. *Diabetes Care* 28:2563-2572.

Chang, C.K., K. Borer, and P.J. Lin. 2017. Low-carbohydrate-high-fat diet: Can it help exercise performance? *Journal of Human Kinetics* 56:81-92.

Colberg, S.R., R.J. Sigal, J.E. Yardley, M.C. Riddell, D.W. Dunstan, P.C. Dempsey, E.S. Horton, K. Castorino, and D.F. Tate. 2016. Physical activity/exercise and diabetes: A position statement of the American Diabetes Association. *Diabetes Care* 39:2065-2079.

Fink, K.S., D.B. Christensen, and A. Ellsworth. 2002. Effect of high altitude on blood glucose meter performance. *Diabetes Technology and Therapeutics* 4:627-635.

Guelfi, K.J., T.W. Jones, and P.A. Fournier. 2007. New insights into managing the risk of hypoglycaemia associated with intermittent high-intensity exercise in individuals with type 1 diabetes mellitus: Implications for existing guidelines. *Sports Medicine* 37:937-946.

Maran, A., P. Pavan, B. Bonsembiante, E. Brugin, A. Ermolao, A. Avogaro, and M. Zaccaria. 2010. Continuous glucose monitoring reveals delayed nocturnal hypoglycemia after intermittent high-intensity exercise in nontrained patients with type 1 diabetes. *Diabetes Technology and Therapeutics* 12:763-768.

Riddell, M.C., and K.E. Iscoe. 2006. Physical activity, sport, and pediatric diabetes. *Pediatric Diabetes* 7:60-70.

Shetty, V.B., P.A. Fournier, R.J. Davey, A.J. Retterath, N. Paramalingam, H.C. Roby, M.N. Cooper, E.A. Davis, and T.W. Jones. 2016. Effect of exercise intensity on glucose requirements to maintain euglycemia during exercise in type 1 diabetes. *Journal of Clinical Endocrinology and Metabolism* 101:972-980.

Tuominen, J., P. Ebeling, H. Vuorinen-Markkola, and V. Koivisto. 1997. Postmarathon paradox in IDDM: Unchanged insulin sensitivity in spite of glycogen depletion. *Diabetic Medicine* 14:301-308.

Valerio, G., M.I. Spagnuolo, F. Lombardi, R. Spadaro, M. Siano, and A. Franzese. 2007. Physical activity and sports participation in children and adolescents with type 1 diabetes mellitus. *Nutrition, Metabolism, and Cardiovascular Diseases* 17:376-382.

Volek, J.S., T. Noakes, and S.D. Phinney. 2015. Rethinking fat as a fuel for endurance exercise. *European Journal of Sport Science* 15:13-20.

Yardley, J.E., and S.R. Colberg. 2017. Update on management of type 1 diabetes and type 2 diabetes in athletes. *Current Sports Medicine Reports* 16:38-44.

Zaharieva, D., L. Yavelberg, V. Jamnik, A. Cinar, K. Turksoy, and M.C. Riddell. 2017. The effects of basal insulin suspension at the start of exercise on blood glucose levels during continuous versus circuit-based exercise in individuals with type 1 diabetes on continuous subcutaneous insulin infusion. *Diabetes Technology and Therapeutics* 19:370-378.

# ——— Index ———

*Note:* The italicized *f* and *t* following page numbers refer to figures and tables, respectively.

# About the Author

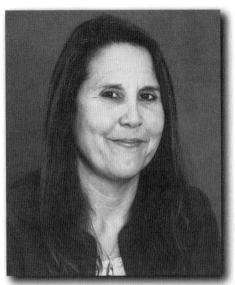

**Sheri R. Colberg, PhD, FACSM,** is an author, exercise physiologist, lecturer, consultant, and professor emerita of exercise science (Old Dominion University in Norfolk, Virginia). In 2016, she was the recipient of the American Diabetes Association's Outstanding Educator in Diabetes award. A respected researcher and lecturer, she has authored more than 400 articles on exercise, diabetes, and health; 28 book chapters; and over a dozen books, including *Diabetes-Free Kids, The 7 Step Diabetes Fitness Plan, 50 Secrets of the Longest Living People With Diabetes, The Science of Staying Young, Diabetic Athlete's Handbook, The Diabetes Breakthrough,* and *Diabetes & Keeping Fit for Dummies.*

A distinguished graduate of Stanford University (BA), University of California at Davis (MA), and University of California at Berkeley (PhD), Colberg consults professionally for the American Diabetes Association (ADA), American College of Sports Medicine (ACSM), Juvenile Diabetes Research Foundation (JDRF), American Association of Diabetes Educators (AADE), and Academy of Nutrition and Dietetics (AND) on numerous committees and projects. As a world-renowned expert and opinion leader, she has developed the exercise guidelines related to diabetes for most of these premier professional organizations, and she is interviewed frequently by various media outlets. In addition, she continues to be involved in consulting and in clinical research on exercise, diabetes, and healthy lifestyles.

With over 50 years of personal experience as an exerciser living with type 1 diabetes, Colberg continues to live a healthy, active lifestyle and serve as a role model for others who want to live long and well with (or without) diabetes. She enjoys working out regularly on conditioning machines, swimming, biking, fitness walking, weight training, and hiking with her husband and family in coastal California.

# You read the book—now complete an exam to earn continuing education credit!

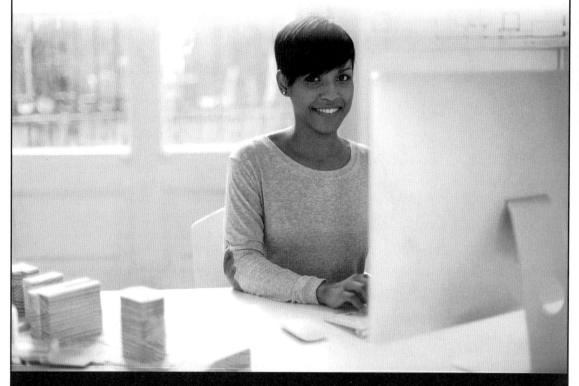

Congratulations on successfully preparing for this continuing education exam!

If you would like to earn CE credit, please visit

**www.HumanKinetics.com/CE-Exam-Access**

for complete instructions on how to access your exam. Take advantage of a discounted rate by entering promo code **AGD2019** when prompted.

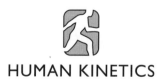

HUMAN KINETICS